THE ECONOMICS, MARKETING, AND TECHNOLOGY OF FISH PROTEIN CONCENTRATE

THE ECONOMICS, MARKETING, AND TECHNOLOGY OF FISH PROTEIN CONCENTRATE

edited by Steven R. Tannenbaum,
Bruce R. Stillings, and Nevin S. Scrimshaw

152937

The MIT Press
Cambridge, Massachusetts, and London, England

Library of Congress catalog
card number: 74-15188

ISBN 0-262-20022-8

PUBLISHER'S NOTE

This format is intended to reduce the cost of
publishing certain works in book form and to
shorten the gap between editorial preparation
and final publication. The time and expense
of detailed editing and composition in print
have been avoided by photographing the text
of this book directly from the author's type-
script.

The MIT Press

CONTENTS

Page

PREFACE, S. R. Tannenbaum,
B. R. Stillings, N. S. Scrimshaw   xi

INTRODUCTORY REMARKS, Harold Olcott   1

PART I   RESOURCES
Fish Protein Concentrate: The
Present and Future Status of
Available Oceanic Resources,
J. Arnold and L. S. Sprague
Chapter I   8

The Response of Fisheries
Management Philosophy to the
Imperatives of Modern Technology,
R. D. Balkovic, R. F. Hutton,
D. R. Moore
Chapter II   33

Raw Material Supply for Fish Protein
Concentrate, W. F. Royce
Chapter III   37

Fish Resources for Production of
Fish Protein Concentrate, FAO
Fishery Resources Division
Chapter IV   44

PART II   PROCESSING
FPC Processes, R. Finch
Chapter V   57

Canadian FPC Research and
Development, L. W. Regier
Chapter VI   102

Aqueous-Solvent Processes,
J. Spinelli
Chapter VII   111

Contents

Page

FPC Approaches and Projects in
Norway, E. Heen
Chapter VIII
122

Liquefied Fish Protein
Concentrate, T. Kinumaki
Chapter IX
125

The Fish Protein Hydrolyzate (FPH)
Process: A Target Design Approach,
M. Rutman and W. Heimlich
Chapter X
135

PART III   NUTRITION
Nutritional and Safety
Characteristics of FPC,
B. R. Stillings
Chapter XI
165

Evaluation of Fish Protein
Concentrate for Infant and Child
Feeding, N. S. Scrimshaw
Chapter XII
212

Evaluation of the Protein Quality
of Fish Protein Concentrate for
Maintenance of Adults, V. R. Young
and N. S. Scrimshaw
Chapter XIII
234

PART IV   UTILIZATION
Utilization of FPC and
Acceptability, V. D. Sidwell
Chapter XIV
255

Enzymatic Solubilization of FPC,
M. C. Archer, S. R. Tannenbaum,
and D. I. C. Wang
Chapter XV
283

Page

Acceptability of FPC Products,
G. M. Dreosti
Chapter XVI   302

The Enrichment of Foods with
Fish Protein Concentrate,
E. Yanez, D. Ballester, and
F. Monckeberg
Chapter XVII   308

Effects of Processing
Parameters on the Chemical and
Functional Characteristics of
FPC,   D. L. Dubrow
Chapter XVIII   318

Utilization of Fish Protein
Concentrate or Marine Protein
Concentrate, A. Bhumiratana
Chapter XIX   328

Studies on the Chemical
Modification of Fish Protein
Concentrate, A. F. Anglemier
and H. J. Petropakis
Chapter XX   330

Fish Protein Concentrate in the
Treatment of Malnourished
Children and in Field, Technology
of Utilization, Preparation, and
Acceptability, J. M. Baertl
Chapter XXI   337

PART V   ECONOMICS
The Economics of Fish Protein
Concentrate, J. A. Crutchfield
and R. Deacon
Chapter XXII   355

Contents

Page

Marketing and Economics: Peru,
Fish Meal and FPC, G. Pontecorvo
Chapter XXIII   439

Factors Affecting the Economics
of an FPC Manufacturing Operation,
E. R. Pariser
Chapter XXIV   446

Some Problems in Marketing FPC,
R. Kreuzer
Chapter XXV   468

Some Aspects of the Fish Protein
Market in Industrialized
Countries: A View from Private
Industry, J. R. Champagne
Chapter XXVI   475

Notes from Nabisco-Astra,
H. J. Watson
Chapter XXVII   480

INDEX   483

PREFACE

This volume is based on papers presented at the International Conference on Fish Protein Concentrate held at Massachusetts Institute of Technology, June 6-8, 1972. Sponsors for the conference were the Committee on Aquatic Food Resources and the Committee on International Nutrition Programs of the National Academy of Sciences/National Research Council; the Malnutrition Panel of the United States-Japan Cooperative Program; the Massachusetts Institute of Technology Sea Grant Program and the University of Rhode Island Sea Grant Program.

While this book is derived from the conference, it is not the proceedings of the conference. Many papers presented are included at greater length, while other contributions do not appear in this volume at all.

We would like to express our appreciation to Drs. C. O. Chichester and James Crutchfield, who helped to plan the conference along with the editors of this volume. We are greatly indebted to Ms. Diana Katz for her tireless and catalytic efforts in putting this book together. We are also greatly indebted to the "team," consisting of numerous individuals from MIT, the National Fisheries Service, and the University of Rhode Island, that made this conference a success.

INTRODUCTORY REMARKS

Harold Olcott
Institute of Marine Resources, University of
California, Davis, California

It is as the present Chairman of the Committee on Aquatic Food Resources of the National Academy of Sciences that I present these introductory remarks. This collection of papers is the result of the gathering brought together by a recommendation made by the Committee under the Chairmanship Dr. B. S. Schweigert that a worldwide appraisal of the status and future outlook for FPC was needed.

I do not intend to review the history of FPC, which was well covered in a recent symposium, a review, and a bibliography.[1,2,3] Many people and organizations have devoted several years to thinking about and working on FPC and are better qualified than I to remind us of what has gone before.

The National Academy of Sciences of the United States has been vitally interested in FPC since it was first asked by the Secretary of the Interior in 1962 to consider three questions. 1. Can a wholesome, safe, nutritious product be made from whole fish? 2. Does a product now exist which is suitable for human consumption? 3. Is there a demonstrable need, either nutritionally or economically, for an inexpensive animal food supplement among people in the United States?

A temporary committee selected by the Division of Biology and Agriculture and the Food and Nutrition Board responded to these as follows: 1. Yes, a wholesome, safe and nutritious product can be made from whole fish. 2. Although laboratory and pilot-plant scale experiments have resulted in acceptable products, no commercially successful plant is in operation. 3. No need for protein supplements in the United States

had yet been demonstrated. The point that
there was indeed a demonstrable worldwide
need for supplementation for selected population groups was not debated.

The same committee also recommended that
the Food and Nutrition Board promptly establish a scientific group to advise the then
U. S. Bureau of Commercial Fisheries on this
project. Such a committee was established
and has continued to meet and make recommendations for the past ten years.

In 1965 the new committee examined the results of the Bureau of Commercial Fisheries
research efforts which had been vigorously
pursued since 1961 and reported that "Fish
Protein Concentrate made from whole hake as
prepared by a solvent process with isopropyl
alcohol is SAFE, NUTRITIOUS, WHOLESOME and
FIT for human consumption."

The situation then was that there was an
acute need for more research effort but the
demand for samples was so heavy that research
effort was being fragmented in the effort to
fill these needs. Publicity about FPC had
been heavy and probably, as we now see, somewhat premature. At any rate the committee
recommended that efforts be made to get fund-
ing for a demonstration plant that could supply sufficient FPC for the demand. These
funds were obtained and the following papers
will include reports of the present status of
that plant.

The concept that the world need for protein could be met by underutilized fish resources seemed simple and unassailable. All
that was needed was a technology that could
make available a stable acceptable product
at low cost. It was a reasonable concept.
The years that have intervened have revealed
factors that were not thoroughly understood
and a world situation that is rapidly changing, but it still seems a reasonable concept.

Certain facts seem unarguable. FPCs have been made from whole fish that are stable and nutritious. They can be added to common articles of diet. Their benefit when added to deficient diets is thoroughly documented. But some of the problems that remain and to which we will devote ourselves include the following: 1. Are there enough underutilized fish? 2. Are the present technologies really adequate? 3. Will the cost be too high? This last question, that of economics, may well be the most serious of the problems to be discussed, since those who need FPC most can afford it least.

Finally we might consider briefly the role of the FDA (Food and Drug Administration) of the United States in this development. In 1962 the FDA decided that FPC for human use was a new product and therefore had to pass the requirements for a food additive. The first petition that it be allowed was rejected on the grounds that the product was unwholesome because it was made of whole fish, and thus fell under the definition of "filthy." After considerable scientific and, I have to believe, some political pressure, the FDA agreed on Feb. 1, 1968, that FPC could be used as a human food but with several restrictions. The restrictions included that FPC must meet a number of specification requirements (as one example, not more than 100 ppm fluoride), that the species of fish used be limited to hake and hake-like fish, and that it be marketed to the public in packages containing not more than 1 lb of product labeled "made from whole fish." As Devanney and Mahnken[4] put it, "...these restrictions were as economically restrictive as direct prohibition."

The matter of the allowable species has since been expanded to include herring of the genus clupea and menhaden but the annoying

situation with the consumer package remained.
The National Academy Committee had protested
the packaging restrictions on several occa-
sions but without evidence of effect. An industry petition filed last year asked FDA to
delete this restriction but it was considered
deficient and was withdrawn in October. At
the time Food Chemical News[5] commented as
follows: "With the withdrawal of the Alpine
petition, the long publicized use of FPC as a
low cost source of protein in food products
appears to be dead in this country unless
some other firm or government agency picks up
the ball and files a petition." Fortunately
another petition was filed early in 1972, and
in July, 1973 the FDA removed the packaging
restriction and permitted the use of FPC in
manufactured foods. Although the U. S. FDA
regulations do not apply in other countries,
they do influence actions in other countries
especially in regard to new concepts and
products such as FPC.

Meanwhile in the past ten years, a billion
babies have been born. Millions in the
developing countries are in the sensitive 2
to 5 year old groups. Even if we assume that
only a small percentage of these are sufficiently protein-deprived to result in some
physical or mental damage, the 10-year delay
means that tens of millions of youngsters
are not as well of as they might have been,
and of these a good many will have died.
Many of us have been inspired and stimulated
by the magnitude of this problem and have
accepted the concept that the world need for
protein can be met at least in part from the
ocean. But the goal is still far off. Hopefully, the papers which follow will help to
illuminate both the path and the obstacles.

References

1. Proceedings, Conference on Fish Protein
Concentrate. October 24 and 25, 1967.
Canadian Fisheries Report No. 10, July 1968.

2. Fish Protein Concentrate. A comprehen-
sive Bibliography, Library of Congress.
Clearinghouse for Federal Scientific and
Technical Information, National Bureau of
Standards, U. S. Dept. of Commerce, Spring-
field, Va. 22151, 1970.

3. Finch, R. Fish Protein for Human Foods.
CRC Critical Reviews in Food Technology,
1971.

4. Devanney, J. W. III, G. Mahnken, Economics of Fish Protein in Concentrate, MIT,
Report No. MITSG 71-3, November 20, 1970.

5. Anonymous. Food Chemical News 33, 11
October 1971, p. 32.

Part I

RESOURCES

I
FISH PROTEIN CONCENTRATE: THE PRESENT AND FUTURE STATUS OF AVAILABLE OCEANIC RESOURCES

John Arnold
Graduate School of Oceanography, University
of Rhode Island, Kingston, Rhode Island 02881
and
Lucian M. Sprague*
International Center for Marine Resource
Development and, Professor of Oceanography,
University of Rhode Island, Kingston, Rhode
Island 02881

In the last few years a rather large number
of analytical studies have contributed very
greatly to our understanding of the limits
within which the growth of fishery harvest
might take place.

Fishery scientists have been notably conservative in their estimates of the limits
of growth, probably because of their awareness of the need for regulatory tools to
limit the physical harvest of specific fisheries. Another factor may be the scientist's
awareness of and response to the layman's
common misconception of the sea as ever fer-
tile and infinitely rich.

For the first time we are beginning to
have a factual outline of the overall productive potential of the seas[1] and consequently the potential total harvest which
might be expected to result from the aquatic
environment.[2] The various chapters of
Gulland's recent work contributed by

----
*Present address: International Bank for
Reconstruction and Development, Agricultural
Industries Division, Washington, D. C. 20433.

regionally knowledgeable authors have greatly
sharpened our ability to place reasonable limits on the potential harvest of aquatic
organisms. At the same time these estimates
provide ample scope for informed differences
of opinion about specifics. Figure 1 shows
the present status of harvest of aquatic species and Figure 2 shows the growth of fishing
power of the developed and developing economies.

Although there has been growing agreement
in the last decade on the need for a framework for limiting the harvest of many marine
animals there is unfortunately little reason
to be optimistic that agreement on the means
to achieve an adequate international management framework is within our grasp.

Clearly because of the finite limits of
aquatic resources and the very rapid pace at
which harvesting technology is outrunning
management tools, any discussion of the potentials of the aquatic regime to supply
protein in any form must assume management,
as at least a goal, and hope that the time
frame within which the management goal is
reached is short enough to prevent massive
dislocations in the system.

Before proceeding further and blundering
into all sorts of hidden assumptions it will
be useful to define what the authors mean
when we speak of FPC (fish protein concentrate). In one framework FPC has been, is,
and will be a major fraction of the form in
which fishery products are consumed. These
FPCs are called smoked and dried fish, or
squid, and, kamaboku, katsuobushi, etc.
However, the thrust of the present discus-
sions assumes that FPC is ideally a product
that is stable, dry, high in protein quality,
free from fishy taste and odors, nontoxic,
water soluble, powdery, and able to be easily used in formulated food products.

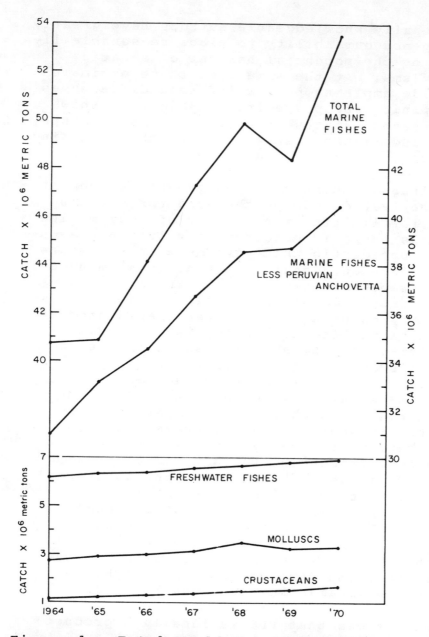

Figure 1.   Total World Catches of Four
Divisions of Aquatic Animals 1964-70[19]

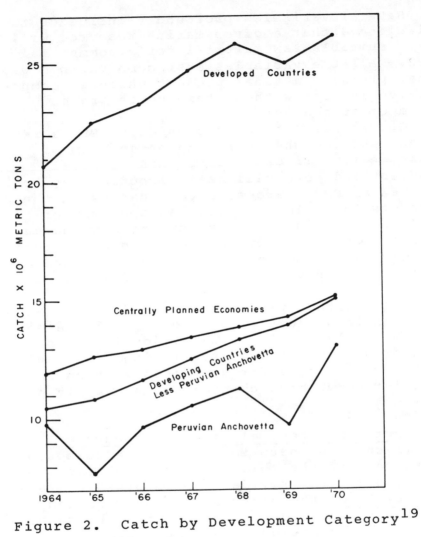

Figure 2.   Catch by Development Category[19]

Several variables profoundly influence the likelihood that a given marine resource will be a suitable raw material for a commercial FPC. All the variables must combine in a way that produces a final product which is competitive in cost with protein concentrates from other sources.

Others have usefully considered FPC a refined and somewhat more expensive form of fish meal.[3] If one adopts this view, all present and potential meal fisheries may be viewed as FPC sources, given changes in the markets for animal feeds. Another way of looking at this might be that market changes are brought about by changes in product technology resulting in FPC or highly refined fish meals which are capable of filling direct consumer demand as an ingredient of formulated food products for human use. Such changes in product technologies, which are quite likely, could have a major impact on the proportion of industrial fish processed into FPC and used for human consumption in the future without changes in the supply of raw material.

Present and Potential Fishery Resources

It is our hope here to set forth a reasonable statement of the ability of the aquatic environment to provide major sources of raw material for the class of products called FPC. It seems to us however that one cannot simply be satisfied with a mere shopping list consisting of a few hundred thousand tons of this and that but that one must also try to set forth the limits of the probable, and improbable.

There are two major classes of underutilized resources. The first class consists of fish that do not find a market because of local food preferences, customary dietary habits, religious proscriptions or because of

competition for hold space exerted by valuable species. This class of underutilized
fish is quite large amounting to perhaps as
much as 5 million tons made up of a very
large number of species. The majority are
poorly recorded in national statistics and
some not at all. They are thus difficult to
assess with any real accuracy. Because they
consist of mixed species of varied usefulness
they are poorly suited for the most part to
provide the raw material for a consistent
high quality product such as FPC.

The second class of resources is known to
occur in very substantial amounts but is not
now the subject of any major fishery for various technological or economic reasons. It
is this latter group that we wish to discuss
in the sections to follow.

Table 1 lists all the main groups that are
believed to be capable of a sustainable yield
in quantities sufficient to provide FPC in
commercial amounts.

It should be noted that some of these
groups, which were on Chapman's[3] shopping
list in 1965-66 as underutilized species of
great abundance, have moved very rapidly to
levels of full or almost full exploitation;
for example, the Arctic capelin, and the
catches of sand eels and West African sardinella.

Full exploitation of stocks is soon to be
expected for additional sardinella stocks in
the Indian Ocean along the Arabian peninsula,
the thread herring in the Gulf of Mexico, and
a variety of mackerel species not yet heavily
exploited, particularly in the Indian Ocean.
Somewhat later in time, very greatly increased catches are expected for coastal
squid along the west coasts of the Americas
and Africa, as well as pelagic herring and
anchovy-like fishes in the southwestern Pacific, eastern Pacific, southwestern Atlantic,

Table 1   Actual and Potential Harvest of Resources for Possible FPC Production

Species	Harvest, year						Potential Harvest		Remarks
	'65	'66	'67	'68	'69	'70	All Oceans $x\ 10^3m$	FPC Raw Material	
Capelin	281	521	513	623	855	1515	2,300	good	Nearly fully exploited on present grounds
Clupeonella	419	455	444	426	352	553	600	good	Fully exploited
Hake	1085	1270	1670	1396	1256	1421	3,400	poor	Table grade fish
Sand eels	254	254	317	356	228	426	2,400	good	
Lantern fish	0	0	0	0	0	0	100,000	?	Excessive harvesting costs
Misc. small Mackerel	2724	2926	3539	3845	4055	4396	9,000[2]	fair	Moderately high harvesting costs
Herring	4600	4611	4295	3734	2885	2804	3,500[2]	good	Almost fully exploited
Sardinella	175	187	253	227	381	764	2,100[2]	good	

Table 1 Actual and Potential Harvest of Resources for Possible FPC Production, Continued

| Species | Harvest, year | | | | | | Potential Harvest | | |
	'65	'66	'67	'68	'69	'70	All Oceans x 10³m	FPC Raw Material	Remarks
Oil sardine	334	307	315	369	251	300	3,500[2]	good	Fully exploited
South African Pilchard	1040	952	1105	1586	1402	672	1,000	good	Fully exploited
Menhaden	784	596	530	625	704	825	900[2]	good	Fully exploited
Thread Herring	9	26	42	42	42	50	1,600[2]	good	Legal-political barriers off U. S. coasts
Anchovy not incl. Peru	1128	1155	1283	1270	1319	1366	10,000	good	Legal-political off W.N. America (4 million mt.)
Peruvian Anchoveta	7681	9621	10530	11272	9709	13053	11,000	good	Fully exploited

Table 1 Actual and Potential Harvest of Resources for Possible FPC Production, Continued

Species	Harvest, year						Potential Harvest[1]		
	'65	'66	'67	'68	'69	'70	All Oceans x 10^3 m	FPC Raw Material	Remarks
Misc. Herring & Sardines	Considerable local harvest						2,000[2]	good	Scattered stocks
Misc. Marine Fish	7610	7850	8440	8760	9090	9580	13,000[2]	poor	Best for animal feeds
Oceanic sharks	410	440	460	480	510	520	500[2]	fair	Plus dog fish and others
Ocean squid	492	472	580	766	583	636	10,000	poor	Harvesting costs high
Red crab							1,000	poor	Direct human consumption
Krill	Research catch only						50,000-100,000	good	

[1]From Gulland unless otherwise noted.
[2]Our estimates based on Yearbook of Fish Stat.[19] U. S. Nat. Marine Fisheries Service, Foreign fishery leaflets and other.

and northwestern Indian Ocean.

Up until about 1960 insufficient resource
information, geographic remoteness, underdeveloped communications, and inadequate processing and transportation infrastructures
set limits on the growth rate of industrial-
grade fisheries. Since then substantial improvements in the information base, a very
rapid development of crucial infrastructures,
and strong demand have led to greatly expanded industrial fisheries. Many industrial
fisheries which can be exploited by present
harvest technologies are fully exploited.
Most industrial-grade fish resources available to present harvest technologies will be
fully exploited by the end of this decade.

Projections of Fisheries Harvest

In Figure 3 we have shown the present total
catch of aquatic animals, this catch less the
Peruvian anchoveta, Chapman's 1969 projection
of total catch, and a stepwise scenario of
future harvest possibilities.[4]

There are five distinct levels which we
believe represent possible patterns for the
future harvest of marine organisms. In order
for substantial harvest to occur in each level, certain prior conditions must be met.
The first level is the present catch. The
four future levels are the catch of the
thread herring, jack mackerel, etc.; the
Antarctic krill; the oceanic squid; and the
lantern fishes (Myctophids).

Given some assumptions presented later in
the discussion section regarding relative
soybean meal and fish meal production growth
rates, all presently known stocks of conventional industrial-grade fishes will be fully
utilized by 1983-1985 or sooner if growth
rates of fish meal consumption are higher
than 4.5 percent. This level of total fisheries harvest will be about 90 to 110 million

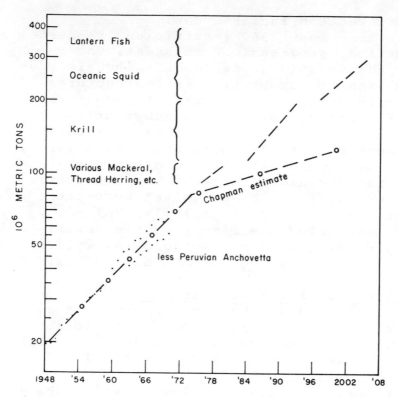

Figure 3.   Percent Catch of Aquatic Animals
and a Possible Future Scenario[4,19]

metric tons for all aquatic species harvested
by present catching technology and processed
by present processing technology.

Low Projection. A low projection for species
from the total fisheries harvest for FPC
would correspond to about 50 million metric
tons. This is based on the assumption that
no economically useful harvesting and processing technologies are developed to go beyond the harvest of present species groups
plus about 20 million tons of known but
underutilized thread herring, mackerel,
anchovies, etc.

We expect that as the level around 100
million metric tons of total fishery harvest
is reached, considerable pressure for higher
prices for refined fish and other protein
meals will develop. If this occurs it will
set the stage for the next level of marine
harvest to develop. But new limits, which
are difficult to assess, are expected to be
imposed on the remaining major fishery potentials by inadequate harvesting and/or processing technologies, conflicts over resource
jurisdiction and use, and in some cases a
deterioration of essential environmental
quality. An additional limit may be price
competition from alternative supplies of high
quality protein.

The groups expected to be constrained by
these limiting factors are principally the
krills, the lantern fishes and in part, the
oceanic squids. One other large marine resource is as yet unexploited, the red crab of
the eastern tropical Pacific, but in our
opinion because of its potential as a direct
high value food product it is unlikely to be
harvested for meal in any form.

Intermediate Projection. Assuming that economically viable harvesting and processing

technologies are developed, we believe the
most immediately valuable and available refined meal resource will be the Antarctic
invertebrate plankton commonly called krill.

If krill are brought into production, and
we believe this to be very likely, the total
aquatic animal harvest will rise to about 200
million metric tons. Of the total harvest,
130 to 150 million metric tons might be
available for FPC manufacture provided that
substantial improvements in processing technology are made. Such improvements might include more efficient, lower cost, and compact systems suitable for shipboard use.

Of the total amount of krill available,
between 10 and 20 percent of the harvest will
be used as cocktail shrimp or some equivalent
high value product; the remainder might be
used as meal or paste.

Krill are small shrimp-like crustaceans,
mostly euphausiids which occur in all oceans
of the world. The most important potential
commercial species is Euphasia superba DANA.
This species has received considerable attention in the last decade because of its great
abundance and relatively large size; adults
are about one to two inches long and may
weigh more than one gram. This species of
krill occurs within the Antarctic convergence
zone. Its area of greatest concentration in
the Antarctic summer (Jan.-March) is shown in
Figure 4.

Estimates of the potential harvest of
Antarctic krill by man range from 30 to 100
million metric tons.[2,5,6] Gulland believes
that the total production could be as much as
200 million metric tons of which a substantial portion is taken by krill predators including the baleen whales, seals, birds,
penguins, and other invertebrates. Man has
taken a significant step in the elimination
of important krill predators by drastically

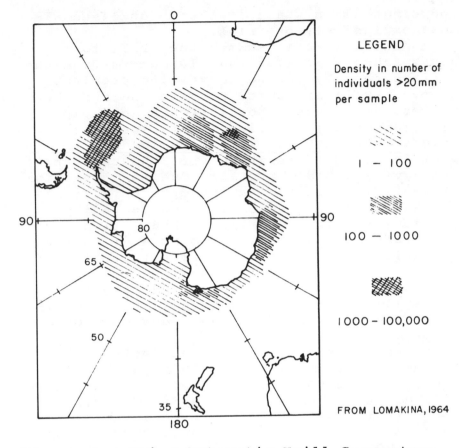

LEGEND

Density in number of
individuals >20 mm
per sample

1 — 100

100 — 1000

1000 — 100,000

FROM LOMAKINA, 1964

Figure 4.   Major Antarctic Krill Concentration[20]

reducing baleen whale stocks which lived almost exclusively on krill.

In the Antarctic summer the krill form
dense schools at less than 10 meters from the
surface thereby easing harvesting problems.[2]
However krill are quite fragile and must be
processed at once. For instance, one expedition reportedly experienced a 16 percent
weight loss when the krill remained on the
deck in 32° F temperature for 3 hours. Krill
spoil very rapidly probably due to the action
of bacterial enzymes having optimum activity
at near freezing temperatures. The edible
portion of krill (1/2-1/3 of body weight) has
a protein content of 19 percent whereas the
inedible portion has a 13 percent protein
content which is mainly bound in the form of
chitin.[8] Therefore, for human consumption,
the shells will probably have to be removed--
a process which has not been developed on a
commercial scale.

Several expeditions have harvested krill
in the last few years. In 1958, an expedition from the USSR trawled 100 kg of krill in
five minutes from one of the denser krill
concentrations they encountered in Antarcti-
ca.[9] In 1963, the USSR vessel, Mukson, harvested 70 tons of krill and used a portion of
this catch to make eleven tons of meal.[7]
More recently, experimental development of
krill fishing by vessels of the USSR has continued to produce cocktail size frozen shrimp
and commercial-grade meal (C. O. Chichester,
personal communication). No data on the
costs of operation or market success of these
efforts is available to us.

High Projection. It seems almost idle to
speculate on events that may give rise to the
demand and economic production of FPC at levels of total fishery harvest in excess of 200
million metric tons. But, two species groups

are available for harvest, oceanic squid and
lantern fish.

Oceanic squid are larger than the smaller
continental shelf varieties which are caught
by the New England, Japanese and other trawler fleets for sale as fresh food, fish bait,
and fish meal. At present oceanic squid are
mainly caught by Japan as a specialty product. Squid have a high protein content,
about 20 percent, which compares favorably
with the fin fishes.[10] The worldwide catch
is relatively small (636,000 mt) but could be
expanded because of their great abundance and
food value. However, available harvesting
technologies would not be adequate for the
development of a refined meal fishery because
of raw material price.

Although statistical data on oceanic squid
are meager, they are believed to be abundant
in all oceans, particularly in areas of upwelling and other productive areas. As
Clarke states, "If a ship stops at night in
any but high latitudes, squid are attracted
to the lights and are often seen in tens of
hundreds within an hour." Based on the
distribution of squid beaks on core samples
taken from bottom sediments, there is a high
correlation between squid concentrations and
regions of upwelling and high productivity.[10]

Gulland states that the total harvest of
oceanic squid could be somewhere between a
few million and 100 million metric tons.[2]
Based on numerous observations similar to
those of Clarke, Sprague believes Gulland's
estimate to be somewhat conservative.

The umbrella jig has proven satisfactory
for harvesting oceanic squid, but this method
is hardly likely to be economically feasible
for the production of raw material for FPC.
If the present Asian specialty market for human use were expanded to include other major
markets, it is unlikely that any significant

fraction of the increase in catch of the
squid resource would become available as raw
material for FPC. We believe that changes in
the market structure for these animals are
more likely than the development of very low
cost harvesting technologies. We believe
further that only a fraction of the available
100 million metric tons of oceanic squid
might be added to prior estimates for resources available to FPC production, say, at
most, 10 percent of production or at full
exploitation, about 10 million metric tons.

Since dried squid are already a form of
FPC and since coastal squid are currently
used for fish meal in small amounts, processing problems do not appear to be a limiting
factor in the future use of squid as FPC raw
material.

In addition to squid, lantern fish represent a future possible resource to FPC use.
Lantern fish, as described herein, include
the Myctophids, Paralepids, Cyclothone, spp,
Gempylidae, Vinciguerra spp, Leptocephalae
and the other small fishes (1 to 5 inches
long) which make up the deep scattering
layer. These fishes are not satisfactory
from the standpoint of taste and texture for
food fish, but their protein content makes
them a possible source for FPC. They were
used by Japan in the mid-1940s when protein
was scarce.[3] Lantern fish are thought to be
very abundant with a potential harvest on the
order of hundreds of millions of tons.[2] However, they would have to occur in dense
concentrations, and few are known, or be
concentrated by as yet undeveloped means to
yield the 10 ton per day catch thought to be
needed to sustain a 50 to 70 foot vessel.[2]
Since there is little data on aggregation of
these animals and economically suitable gear
has not been designed, we believe that these
fishes will be the last to be harvested.

Figure 3 shows possible production levels which might be reached if lantern fish were harvested.

Projection Summary. In the lower level including meal fisheries as potential supplies of FPC and future stocks of thread herring, mackerel, etc., potentials are about 50 million metric tons.

In the intermediate level which includes krill, an added 90 million metric tons for a total of about 140 million metric tons are potentially available.

In the high level perhaps part of the squid catch to a total of about 10 percent of production or 10 million tons as a maximum is available and of lantern fish, quantities deserving the sobriquet vast are available, but under present or forseeable harvesting and processing conditions these quantities are of little practical importance for FPC manufacture.

Effects of Alternative High Quality Protein Supplies

The most important alternative sources of low cost, high quality proteins are the vegetable meals. The relationship between vegetable meals rich in essential amino acids and fish meals is an important one. The price, supply, and demand for meals, particularly soybean meal, affects the demand for fish meal and its price, and the rate at which vegetable meals are placed on the market may have a profound effect on the rate at which presently underutilized marine resources are brought into production.

The most important substitute for fish meal is soybean meal. It is the best plant protein feed supplement for dairy and beef cattle, and because of its generally high quality protein profile it ranks ahead of all

other common vegetable meals for feeding
swine and poultry.

Soybean meal lacks methionine and vitamins
and is low in lysine, phosphorous, and calcium content. Complete animal feed formulations may be achieved by adding vitamins,
methionine, lysine, and minerals or by mixing
soy meal and fish meal together. Because
high quality fish meals contain "unidentified
growth factors," in addition to methionine,
lysine, and minerals, the latter may often be
preferable.

The same pattern of formulation is very
likely to emerge in the high quality meals
designed for human consumption, namely, that
the ultimate product will not be solely FPC
but will be a blend of high quality meals
each chosen for its unique contribution to
the nutritional quality, ease of use of the
final product, and its contribution to the
final product price.

In other words a simplistic solution to
the problem of supplying protein-rich high
quality meals is not likely to be found in
FPC or in any other single meal source.
Since each meal has its unique advantages
and disadvantages it seems appropriate to
combine them; a fact known, we are told, to
the industry for some time.

The recent growth rates in production and
consumption of vegetable meal and fish meal
show substantial increases. In the period
1955-1957 through 1963-1965, fish meal production increased 12 percent annually compared with a 4 percent rate of increase for
all vegetable meals. In the 1963-1965 period, annual fish meal production was about
3.3 million tons or 8 percent of total meal
production, which was about 45.5 million
metric tons. By 1970 fish meal production
was about 5.4 million metric tons of total
meal production which was 57.6 million

metric tons. Rates of growth during 1963-
1965 to 1969-1970 were about 8 percent per
annum.[11]

These rates of growth in fish meal production are expected by some to slow somewhat
to about 4.5 percent per annum such that by
1975 about 6 million tons of fish meal are
projected based on present rates of growth
and present price ratios of about 1.6 to 1.7
of use of soybean meals to fish meals.[12,13,14]
The picture presented by Alverson and Broadhead and shown in Figure 5 illustrates the
recent history of meal production.[15]

The present demand for meals is generated
almost entirely by animal feeding programs
which are at present most highly developed in
the United States, Western Europe, and centrally planned countries, although the consumption and rates of consumption are growing
rapidly in some developing countries.

In addition to soy protein, considerable
recent attention has been directed toward
single-cell protein (SCP) grown by fermentation processes on a variety of substrates
including methane, petroleum and molasses.

Although substantial plans are under way
in the centrally planned countries to produce SCP supplements, their use in animal
feeds or human nutrition is not yet far
enough developed to determine what if any
effect SCP might have on the development of
fishery-based protein supplies. It is also
not possible here to assess the relative
importance of urea as a cattle food supplement although according to FAO reports the
use of urea may be increasingly important.[16]

Need for Resource Management and Research
With the exception of stocks in the Indian
Ocean, the southeast Atlantic, and selected
areas in the South China Sea and the Indonesian archipelago, most of the world's table

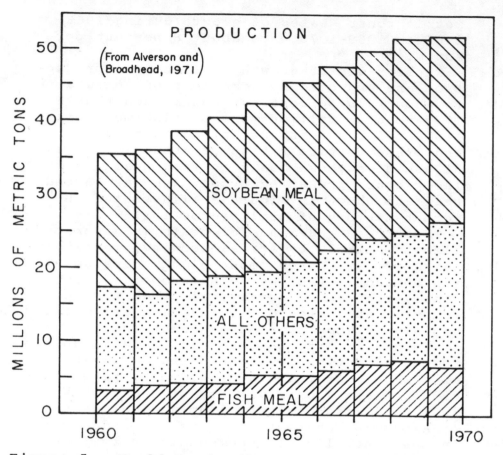

Figure 5.   World Production of Oilcake Meal
44% Soybean Meal Equivalent and Percent
Contribution by Major Components 1960-1969[15]

grade fisheries resources are now being
harvested at or beyond their maximum sustainable yield. Many of the industrial-grade
species from traditional fishery areas are
also being heavily exploited.

We believe that effective national and
international mechanisms are needed at once
to prevent serious changes in the biological
composition of species available for harvest,
as exemplified by the history of the California sardine fishery. Effective management
mechanisms are also needed to prevent very
serious economic dislocations which would
follow in the not unlikely wake of additional
major failures in important fisheries of
which haddock, whales and sardines are examples.

If prior conditions are fulfilled, leading
to the major harvest of krill, oceanic squid,
and lantern fish, we will be in serious trou-
ble. These troubles will extend to areas beyond the scope of this paper but not your
imagination. One may seriously question the
wisdom of harvesting the food web of the sea
so intensively as to possibly destroy the
various linkages which must exist within the
web.[17]

For example a harvest of the krill population at levels approximating 100 million
tons would almost certainly preclude the recovery of the Antarctic baleen whale populations even under conditions of a moratorium
on the harvest of whale stocks. Other highly
adapted species in the Antarctic that depend
directly or indirectly on the krill might also be reduced or eliminated.

There is increasing evidence that species
diversity per se is a measure of and a necessary condition for what might be termed the
biological quality of life.[18] And in view of
the fact that we so poorly understand the
implications for human populations of changes

in the global food web, we believe that it
would be unwise to press vigorously for the
harvest of the <u>greater part</u> of the potential
marine resources available for FPC manufacture prior to mechanisms for: 1. limiting
the catch at levels sufficient to sustain the
fished populations as well as other populations known to depend upon the fished populations for their livelihood; 2. limiting
economic and political conflicts in regard to
the harvest of resources beyond national
jurisdiction; and 3. providing sources of
funds from the use of present and future resources to support resources research primarily for management purposes.

A generous estimate places the present
level of living marine resources research
(not including "oceanographic" research) at
somewhat less than one percent of the ex-
vessel value of the fisheries harvest of the
oceans. It seems almost certain that increased expenditures on resources research
leading to better management and sustained
harvest would be more than recovered by an
increase in average yields and a more stable
investment climate for fisheries. Well-
designed systems of limited entry appear to
be a necessary corollary to both the research
and the capital investment needed if ocean
resources are to be used for the maximum
benefit to man at minimum environmental degradation.

References

1. Cushing, D. H. 1969. <u>Upwelling and Fish
Productions</u>. FAO Fisheries Technical Paper,
No. 83, June. FAO, Rome.

2. Gulland, J. A. 1970. <u>The Fish Resources</u>

of the Ocean. FAO FIRS/T97, pp. 307-319.
Rome.

3. Chapman, W. M. 1967. Fish potential of
the world ocean for the manufacture of fish
meal and fish protein concentrate. Paper
read at the 9th Annual Fisheries Symposium
National Fish Meal and Oil Assoc., Washington, D. C.

4. Chapman, W. M. et al. 1969. Fishing in
the future. Ceres II 3:22-26.

5. Kasahara, H. 1967. Food production from
the ocean. Ms. p. 43.

6. Marr, J. W. S. 1967. The natural history and geography of the Antarctic krill
(Euphausia superba DANA). Discovery Report
32:33-464.

7. Idyll, C. P. 1970. The Sea Against
Hunger, New York: Crowell.

8. Mauchline, J., and Fisher, L. R. 1969.
The biology of euphausiid. In Advances in
Marine Biology, vol. 4, pp. 1-454, eds.
F. S. Russel and M. Yonge. New York:
Academic Press.

9. Solyanik, G. A. 1964. Mass catch of
Euphausia superba with a variable-depth trawl
from a whaling ship. Soviet Antarctic Expedition, vol. 2, pp. 124-125. New York:
Elsview.

10. Clarke, M. R. 1966. A review of the
systematics and ecology of oceanic squid. In
Advances in Marine Biology, vol. 4, pp. 91-
300, eds. F. S. Russel, and M. Yonge. New
York: Academic Press.

11.   World supply of demand prospects for oilseeds and oilseed products in 1980.   1971. Foreign Agriculture Economic Report No. 71, U. S. Department of Agriculture, Marcy.

12.   Commodity Review and Outlook, 1968-69 and 1969-70.   Rome: FAO.

13.   Monthly Report   1970.   Fish Meal Exporters Organization, August.

14.   World Agriculture Production and Trade, 1970.   U. S. Department of Agriculture, August.

15.   Alverson, G. and Broadhead, W. C.   1971. International Trade - Fish Meal, IOFC/DEV/71/ 17, FAO, Rome.

16.   Agriculture Commodity Projections 1970-1980, 1971.   Vol. 1, p. 164.   FAO, Rome.

17.   Steele, J. H.   1970.   Marine Food Chains.   Berkeley: U. of Cal.

18.   Patrick, R.   1968.   The structure of diatom communities in similar ecological conditions.   American Naturalist 102 (924): 173-183.

19.   Yearbook of Fishery Statistics   1972. Vols. 30 and 31.   FAO, Rome.

20.   Lomkina, N. B.   1966.   The Euphausiid fauna of the antarctic and notal regions. In Biological Reports of the Soviet Antarctic Expedition, 1955-1958.   Vol. 2, eds. A. P. Andviyashev, and P. V. Ushakov.   Moscow, 1964, published for the National Science Foundation by the Israeli Program for Scientific Translations, Jerusalem, 1966.

II
THE RESPONSE OF FISHERIES MANAGEMENT PHILOSOPHY TO THE IMPERATIVES OF MODERN TECHNOLOGY

Robert D. Balkovic
Robert F. Hutton
Denton R. Moore
Office of Resource Management, National
Marine Fisheries Service, NOAA, Department
of Commerce, Washington, D. C.

"Modern fisheries are changing and developing
so rapidly that the traditional procedures
for the scientific assessment of the stock
and for the implementation of management
measures are no longer entirely appropriate.
Management authorities should be prepared to
take early action, and usually cannot afford
to wait for complete scientific evidence.
Equally, the scientific community must be
prepared to give early advice even when the
data are very scanty. At the same time
arrangements should be made to continually
revise the advice as new data become available."[1]
     Gulland's statement is an appropriate
introduction to the following discussion.
We will begin with some comments on some of
the statements in the paper presented by
Sprague and Arnold and then provide some insight into the role of the National Marine
Fisheries Service in discharging its responsibility for the management of living marine
resources.
     First, we cannot entirely agree with
Sprague and Arnold that there is little reason to be optimistic that means to achieve
an adequate international fisheries management framework is within our grasp. While
results may not be immediate, there is clear

evidence that steps toward such a framework
are being taken and will accelerate during
the next two years. Political interest is
being stimulated as both the domestic and
international fishing intensity increases on
both traditional and underdeveloped stocks
and as the coastal countries become increasingly interested in reserving resources near
their shores for their own fishermen.

Our work with the various international
fisheries commissions to which the United
States is a party, with the FAO, UNESCO, and
other international bodies, is continuing.
We expect significant international fisheries
management philosophies to be agreed upon
during the forthcoming Law of the Sea Conference. Other management arrangements will
develop through bilateral agreements, and
unilateral measures affecting specific resources can also be expected.

However, past experience has shown that
the success of international negotiations
concerning fisheries has been directly related to the quality and completeness of
scientific knowledge and the effectiveness
of domestic management systems.

Secondly, it is abundantly clear that the
serious conditions existing in some of our
traditional fisheries have resulted from
either improper management systems or their
absence. We cannot permit these conditions
to develop in other fisheries which have retained their viability but which are being
fished at or near-- or perhaps even beyond--
their maximum sustainable yields. It is in
those fisheries that we believe immediate
steps must be taken to implement appropriate
management systems before it is too late.

Finally, we cannot deny that many of our
coastal fisheries resources have broad
national importance, for several reasons.
Not only do they provide valuable food, but

they also yield raw materials for a number of
industrial products and they serve as potential raw material for FPC (fish protein concentrate) production. They also furnish
important economic returns for many coastal
communities, some of which are already hard-
pressed as a consequence of depletion of specific fisheries, and they provide unique and
irreplaceable recreational opportunities for
millions of our citizens.

In this context an unavoidable broad
national interest emerges. The National
Marine Fisheries Service recognizes that national interest and the responsibility it
carries with it. In the discharge of that
responsibility, we are beginning, in cooperation with the states, to design management
systems which recognize the multitude of
legitimate interests, so that all of the
concerns--the biological health of the resources themselves, the economic and social
health of dependent fishermen and their
communities, and the psychological satis-
factions of millions of U. S. sportsmen--
will be met. This task is far too complex
for the states or the federal government to
do alone within their respective jurisdictions. There must be coordination among the
various jurisdictions involved.

A new program, the State-Federal Fisheries Management Program, was formally
established within the National Marine Fisheries Service in 1971.

Its goal is to establish coordinated
State-Federal programs designed to improve
the management of fish resources in order to
achieve the appropriate allocation of these
resources among competing users and to provide the legal-institutional environment for
the development of a viable commercial fishing industry and maximum recreational
opportunities. This program contemplates

limited entry where necessary to conserve
resources and assure the maximum use of capital and labor. The harvesting segment of
some of the commercial fishing industry has
experienced economic difficulty over the past
two decades. The fleets in certain of our
important fisheries have deteriorated to the
point where the vessels can no longer be considered efficient, seaworthy fishing units.
Symptoms of the existing situation in many
parts of this industry have been low returns
to labor and capital. The result, too often,
has been antiquated vessels operated by old
crewmen.

Subsidies, technical assistance, and other
direct aid programs which attack only the
symptoms and not the basic problems cannot in
themselves ensure a viable commercial fishing
industry and maximum recreational opportunities. Rather, it is necessary to solve the
twin basic problems associated both with
generally free international and domestic entry into any fishery, and obscure, ambiguous
fisheries jurisdictions.

References

1. Gulland, J. A. 1971. Science and
fishery management. Journal du Conseil
International pour l'Exploration de la Mer
33 (3):471-477.

III
RAW MATERIAL SUPPLY FOR FISH PROTEIN
CONCENTRATE

William F. Royce
National Marine Fisheries Service, National
Oceanic and Atmospheric Administration,
U. S. Department of Commerce, Washington,
D. C. 20235

The special values of fish protein in human
nutrition and the theoretical usefulness of a
stable dry powder made from fish and known as
Fish Protein Concentrate has been of interest
for some time.* In examining the problems
and assessing the future potential of allevi-
ating human nutritional problems with FPC,
some of the restraints on its production,
especially with respect to raw material,
should be identified.

Raw Materials for FPC
Theoretically, FPC can be produced from any
high protein aquatic animal that is nontoxic.
The possibilities include hundreds of kinds
of fish, molluscs, and crustaceans, that are
the groups commonly caught by the fisheries.
The possibilities also include the parts of
animals left after filleting or dressing and
the animals discarded after the more valuable
ones are sorted out.
    In practice, however, the potential raw
materials are severely limited. These limitations, which are discussed below, are related to quality, uniformity, conservation,
steadiness of supply and above all, cost.
    In the U. S. the required quality of raw

----

*This article draws heavily on the excellent
review by Finch, 1970.[1]

material for FPC is, according to the Food
and Drug Administration, "...species of fish
handled expeditiously and under sanitary
conditions in accordance with good manufacturing practices recognized as proper for
fish that are used in other forms for human
food." Species presently approved for FPC
manufacture include hake and hake-like fish,
menhaden, and herring of the genus Clupea.*
Just how much loss of quality is technically
tolerable is not clear but presumably there
could be no substantial degradation of the
protein quality or development of undesirable color, flavor or odor that would remain
in the final product.

With existing technology, the quality of
the raw material as landed is directly related to hours, not days, on board the vessel
after capture, because the price and volume
to be handled almost surely preclude the use
of cooling equipment. In tropical waters
this probably means 12 hours, in northern
waters not more than about 24 hours between
the time of capture and the time the fish enter the drying process, if the quality is to
approach that of fish used in other forms of
human food. The alternative is new technology that permits low cost cooling or chemical
preservation for longer periods.

One important aspect of quality other than
sanitary handling is the control of certain
materials in the final FPC. These may be
trace elements such as fluoride and lead,
which tend to concentrate in bones and
scales. They may be reduced to tolerable
levels by skinning and deboning. The material may be an organic toxin that causes
ciguatera or paralytic shellfish poisoning.
Either the process must remove or destroy the

----

*California anchovy (Engraulis mordax) was
approved in July 1973.

toxin or animals containing the toxins must
be avoided.

Another important characteristic of the
raw material is uniformity. Economical processes require uniform raw material and any
substantial variation in oil, minerals, or
nonprotein nitrogen will require adjustment
in the process and perhaps cause a substantial change in the quality of the product.
For this reason the use of discarded fish of
diverse species could present technical and
economic problems.

The requirement of conservation may
eliminate the use of young fish of a species
that later in life will bring a higher price.
If these cannot be avoided or released alive
by the fishermen, their use will probably be
prohibited.

The manufacturing process for FPC will be
more economical if the supply of raw material is steady. Ideally, a constant amount of
raw material should be delivered each day.
If too much is delivered it must be stored
with adequate preservation. If too little
is delivered the process is interrupted.
Such continuity is difficult at best and impossible in fisheries for many species.
Some species vary in quantity during their
seasonal migrations, others according to the
relative success of their spawning. Fishing
is affected by weather and, in temperate or
northern areas, frequently interrupted.
Such problems can probably be alleviated by
new technology of preservation.

Finally, the raw material as delivered to
the processing machinery must not cost more
than about $.05 per kg. The minimum possi-
ble is probably the price of the Peruvian
anchovy which was landed for about $0.014
per kg in 1970. Other average prices worth
noting for the year 1970 are $0.037 per kg
for U. S. menhaden and $0.31 per kg for

Norwegian capelin* both of which are produced in quantities around one million tons.

Despite the actual cost of production the value of the raw material must not be greater for any other use. If, for example, a fishery were established to supply an FPC plant and the species became marketable at a higher price as frozen fillets, then obviously the supply or price of the FPC plant would be affected.

With these restraints a large proportion of the world's fisheries could not supply an FPC plant with suitable raw material at a suitable price. The fisheries of the lesser developed countries tend to catch diverse kinds of small quantities per person at widely scattered ports. It seems highly unlikely that any of these fisheries could supply an FPC plant, and therefore we are left with the more sophisticated and highly mechanized fisheries. Among these fisheries, those using traps, hooks, gill nets, and even bottom trawls are probably eliminated from supplying FPC plants because of their inability to catch fish cheaply enough or because they can earn more by fishing for more valuable species. This leaves only the purse seine or midwater trawl fisheries as the ones likely to supply FPC plants.

The cost restraint can be used to estimate the productivity levels that will be necessary in FPC fisheries. If we assume a nearly year-round operation, a price of $.05 per kg and half of the price to the fisherman (half to the vessel), then a vessel must catch 400 tons per man per year to provide a fisherman with $10,000 per year, which is close to the minimum for a U. S. fisherman. By compari-

---

*Data on prices are from U. S. and FAO fishery statistics.

son, the best Peruvian seiners catch about
1,000 tons per man per year and most of them
average more than 300 tons per man per year
of anchovies.

Such generalities do not mean that a profitable venture cannot be developed around,
say, bottom trawl fisheries under special
circumstances. But suitable circumstances
must be regarded as an exception rather than
a rule. Similar considerations apply to the
use of previously discarded species or parts
of fishes. The costs of sorting, special
handling, trans-shipment to an FPC plant or
loss of vessel time may prevent the use of
these materials. It also is possible such
fish may not be acceptable for esthetic
reasons.

When we put these restraints together we
find that we must seek an abundant species
of fish catchable by purse seine or midwater
trawl within about 100 kilometers of port.
This species must be regularly available
during most of the year and must not be readily marketable in a more valuable form.

With these restraints the known stocks of
fish that are likely to form a ready supply
of raw material for FPC are restricted to
those that are now supplying raw material for
fish meal. Examples are U. S. menhaden,
Peruvian anchovy, South African jack mackerel, and North Sea capelin. These stocks are
relatively well known and the diversion of
parts of the catch into raw material for a
human grade of FPC should be relatively easy.
Further, the cost of doing this should be
calculable with greater precision than the
cost of developing a fishery on any other
stocks that are less well known.

If we consider stocks of fish that are not
now being harvested, the potential sources
of raw material for FPC are highly specula-
tive (an exception to this is the California

anchovy). The stocks that are most likely to
be available in quantity according to
Gulland[2] are likely to be those of the anchovy and herring families, the cephalopods, the
lantern fish or the euphausiid crustaceans.
The last three are sources of protein that
are probably larger than all of the stocks of
fish now being intensively harvested. We
know very little, however, about the location
and abundance of these stocks and the technology of using them.

It seems safe to conclude, therefore, that
the most promising opportunities for producing FPC on a large scale with existing technology lie almost entirely in the diversion
of existing stocks of the shoaling pelagic
fishes from fish meal to FPC. Even this will
not be easy, however, because of the requirement for handling the fish under "sanitary
conditions and accordance with good manufacturing practices recognized as proper for
fish that are used in other forms for human
food." This requirement will mean major
technical changes in the methods of handling
the fish and the methods of preservation--
both of which may increase costs.

If we accept the validity of these arguments and urgency of relieving human nutritional problems by using fish, let's look at
a broader spectrum of possibilities. These
possibilities are FPC in the broad sense and
include any product, wet or dry, made from
fish which contains a larger proportion of
protein than the raw fish. Such products are
those from which we remove moisture, bones or
viscera. The products include a variety of
minced fish flesh products and the cooked,
smoked and dried fish that are already so
widely distributed in many countries.

In summary let us take a more flexible
approach toward developing low cost fishery
products. Let us consider that new products

are expensive at first and become low in
price after we apply our technology, develop
markets and increase the volume. The number
of possible products is very large.

References

1. Finch, Roland A. 1970. Fish Protein for
Human Foods. CRC Critical Reviews in Food
Technology, pp. 519-580.

2. Gulland, J. A. (Editor) 1970. The fish
resources of the oceans. FAO Fisheries
Technical Paper No. 97, p. 425.

IV
FISH RESOURCES FOR PRODUCTION OF FISH PROTEIN CONCENTRATE

FAO Fishery Resources Division

(Updated version of a summary prepared by
L. K. Boerema, FAO, and A. C. Burd, Fisheries
Laboratory, Lowestoft, U. K., at the meeting
of the FPC Working Group of the FAO Protein
Advisory Group, held in London, November
1970)

Introduction
It would appear that for production of FPC
(fish protein concentrate) of whatever type
at a reasonable price, substantial factory
throughput per day of low-priced fish is en-
visaged. Therefore, the raw material to be
used for this purpose consists in the main of
pelagic and other shoaling fish species. The
concentration of these fish in shoals allows
high catch rates, resulting in relatively low
catching cost. Hence, the resource requirements are the same as for conventional fish
meal production, with which in the present
situation, production of FPC for direct human
consumption would compete for raw materials.
Furthermore, a large FPC industry might compete for its raw materials with the use of
fish for direct human consumption in any
other form. The presence of little exploited
resources, e.g., in areas of developing countries, would therefore not necessarily mean
that these should become available for protein concentrate production when a fishery on
these resources develops.
     The present paper gives a short summary of
the available knowledge of the world's marine
fish resources and their state of exploita-

tion. The scope of this paper does not allow
going into any details of the availability of
little exploited resources along the coast of
individual countries, and the information on
the magnitude of little exploited resources
in particular in the developing areas of the
world, is in most cases rather scanty. Most
of the material used as a background for the
present document has been taken from an FAO
area review of fish resources, prepared for
the FAO Indicative World Plan for Agricultural Development.[1] The catch figures for 1970
have been taken from the FAO Fisheries Yearbook.[2]

Regional Supplies of Appropriate Species, with Future Projections

By 1970 the total world catch of marine fish
was 61.7 million tons. Pelagic species
accounted for 26 million tons, of which 23
million tons was reduced to fish meal. In
addition, 2 million tons of non-oily fishes
were processed for meal. Of the 2 million
tons of non-oily fishes, 0.3 million tons
were derived from waste fish from processing
in the United Kingdom. Japanese catches
accounted for some 0.6 million tons and, in
the main, cod and hake catches accounted for
the remainder.

The catches of oily fishes are dominated
by the Peruvian/Chilean anchoveta catch of
13 million tons in 1970. Herring and mackerel catches accounted for about 6 million
tons, mainly from the North Atlantic. About
1.5 million tons of pilchard, anchovy and
horse mackerel were taken off South and
Southwest Africa and Angola.

As indicated in the FAO Indicative World
Plan for Agricultural Development, the potential yield of the marine fish resources has
been estimated to be of the order of 100 million tons, not including molluscs (e.g.,

squid) and crustacea. The potential pelagic
yield is estimated at 58 million tons. These
figures are theoretical potentials and it
would not be feasible to exploit all the
stocks to their maximum sustainable level.
The potential yield of some open ocean pelagic species, such as myctophids, is not included in these figures as no technique for
economically harvesting them is yet available. There are also believed to be extensive resources of saury. These species may
occur in large quantities but are also very
widely spread, and no estimates of their potential are available for most areas.

In practice, because of the difficulties of
managing fisheries so that each species is
fully exploited, it would not be expected
that more than about 80 percent of the total
potential of an area would be harvestable.

In reviewing the potential yield of marine
fish resources, mention should also be made
of the resource requirements for an FPC industry. A relatively large FPC plant might
have a capacity to process 200 to 400 tons of
fish per day. If operated for 250 days of
the year, which may be a high estimate, the
total resource requirement would range from
50 to 100 thousand tons annually.

North Atlantic. In the North Atlantic, conservation action is under discussion for herring and mackerel stocks. In the short term,
a reduction in yield of these species is expected. The potential of the capelin fishery
is uncertain. High variability in the abundance of the unfished stock has been recorded. Very high yields have been obtained
in recent years with an intensive fishery,
but the ability of the stock to withstand it
is in doubt. At present, unexploited stocks
of blue whiting and polar cod exist and expansion of fisheries on horse mackerel, sand

eels, hake, and perhaps sauries is expected.
     It would seem that no expansion in total
yield from the area can be expected and indeed the catch for conversion to meal might
well be reduced in the near future.

Central Atlantic. The total catch from the
Central Atlantic in 1970 was 4.1 million
tons. Of this 1.5 million tons came from the
western half of the area (west of 40° W).
The potential yields for the western and
eastern areas are estimated at 5.5 million
tons and 3.0 million tons respectively, somewhat more than half consisting of pelagic
species. Large pelagic species such as tuna
are excluded from the latter estimate.
     Since these estimates were made, a con-
siderable development in exploitation of
sardinella stocks in the eastern area has
taken place. Catches of the order of several
hundred thousand tons have been reported.
Until detailed statistics are available it is
impossible to estimate the potential with
precision.
     Little-exploited stocks of anchovy and
thread herring occur in the Caribbean area
and the Gulf of Mexico. Pelagic stocks potential is given as 0.5 to 1 million tons in
the Caribbean and about 1 million tons for
the Gulf. In addition, in this latter area,
a potential yield of 1 to 1.5 million tons of
demersal fish is possible, consisting of a
wide range of species. An estimated catch of
0.6 million tons is already taken as by-catch
in the shrimp fishery. Some of the species
taken in these mixed catches may be poisonous
and the incidence of occurrence of these
should be examined prior to any development
in the utilization of the by-catches.

South Atlantic. The 1970 catches from the
South Atlantic region amounted to about 3.5

million tons. About 2.5 million tons were
taken off the African coast and consisted of
about 1.5 million tons of pelagic species,
the remaining catch consisting mainly of
hake. The pelagic catches consist of pilchard, horse mackerel and anchovy. In recent years there has been a considerable
decline in the catches of pilchard while the
anchovy catch has increased. With the advent
of the recent increased effort due to the
offshore fishing by factory vessels there is
some concern that the stocks may not be able
to sustain the present catch levels.

An estimate of the hake potential for the
area has been given as 1.5 million tons,
based on data obtained after the recent expansion in the fishery. Annual catches of
this order have already been reached.

The Southwestern Atlantic region is generally underexploited. The major resources are
anchovy (1 to several million tons), Falkland
herring (perhaps 1 to 1.5 million tons),
hake, poutassou and various other demersal
species (1.5 million tons). These refer to
the region off Argentina and Uruguay. Little
is known of the potential off Brazil.

North Pacific. The North Pacific catch in
1970 was 16.6 million tons. The potential
for the area is given as 18 million tons.
(This figure differs from figures previously
cited due to a change in the statistical
boundaries.) There is still some potential
increase in yield for some pelagic species
(saury and sand eels). Others may be in need
of conservation, which would imply a reduction in the near future compared to the present total catch.

Central Pacific. The western Central Pacific
area includes very varied areas of shallow
water where exploitation rates range from

subsistence fisheries in the island areas to
fairly heavily exploited regions off the
Philippines, and in the Yellow and East China
Seas. The Gulf of Thailand may be already
overexploited for demersal species.

The total estimated catch in 1970 was 4.8
million tons. A potential yield for the area
was estimated at 16 million tons, of which 7
to 8 million tons were shoaling pelagic species. These estimates are extremely rough.
Due to the large shelf area, the potential
for the catch per unit area is thought to be
rather low, and there is a wide variety of
species.

A minimum catch of 0.9 million tons was
taken in 1970 from the east Central Pacific.
A pelagic fish potential yield of 4 million
tons is estimated. Two million tons of anchovy could be taken off California and Mexico. The thread herring and anchovy resources
off Central America would perhaps support
catches of about 1 million tons annually but
may be widely distributed. The hake stocks
off the west coast of the United States are
estimated at 0.2 million tons potential annual yield. Trash fish catches in shrimp
fisheries at present amount to about 0.3 to
0.8 million tons.

South Pacific. The present catches from the
Southwest Pacific amount to about 0.2 million
tons per annum. The potential is estimated
at 0.6 million tons, though little is known
of stocks in the area.

In the Southeast Pacific area 14 million
tons, mainly of anchoveta, were taken in
1970. The hake catch from the area was 0.1
million tons. The anchoveta is fully exploited. Potential yields have been estimated as 0.2 million tons of hake, 0.2
million tons of grenadier and several hundred
thousand tons of mackerel, jack mackerel and

Falkland herring.

Indian Ocean. The 1970 catch from the Indian
Ocean was estimated at 2.8 million tons, of
which pelagic fish form a substantial part.
Potential yields for the western region are
4.5 and 4.0 million tons for demersal and
shoaling pelagic fish, respectively. In the
eastern region, potential yields for these
two resources are 3.0 and 2.0 million tons.
     The distribution of the pelagic resources
is patchy, with high stocks in the Arabian
Sea and Gulf of Aden (sardines) and possibly
off Indonesia. Some other areas may have low
potential. Even in the high potential areas
the localized distribution of the pelagic
species may well be highly variable, as their
availability is related to the effects of the
monsoons.

Other resources. As stated, the above resources refer only to fish, and do not include cephalopods (squid), crustacea, etc.
It is known that squid is abundant in several
sea areas, but little is known about the potential of these resources. The total squid
potential is guessed at probably over 10 million but less than 100 million tons. The
unexploited squid potential of Peru is estimated at 0.5 million tons. The resources of
common squid off the Japanese coast seem to
be fully exploited at the present catch level
of 300 to 500 thousand tons annually. The
total world catch of cephalopods in 1970 was
0.9 million tons.
     The resources of Antarctic krill are very
large, with an estimated potential of over 50
million tons. Catching this krill in sufficient quantities presents difficulties, however, and the technology of catching and
processing will have to be developed before
industrial exploitation of this resource can

materialize. Its development is well under
way in some countries, particularly in the
U.S.S.R.

Seasonal Considerations in Fisheries
The duration of the period of high catch
rates of different pelagic stocks is variable, depending on the particular migration,
spawning and behavior patterns of the species. For example the sand eel fishery in
the North Sea is limited to a period of about
eight weeks. On the other hand, as a result
of improvements in fishing tactics, the exploitation of the Atlantic-Scandian herring
stock was extended from the immediate pre-
spawn and spawning period of about three
months to the whole year. Even though a species may be fished over a long period, it is
usual that peak catches occur at certain seasons. Peruvian anchoveta give high catch
rates over about four months, but can be
fished in reasonable quantities over another
five months.
   The seasons of abundance of the presently
exploited species are well documented. In
some cases, high catch rates may be maintained over a longer period of the year by
switching the fishing operation from one species to another, The alternation of the
exploitation of North Sea herring and mackerel by the Norwegian purse seine fleet is an
example. On the other hand, in the South
African fishery the various species appear to
be caught at about the same period.
   Relatively little can be predicted on the
variability in catch rates of the presently
unexploited resources. The Argentine anchovy
is known to occur very close to the coast
during several months from August on. After-
wards they migrate northeasterly towards the
edge of the shelf. Fleets capable of following the migration have the opportunity of

exploiting the stock over a great part of the
year.

In the Arabian Sea the availability of the
fish appears to be related to the monsoon
period.

The hake stocks off Chile, Peru and Argentina appear to have a relatively limited migration. They could be exploited over a
fairly long period by suitable vessels.

Sardinella stocks off West Africa are
known to be sharply seasonal in their migration and the abundance in certain regions.
Present investigations in the area will provide information on the problem of availability.

The general seasonality in abundance of
pelagic species means that the maintenance
of input to factories will be to some degree
dependent on the type of catching fleet.
The dependence of a large plant on the
catches of a small-vessel fleet would make it
more vulnerable to changes in availability of
the fish due to migrations than it would be
where the fisheries were exploited by large
sea-going vessels. An understanding of the
seasonal changes in availability and distribution of the stock is essential for the proper planning of the utilization of the resource.

General Considerations on Resource Supplies
At first sight the resource potential would
appear to allow for a substantial further
development of the fishing industry. However, when we examine the states of specific
stocks it can be seen that many which have
supported the industrial fisheries in recent
years are fully or even overexploited. To
maintain the present yield, fishing fleets
must shift their efforts to new resources.
Many of the new resources are in distant waters or in remote areas. In some cases new

techniques of capture may have to be
developed. It might well be difficult to
substantially increase or perhaps even maintain the present level of catch for fish meal
production in the near future.

Reviewing the above information on the resources and their present catch in the various areas, it would appear that the major
areas in which important unexploited or
underexploited stocks are still available are
the Western Central Atlantic (in particular
the Gulf of Mexico), the Southwest Atlantic
(off Argentina and Uruguay), the East Central
Pacific (South California and Mexico), the
southern half of the West Central Pacific
(offshore areas in the South China Sea), and
various areas in the Indian Ocean (e.g., Indonesia, Arabian Sea). In only a few of these
areas is the magnitude of some major stocks
and the occurrence of these fish in commercial densities fairly well documented, e.g.,
as in the area off Argentina and Uruguay. In
some other areas the potential stock may as a
total be quite high, but spread over a large
area and hence occurring in low densities, as
seems to be the case in the offshore areas in
the South China Sea. In still other areas,
e.g., parts of the Indian Ocean, the southern
part of the East Central Pacific, etc., the
figures have been based more on indications
and conjecture than on real measurements.

Whereas some of the estimates given above
may well be considerably too high, others may
be substantially too low, but in any case
they are believed to represent the best estimates presently available.

With the increase in world fish demand and
the probable decline in the established supplies of fresh and frozen fish for human consumption in developed countries, an increased
market for suitable alternative fish supplies may emerge. In view of the much higher

value of such fish, diversion of supplies
such as hake to this market would result in a
reduction of supplies of fish meal and FPC
production.

   Availability of raw material for FPC production may be influenced by more demanding
care of the catch than is customary in normal
fish meal production. In view of the better
quality of the fish required, an alteration
in vessels and equipment might be necessary,
increasing the cost of prime material. A
change in fishing tactics, such as the limiting of the effective area of fishing, might
also result.

   Where the utilization of yet unexploited
resources is considered in plans for FPC production, the problem involved in simultaneously developing a fishing fleet, training
fishermen, establishing shore facilities,
establishing plants and developing a market
for such a novel product will need consideration, and they should be compared with the
problems of developing fisheries for the more
traditional products for which the same resources can be used.

References

1. Gulland, J. A. 1970. The fish resources
of the oceans. FAO Fisheries Technical Paper
No. 97, p. 425.

2. FAO Yearbook of Fishery Statistics.
1970. Vol. 30.

Part II

PROCESSING

V
FPC PROCESSES

Roland Finch
National Marine Fisheries Service, National
Oceanic and Atmospheric Administration, U. S.
Department of Commerce, Washington, D. C.
20235

The general and technical requirements for a
satisfactory process for making fish protein
concentrate (FPC) are discussed. Solvent extraction processes, especially those using
isopropyl alcohol (IPA), have been most widely examined. Stages in the extraction of
fish with IPA as a prototype method are reviewed. Variations in solvent processes,
modifications to simplify them and to retain
functionality in the end products, and nonsolvent methods including enzymic digestion
are discussed. Future developments are considered.

Introduction
The present paper reviews briefly some general process considerations for producing FPC.
Information about isopropyl alcohol extraction of fish on a large scale is now available, and this will serve to focus attention
on certain practical problems involved in
commercial production. Variations on solvent
and other processes will be considered
followed by a comment on future potentials.
   A great deal is known about many scientific
and technical aspects of making FPC,[1,2] yet
we are still largely unable to judge the potential commercial application of the various
processes and products because of our insufficient knowledge about the economics of
these processes, and the characteristics,
uses, and acceptance of the products in the

market place; we are therefore unable to
judge whether the business of making and
selling them offers an attractive investment.

There is an old story in the folklore of
FPC that, given a bottle of gin and a herring, one can make FPC. However, it is poor
quality FPC, tasting of juniper berries; it
is very expensive FPC; and furthermore, it
ruins the gin. A process which makes an
unacceptable or even a marginally acceptable
product is not satisfactory. Nor is one
which makes a product too expensive to use,
and an extraction process which renders the
solvent unusable cannot hope to succeed.
What, then, are the product characteristics
of a successful process?

The first characteristic for any food
product is safety. It must be safe for human consumption under its end conditions of
use. Precautions must be taken against undesirable substances which may form in any
process of production and against the possibility of concentrating to an unsafe point in
the end product naturally occurring substances such as fluorine, or contaminants
such as pesticides.

Second, the products should possess
characteristics which render them acceptable
and valuable. The term FPC covers a variety
of products which can differ considerably in
color, odor, flavor, composition, and physical (functional) and nutritional properties.
These characteristics determine the ways in
which different FPCs may be used in different
food systems, the benefits they confer on the
food systems into which they are incorporated, and in consequence, their value in any
particular application.

The third factor important to a successful
process is cost. An FPC should be produced
and distributed at a cost which will enable
it to compete in markets with like products

and provide an adequate return on the investment in the operation.

Finally, the question of supply is important. FPC must be available continuously in
sufficient quantity to keep users supplied
without undue delay.

General Process Considerations

The recently revised FAO guideline for fish
protein concentrate for human consumption de-
fines the product as follows:

"Fish protein concentrate (FPC) is a stable
product suitable for human consumption, prepared from whole fish or other aquatic animals or parts thereof. Protein concentration
is increased by the removal of water and in
certain cases of oil, bones and other materials. Traditionally-dried or other tradition-
ally preserved products do not fall within
this guideline."[3]

This is a broad definition and in various
countries more specific requirements exist.
For example, the U. S. Food and Drug Administration limits the species which may be used
(hake and hakelike fish, menhaden and herring
of the genus Clupea), the processes which may
be used (extraction with isopropyl alcohol or
extraction with ethylene dichloride followed
by isopropyl alcohol), and requires the product to meet certain chemical and nutritional
specifications.[4,5] A similar example is the
Canadian regulation on fish protein.[6] Many
processes have been proposed for making forms
of FPC which meet the broad FAO definition.
They have in common the concentration of protein; the stabilization of the fish product
against the growth of microorganisms, mostly
by reduction of the water level; and its
stabilization against chemical change, especially lipid oxidation, by removal of most of

the lipids. Given the right combination of
conditions, all or most of the nutritional
value of the original fish protein can be retained. FPC processes therefore consist of
stages of separation and concentration.
     In order to consider likely differences
between alternative methods for making FPC,
it is necessary to review the composition of
fish and to determine how the different fractions of the fish may be affected by the process.[7,8] Most of the information available
on the composition of fish refers to the mus-
cular tissue which represents in most cases
the major fraction by weight of the fish. It
is obvious that the whole fish containing also the bones, head, viscera, etc. will have a
substantially different chemical composition.
Table 1 illustrates this with a comparison
between the composition of the muscle tissue
and that of the corresponding whole fish for
butterfish (a fat fish) and red hake (a lean
fish) calculated on a dry basis. The difference between whole fish and fillets is apparent. It is interesting to note that a fish
considered lean because of the low fat level
in the muscle may contain considerable vis-
ceral fat, and its total composition may not
be low in lipids. One important difference
is the high ash in the whole fish due to the
bone content. The bone consists largely of
calcium and phosphorus but it also contains
most of the fluoride found in fish. Levels
in FPC made from whole fish have been reported from 58 ppm using capelin and ocean pout
as raw material, to 761 ppm using dogfish.[1]
Fluoride in FPC is limited to a maximum of
100 ppm in the United States and 150 ppm in
Canada. This means some degree of bone removal is needed to reduce fluoride to these
levels in some species. Whole menhaden-FPC
may contain less than 100 ppm and so not require any bone removal, whereas herring-and

Table 1. Proximate Composition of Fillets and Whole Fish (Percent, Dry Basis)

	Butterfish (Porotornus tricanthus)		Red Hake (Urophycis chuss)	
	Fillet	Whole fish	Fillet	Whole fish
Protein (N x 6.25)	73.9	76.9	90.3	68.6
Oil	20.8	11.3	3.2	19.2
Ash	5.3	11.8	6.5	12.1
Fillet yield (av.)	33.1		24.7	

Calculated from the data of Brooke et al.[9]

anchovy-FPC contain around 150 ppm. Red
hake-FPC contains about 200 ppm and Pacific
hake-FPC, up to 500 ppm.

The composition of fish lipids consist
primarily of triglycerides, but amounts up to
1 percent of the tissue weight are in the
form of phospholipids.[10] The fatty acids in
these compounds are highly unsaturated and
therefore readily oxidized. Free fatty acids
commence to form by hydrolysis soon after the
fish are caught and may reduce extractability
of the protein with salt solutions.

Sphingolipids and sterols are also found
in fish lipids, and hydrocarbons such as
squalene and wax esters occur in a few species. In general, nonpolar solvents such as
hexane will remove triglycerides very efficiently and are widely used commercially for
oil extraction, as in the defatting of soya,[11] although the flammability of hexane is
a cause for concern. Trichloroethylene was
used at one time to reduce this risk but was
abandoned because of the undesirable effect
of small residues upon animals to which the
extracted cake was fed. However, nonpolar
solvents do not readily dissolve phospho
lipids and unless this lipid fraction is removed, oxidation of the residue and reversion
will occur.[12] Polar solvents such as the alcohols and acetone will remove phospholipids
more completely. However, alcohols are not
particularly good lipid solvents, especially
at room temperature, so they present a possible conflict between rapidity and completeness of removal of lipids. They appear to be
more stable than acetone which can react with
minor tissue constituents to give distinct
off-odors in the finished product.[13]

Proteins in fish comprise some 80 to 90
percent of the total nitrogenous compounds,
although in the case of the elasmobranches,
this is about 20 percent lower. Muscle

proteins are usually divided into three prin-
ciple fractions: the fibrillar or insoluble
muscle protein comprising about 65 percent of
the whole muscle; sarcoplasmic proteins,
which are soluble in weak salt solutions and
amount to about 20 to 30 percent; and connective tissue proteins comprising about 3 percent of the total protein, a level which is
much lower than that typical of land mammals
(about 17 percent) and which probably ac-
counts for the relative softness of fish tissue. These different fractions will behave
differently in different solvents or even in
a single water miscible solvent as it is diluted. Dambergs[14] measured the amount of
lipids, protein and nonprotein water solubles
extracted from cod by different concentrations of boiling IPA (isopropyl alcohol) and
of acetone. He found that as the concentration of IPA decreased, the amount of crude
protein and water solubles which were extracted increased considerably. Thus as the
IPA:water ratio decreased from 100:0 to 50:
50, the amounts of lipids extracted decreased
from 4 to 2 percent; the soluble solids extracted increased from 4 to 15 percent; and
the protein extracted increased from 0 to 11
percent. Thus the concentration of IPA used
greatly influences the composition of the extracted material, and hence of the extract
fish cake. Less polar solvents such as
ethylene dichloride and hexane will extract
considerably smaller amounts of nonlipid
material.
    The amount and nature of the nitrogenous
compounds originally present in the whole
fish which remain in the final product affect
not only the yield but also the characteristics of the FPC. Protein in the bone and
skin fraction is lower in nutritional value
than that in the muscle. Thus the PER (protein efficiency ratio) of samples of FPC made

by isopropyl alcohol extraction of whole
Pacific hake (Merluccius productus) averaged
105 percent of casein. The PER of FPC made
from deboned samples of the same species
averaged 113 percent of casein. Hallgren[15]
found that the water soluble fraction of fish
protein was lower in some essential amino
acids and higher in glycine than the insoluble fraction. The PER of whole fish protein
was 105 percent of casein while that of the
insoluble fraction was 119 percent casein.

However, Dubrow et al.[16] found that the
PER of FPC made from three samples of whole
red hake was essentially the same as that of
the same lots of hake freeze-dried. In a
further sample, the PER of the freeze-dried
fish was found to be significantly higher.
Removal of the water soluble fraction may
then increase the nutritional quality but
will certainly decrease the yield. The removal of water solubles also increases the
stability of the product.[14]

Another factor which needs to be considered in the process is the fate of various
microconstituents through the FPC process.
Since the process is one of concentration,
many of the constituents will be present in
FPC in larger amounts than in the corresponding raw fish. This is of potential concern with respect to heavy metals, pesticides, etc., although it should be remem-
bered that FPC is not eaten directly as a
food. The amounts of FPC consumed would be
relatively small, and since the total weight
of microconstituents ingested would not be
more than in the corresponding amount of raw
fish, the higher concentrations would be of
less consequence. Little data are available
about the concentration in most processes
and of most substances. Mercury is an ele-
ment of some concern since it exists in many
species in the form of the highly toxic

methyl mercury. Work by the NMFS indicates
that, although the IPA extraction process
concentrates fish some sevenfold, mercury is
concentrated only about fourfold[17] so that
some appears to be removed in the process.
With most species of fish, the final levels
in FPC are below 0.5 ppm. An inexpensive
partial removal even of this amount is possible by the addition of small amounts of cysteine hydrochloride to the first extraction
stage of the IPA process. Reductions of over
50 percent in the final level of mercury have
been achieved in the Aberdeen demonstration
plant. However, it is not clear whether this
could be carried out continuously. It is
found that only about one-sixth of the amount
of arsenic present in the raw fish is left in
the FPC. Chlorinated pesticides such as DDT
are largely extracted. Some elements are
concentrated in the bone of the fish, the removal of which, prior to extraction, reduces
the level in the FPC compared with that in
FPC made from whole fish. Samples of
anchovy-FPC were found to contain 8.3 ppm
lead when made from the whole fish but only
3.5 ppm when made from the deboned flesh.
Table 2 shows some preliminary data on the
concentration of some elements by the IPA extraction process, but this represents a
single sample and should be considered only
indicative.
     Sanitation in processing is an important
consideration. Fish carry numerous microorganisms especially on the skin and in the
intestinal tract. The count will increase on
transport and storage, especially under poor
conditions. The action of solvents, particularly alcohol, will generally reduce the number. When menhaden samples with an average
TPC (total plate counts) of 70,000 were converted to FPC, the average TPC fell to 300.[18]
When raw hake with an average TPC of 10,000

Table 2. Concentration of Some Elements in a Single Sample of FPC made from Swordfish (ppm)

Element	Concentration in Raw Fish	Expected Concentration in FPC (based on 7.5:1)	Concentration in FPC	Actual as Percent Expected
Arsenic	0.7	5.2	0.25	5
Chromium	< 0.23	1.72	2.28	132
Copper	0.32	2.40	4.69	195
Cobalt	0.07	0.52	0.17	33
Manganese	0.09	0.68	1.12	165
Selenium	0.61	4.57	2.70	59
Zinc	17.30	130	114	88
Mercury	1.22	9.15	7.63	83

was converted to FPC the average TPC fell to
200. Flavobacterium and Pseudomonas were
predominant in the raw fish whereas bacillus
predominated in the FPC. The levels of
Salmonella montivideo and S. aureus innocu-
lated into FPC did not survive on storage at
35° C for four months, especially at high
storage humidities.[19] Bacillus species declined more slowly whereas molds grew well
at and above 84 percent R. H. These tests
were made in laboratory systems and, as will
be noted later, high counts can occur in the
drying and other stages in plant operations.

Extraction Process

Most of the research into processes for making FPC has concentrated on solvents extraction with special reference to the use of
isopropyl alcohol, which has been most widely
used. However, in addition to the more or
less standard extraction processes, subsidiary manipulations have been suggested to alter the composition and the characteristics
of the FPC or to effect economics in the process. These include evisceration, removal of
part or all of the bone, preremoval of water
and/or lipids, segration of some protein
fractions, modification of the protein, and
chemical treatment to modify odor and flavor
or to partially remove constituents of the
raw fish. With the exception of the enzyme
process, which will be dealt with separately,
and a proposed method for removing lipids
with surfactants, the above largely center
around solvent extraction methods. The discussion will therefore first review extraction processes, from fish to FPC, and then
some of the variations and additions which
have been proposed.

Raw Material. The cost of fish is a principal item in the cost of the finished FPC and

must be low in cost. This means that species
must be used which are not in demand for direct use as food. FPC must also be made from
species that are available in volume for a
considerable part of the year so that fixed
plant costs can be spread over the maximum
possible number of days operation. Finally,
FPC should preferably be made from high oil
species to provide a maximum by-product value
and so further reduce the FPC cost. Much of
the original work on IPA extraction in the
U. S. was carried out on hake since underutilized stocks were available, and it was
believed that it would be simpler to work out
a process involving extraction of most of the
lipids from low fat fish.

However, fatty species such as menhaden,
anchovy and herring fill the requirements of
availability and cost mentioned above. One
disadvantage of fatty species is their generally darker color due to a higher level of
heme pigments. A second disadvantage is that
heme pigments catalyze the oxidation of the
highly unsaturated lipids in the fish with a
net result that the FPC tends to have a darker color and stronger residual odor and flavor, although the effect varies with the food
to which it is added, as shown in Table 3.
Nevertheless fatty fish are likely to provide
the main source of raw material for FPC. A
subsidiary supply in some cases may be waste
from fish filleting operations, which is permitted within certain limits in Canada but
not in the U. S. It would not be profitable
to use fillet waste as a sole source of raw
material.

Handling and Preparation Stages. About one-
third of the world catch is converted to fish
meal and most of this is handled in bulk.
However, the fish are not stored and unloaded
according to the standards required for human

Table 3. Taste Panel Scores on Foods Continuing FPC Made from Various Fish (5-point hedonic rating)

Food Base	Attribute	Red Hake	Menhaden	Anchovy	Herring
Pasta	Appearance	3.0	2.6	1.0	1.8
	Flavor	3.0	3.0	2.5	2.9
Bread	Appearance	2.8	2.1	1.5	2.3
	Flavor	3.0	2.5	2.4	2.8
Cookies	Appearance	2.9	3.1	1.6	2.2
	Flavor	2.8	2.7	2.6	2.4

foods. The revised guideline for FPC proposed by the Protein Advisory Group specifies
that the quality of the raw material and the
handling practices shall be equivalent to
those used for fish for processing for human
consumption. It also indicates that the fish
may be preserved prior to processing in a
whole or ground form by means of dehydration,
chilling, freezing, or immersion in the solvent used for extraction. An important aspect of sanitary handling requirements is
their effect upon the cost. Fish for reduction are valued at 1.0 to 1.4¢ per pound in
the U. S., but the cost would be substantially increased through the provision of vessel,
unloading and storage facilities which are
suitable for food use. Sufficient storage
capacity must be available to enable a plant
to operate continuously. Since the end-
product cost is an inverse function of the
number of hours the plant operates yearly, it
may be advantageous to install additional
storage capacity to extend the operating season and reduce costs, but the increased capital investment would need to be taken into
account in assessing a particular situation.
    If refrigerated storage is to be used, it
would be important to assess the losses
which might be incurred. Thus, it has been
shown that the storage of Pacific hake
(Merluccius productus) in 5 percent chilled
brine causes a reduction of the protein level
contained by 0.3 to 0.4 percent daily. This
is due to solubilization rather than an increase in water content. In this case, an
initial protein level of 14 percent will drop
to around 13 percent in three days with a
consequent lower yield. This loss may be due
to the highly proteolytic Kudoa spp--organ-
isms known to infest Pacific hake and to give
rise to softening of tissue, associated at
times with a dramatic fall in protein level

in the raw fish.[20] It is parallel to a
similar effect noted in pilchards used for
canning.[21] This loss of protein on brine
storage may not be as important for all species. Koury et al. found the muscle of herring to be quite stable against autolysis on
storage as compared with that of hake. When
mixed with herring intestinal material or
with hake muscle tissue, the protein rapidly
solubilized.[22] The yield of FPC made from
the treated material bore a close inverse relation to the degree of autolysis. In any
case, fish can only be stored in ice or RSW
(refrigerated sea water) for a limited period. The use of carbon dioxide to saturate
RSW can greatly increase storage life.
While the carbon dioxide is inexpensive in
itself, its use increases capital costs due
to the need to provide suitable noncorrosive
surfacing, especially in the heat exchangers.
Preliminary experiments with titanium coils
indicate that they will resist corrosion and
function well.[23] Dubrow et al. examined FPC
made from red hake processed after storage on
ice up to eleven days. The PERs of the samples did not change over this time although
the raw fish was considered to be edible only
for the first eight days.[24]
   Storage of ground fish in isopropyl alcohol has been proposed as an alternative to
refrigerated storage. In such a procedure,
the fish would be passed through a grinder at
sea or on arrival in port and mixed with isopropyl alcohol or another solvent which will
inactivate microorganisms and if present in
sufficient quantity, will presumably under-
take the first extraction stage. In a
counter-current system the miscella from the
second extraction stage could be used. There
would be obvious design and insurance problems to be overcome with a seagoing operation, but the idea has potential economic

advantage. Storage experiments with ground
cod scrap[25] and whole red hake[26] which were
mixed with IPA and stored, indicate that the
alcohol reduces the bacterial count to insig-
nificant levels. In the case of red hake,
slight losses of nitrogen and yield were
found after eleven days. Since there was no
bacterial activity, this was attributed to
native enzymes in the fish.

Deboning and comminution. Deboning is considered part of the regular process since the
fluoride levels of many species of fish makes
this operation necessary to meet U. S. and
Canadian requirements. Studies have been
made on reducing the bone content of fish
both in the wet state before extraction and
in the finished state by air separation of
screening. Equipment available for wet deboning is of two types. The first is typi-
fied by the Beehive machine* used extensively
for deboning chicken. It consists of a continuous screw press which forces the muscle
tissue through a screen, while the bone and
scale, etc. pass on around a pressure plate.
This type of equipment needs very careful
adjustment for each set of conditions to
achieve and maintain good operation. When
properly adjusted it operates well at a high
volume. The second type of equipment, manufactured principally in Japan for the preparation of comminuted fish products, uses an
adjustable moving plastic belt to press fish
against a rotating perforated horizontal cylinder. The belt and cylinder move in the
same direction but at different speeds. The
fish is rolled against the drum and the
muscle tissue forced through the holes to the

----

*The use of trade names implies no endorse-
ment.

inside of the drum from which it is discharged. The scales, skin, bone, etc., do
not pass through the perforations. They are
carried past the drum and ejected separately.
These devices only give an approximate separation and to obtain good yields it may be
necessary to use a second machine to recover
additional fish flesh from the scrap stream.
Fish may require prebreaking or comminuting
before feeding to these machines, or thawing
if frozen.

The separated fish flesh may present problems at subsequent processing stages. For
instance, it may be too finely ground for
efficient extraction and drying. The comminuted fish may be more difficult to handle
than whole fish in a continuous cooking and
pressing operation. In the Astra process,
the fish is cooked before it is deboned and
this may give a better separation.[27]

Some experimental work has been carried
out on dry deboning. Its success is likely
to depend a good deal on the condition of
the product as it emerges from the drier.
So far it is not very efficient, and losses
are heavy. The plant would have to be sized
to solvent extract and dry more material
than that which was finally used, i.e., extract both the flesh and the bone. However,
the separated bone fraction would be stable
without further treatment. Deboning reduces
the yield of FPC, however not only the direct
yield but also the composition of the resulting FPC has to be taken into account. Whole
hake-FPC normally has a crude protein content
of about 80 percent. Deboned Pacific hake-
FPC is over 90 percent. Corresponding ash
figures for a series of samples of FPC made
from Pacific hake were from 14 to 20 percent
on the whole fish, but 3 to 6 percent on FPC
made from deboned fish. Moreover, the PER of
FPC made from deboned fish is higher than

made from whole fish, at least in the case of
hake. However, deboning is a complicating
step and leads to some cost increase.

Comminution is an important step which has
an effect on each of the subsequent processing steps of extraction, separation, drying
and steam stripping, and dry deboning. However, it is not possible to be specific about
the effects since they will vary with the
equipment in use, except to note that particle size is likely to be a more critical factor in extraction when screens and pulp
presses rather than centrifuges are used due
to possible losses of fines from the press
cake.

Extraction. Extraction processes are used to
remove lipids or both lipids and water and
may be carried out continuously or in batches
using a counter-current process to ensure
efficiency.[28,29,30] Three counter-current
stages are adequate to extract hake, but more
may be needed for fatty fish.

A wide variety of solvents and combinations has been proposed for extracting lipids
from fish including methyl alcohol,[31] ethyl
alcohol,,[32,33] isopropyl alcohol,[28,34] tertiary butyl alcohol,[35] acetone,[36] cellosolve,
hexane, dioxane,[37] and ethylene dichloride.[38]
Solvents may not only have differing efficiencies in extracting but may differ in the
case with which last traces can be removed
from the FPC. They may give different physical properties to the FPC although these
will also be affected by a number of other
factors.

Ernst has described the layout of an
Experiment and Demonstration Plant operated
for the U. S. Government by Ocean Harvesters,
Inc., which uses a four-stage counter-current
IPA extraction process.[39] Separation of the
extracted cake and the miscella can be done

by filter, vibratory screen, with or without
the addition of a pulp press to increase the
removal of miscella, or by centrifuges.
Screens and pulp presses may prove limiting
if considerable quantity of fines are generated in the process, since fines may pass
through with the miscella making complica-
tions in the oil separation and solvent recovery stages[40] and also reducing the yield.

In the VioBin process,[31] ground fish is
heated with EDC (ethylene dichloride) in a
reaction vessel, and the azeotrope of EDC and
water distills at 71° C. The condensed mixture separates into two phases in a decanter
and the solvent is returned to the extractor.
As the granules of fish lose moisture they
become denser and settle to the bottom of the
conical reactor where they are removed continuously. At the same time the solvent extracts lipids from the fish. The solids are
washed with further solvent to reduce the
lipids to a low level and dried. The resulting product is a high quality, a low fat fish
meal. It is somewhat darker, and stronger in
odor and flavor than conventional FPC, but
has nevertheless been used extensively in human feeding studies. This product can be
further extracted with IPA to remove the
small amount of residual color, odor and flavor,[41] and to bring the EDC level down to the
level of 5 ppm required by present U. S.
regulations. During the EDC extraction stage
little water soluble material is removed and
yields are correspondingly higher. As noted
previously the retention of solubles could be
a disadvantage, but the following IPA extraction will remove at least some of soluble
matter.

Although the VioBin process appears to be
the only azeotropic process used in commercial practice, others have been described.
One of the earliest was that of Ash, who

proposed treating fish as fish waste with
xylene vapors to distill off the water and
extract the fat.[42] A patent by Blaw Knox
describes the use of octane as an azeotropic
separation method, followed by vapor extraction of the dried product using the same
solvent.[43] Hevia et al. have described the
experimental use of isobutanol for azeotropic
distillation of fish.[44] Thijssen has developed a pilot plant operation using IPA in
which water is removed as a solvent azeotrope
from the top of an extraction column filled
with perforated plates down which a suspension of groundfish in solvent descends. The
suspension of dried extracted fish is withdrawn from the bottom of the column, centrifuged and the separated product is further
washed with fresh solvent to remove residual
lipids. The advantages claimed for this process are the use of a single solvent and a
reduction of the amount of energy needed.
The examples given use IPA as the solvent.[45]

Drying and desolventizing. Drying may be
carried out in batch driers or continuously.
Temperatures must be kept low enough to avoid
damage to protein. Early laboratory studies
showed that mild drying conditions such as
drying in air at 100° F to 110° F for 24 to
36 hours,[34] at 71° C to 66° C at reduced
pressure for 18 to 22 hours,[46] and at temperatures of 43° C to 66° C for six hours[28] had
no effect on protein quality. Dubrow and
Stillings subjected FPC to dry and moist heat
and measured PERs. Using dry heat they found
virtually no change in four hours at 120° C
but after two hours at 150° C there was a
serious drop in the PER. Using moist heat
there appeared to be no change in four hours
at 100° C or two hours at 120° C but some
fall in four hours at 120° C.[47] Hallgren
found FPC stable at temperatures below 140° C

based on measurement of available lysine.[15]
Thus time-temperature conditions for drying
do not appear to be critical from a nutritional aspect, within the bounds of typical
food drying practice.

Dubrow prepared FPC by extraction of red
hake and menhaden with IPA at room temperature. Increasing the drying temperature from
between 40° C to 50° C to between 110° to
120° C decreased the protein solubility of
the FPC from 30.7 percent to 12.5 percent.
The functionality of the product as determined by the stability conferred on an oil/
water emulsion was satisfactory at drying
temperatures up to 90 to 100° C but not at
110 to 120° C. Desolventizing dry solids or
alcohol wet solids by steam stripping caused
a dramatic loss in soluble protein and emulsion stability.[48]

Provision must be made for recovering the
solvent since as much as 10 percent entering
the extraction system may be carried into the
drier. When IPA is used as a solvent it cannot be removed completely by direct drying.
Residual levels of 0.6 to 1.9 percent of the
FPC remain even when drying is prolonged.
This amount represents approximately 0.1 percent of the whole amount used and its recovery is not economically essential. However,
U. S. regulations require that IPA residues
be reduced to no more than 250 ppm in the
finished FPC.[4]

Differing arguments exist as to the reason
for the retention of these solvent residues.
IPA can be removed by wetting or steam treatment followed by further drying. This suggests that the solvent binds to the protein.
Thijssen and Rulkens have demonstrated that
low moisture contents greatly reduce the
rates of diffusion of solvents from the center to the surface of food particles[42] and
consider that this phenomenon is responsible

for persistence of the residues. Ackman and
Odense believe that a sieve effect is responsible which restricts the passage of solvent
from FPC particles below limiting water
levels.[49]

At the NMFS' College Park Laboratory, IPA
is removed under vacuum in a conventional
batch drier, followed by steam sparging and
redrying. Ocean Harvesters dry continuously,
employing a four-stage horizontal jacketed
drier with countercurrent steam injection into the first stage.[40] Control of the drying
operation has proved quite critical in reaching the required solvent residue although it
seems to be quite easy to get down below 1000
ppm. A better solution, and one which might
permit simpler drying systems, would be to
modify the present FDA regulations to permit
a higher residual level. Since the original
regulations were published, work by Wills et
al. has established that relatively high levels of IPA can be consumed safely by man and
this should provide a basis for reconsidera-
tion of the permitted maximum.[50]

Other problems experienced by Ocean Harvesters with the continuous drying system
were high microbial counts apparently due to
partial balling of moist product in the drier
and the use of conveyor systems which were
inaccessible for frequent cleaning. Since
IPA is removed in the first drying stage in
this system, it can exert no protective effect against the growth of microorganisms.
The problems were largely overcome, but particle size, residence time, venting, etc.,
must be taken into account when designing a
drying system for continuous operation.

An advantage of the multiple batch drying
system as used by Alpine Marine Protein Industries, Inc. in their New Bedford plant is
accessibility and the option to pull out one
unit for repair without closing down the

whole system.

Milling. For use in certain foods it is
necessary to mill FPC to 200 mesh (74 mic-
rons) or a sandy mouth feel is imparted to
the food. In order to mill FPC to this degree of fineness using a Model 60 ACM Mill,
the initial moisture content of the FPC
should not exceed 10 percent. The milling
operation furhher reduces the moisture by
about another 2 to 4 percent.[40] Fluid energy
milling has been found to be satisfactory.

Solvent recovery. Fairly complete solvent
recovery is required for an economic operation. A loss of 1 percent of IPA at 6.5¢ per
pound will cost nearly 1¢ per pound of FPC.
The quality of the recovered solvents is also
important. The solvent will extract odor-
and flavor-bearing substances from the fish
and these must be removed during the recovery
stage so that do not build up in the solvent
and impart flavor to the FPC. The factors
involved in the material balance for odors
and flavors in the system are the level of
odors and flavors in the raw fish, the operating conditions in the steam stripping
stage, the design and operation of the solvent recovery system and the total losses of
solvent from the system. If the losses are
high, the system will be purged and kept
clean at the expense of high solvent losses.
A single column system using 25 trays was
selected for the Ocean Harvesters plant, with
phosphoric acid injection to retain volatile
bases in the still bottoms. There did not
appear to be a build up of odors in the IPA
over one season's run, or at least to the extent which affected the product, but solvent
losses were initially high although later reduced to about 3 percent and probably capable
of further reduction. Most of the solvent

was lost through evaporation in the extraction and drying stages with smaller amounts
leaving via the sludge and still bottoms.
Originally, consideration of solvent losses
was limited to those resulting from the recovery stage. However, losses can also occur
through spillage, open equipment, and loss in
still bottoms, recovered oil, sludge and drying air. Figure 1 shows a simplified material balance for the circulation of IPA (calculated as anhydrous) based on one operating
run of 95.9 hours in the demonstration
plant.[34]

Oil recovery. Recovery of oil is essential
to keep the cost of the main product down.
As much as a half pound of oil may be recovered for each pound of FPC over a season.
In the IPA extraction process, oil leaves
with the miscella from the first stage.
Since the incoming fish cools and dilutes the
solvent at this stage, relatively small
amounts of oil remain dissolved. It will
pass into suspension and may be separated by
continuous centrifugation. The density of
IPA under those conditions is slightly lower
than that of the fish oil, which tends to
settle downwards with the suspended solids
from the first miscella. This can cause
difficulty in separating a clean oil. The
suggestion has been made that dilution of the
miscella with water will raise the gravity to
a point at which the oil will rise and be
readily separated. Drozdowski and Ackman
examined lipids extracted from herring with
70:30 IPA:water, followed by two extractions
with 99 percent IPA.[51] They found that phospholipids were extracted without obvious degradation, together with free fatty acids in
the IPA phase of the first miscella, whereas
the separable oil consisted predominantly of
triglycerides. The quality of the oil

separated is expected to be quite high since
the heating is minimal. It will, however,
carry dissolved IPA, which can be removed by
water extraction.

Waste streams. Streams of materials other
than FPC will depend on the nature of the
process but may include the following:
1. waste fish which is not up to the required
standard of wholesomeness for use in foods;
2. skin and bone waste from the deboning
operation; 3. solids carried over in the miscella and removed in the centrifuging operation. The composition and amount of these
will depend upon the efficiency of separatory
operations and the composition of the fish;
4. still bottoms containing soluble nitrogenous solvents, considerable amounts of water; and 5. various liquid streams including
fish fluming and washing water, storage
brine, clean-up-water, and spills.
     Present requirements in the U. S. require
that liquid wastes are treated before discharge. In some areas waste could be
screened to separate solids followed by discharge into a sanitary sewer. Preliminary
indications are that still bottoms, wash water, etc., can be successfully flocculated
and the BOD largely reduced by flotation.
Some streams such as still bottoms, sludge,
and the bone fraction could be handled
effectively in a regular fish meal plant.
However, it would be preferable to recover
as much as possible of the various by-products.

Other Processes and Modifications of
Nonsolvent Processes
The removal of lipids from fish is one of
the two major requirements for stability.
Solvent extraction is an obvious approach,
but its necessarily complex requirements

have lead to alternative proposals for removing lipids, or at least substantially removing them and stabilizing the remainder. Moreover, the elimination of solvents from a process may offer an increased opportunity to improve functionality since solvents, especially hydrophyllic solvents, tend to denature proteins. None of these processes have reached commercial production, and it is questionable whether lipids can be removed to an extent necessary to achieve stability without using solvents at some stage.

A logical way to free oil from the highly emulsifying fish tissue is to dissolve protein with alkali then reprecipitate with acid.[52,53,54,55,56] Rogers produced a heat coagulable protein by simple water extraction of ground fish at room temperature or lower. The yield was increased when 1 to 5 percent sodium chloride solution was used; the salt was removed by subsequent dialysis.[57]

Surface active agents have been proposed as an alternative to the use of alkali as separation, but all the procedures noted have serious problems.[58,59]

Pigott and his collaborators have carried out a series of studies on the extraction of protein by acidified brine and of treating the different waste streams to define alternative systems for a more complete utilization of fish and fish by-products. The pilot system is also used to indicate how different waste control systems may be applied to fish processing operations.[60]

Modification for functionality. Another cause for seeking to modify the processing of fish protein is to make the final form of protein more functional. The action of many solvents and of heat or drying on fish protein is to denature it so that it becomes nonfunctional. While it remains valuable as

a nutritional supplement, because it does not
change the characteristics of the food to
which it is added, it has no functional properties which would make it additionally valuable for use in food formulation.[61] Some of
the alkali treatments referred to earlier
have this objective as indicated by claims
for whippability, etc. Spinelli et al.[62,63]
and Rutman et al.[64] have described somewhat
similar processes in which ground fish tissue
is washed with water then subjected to a mild
enzymatic treatment which appears to stabilize the protein against denaturation. Rutman then converts the protein into a stable
milk substitute by emulsifying it with oil
containing an antioxidant. Spinelli checks
the enzyme action by precipitating the modified protein as a protein phosphate complex
followed by IPA extraction of residual lipids. The resulting product retains its functionality up to 70° C.

Tannenbaum et al. have investigated modification of FPC made by IPA extraction using
alkalies.[65,66] These products could be used
in foods, but the economics of a process
commencing with FPC might be unfavorable.
Similar studies have been conducted by
Anglemier.[67]

Modification to simplify processing. The
removal of water by extraction with water
soluble solvents required large solvent volumes, a factor which increases the cost of
plant construction and operation. Moreover,
ethyl and isopropyl alcohols are not very
good lipid solvents at low temperatures, especially in the first stage of a counter-
current operation when they are diluted by
the water from the incoming fish. According-
ly, proposals have been made to reduce water
and/or lipids before extraction. One obvious
route is to process fish by the cooking and

pressing stages used in the conventional reduction of fish to meal. This substantially
reduces the water content from four pounds
per pound of solids in lean fish, and two to
three pounds per pound of solids in fatty
fish, to around one pound water per pound of
solids. In fatty fish, the oil content is
also substantially reduced. Dubrow and
Stillings have shown that cooking fish prior
to extraction did not affect the PER provided that the temperature does not exceed
109° C.[68] A further variation is the complete reduction of fish to meal followed by
solvent extraction of the meal. This combination is similar to the extraction of
press cake except that press cake is dried
in advance of extraction and so the amount
of solvent required is reduced. However,
performing the drying operation prior to removal of the oil and soluble fraction may
increase the proportion of undesirable solids which may be unextractable and remain in
the product. For instance, the heme pigments
will denature and resist extraction giving a
darker end product. Production and extraction of fish meal with ethyl alcohol and hexane were used in a UNICEF pilot plant at
Quintero, Chile.[69] Verrando extracted fish
meal in a patented system using hexane vapor
and liquid.[70]
    Acceptance is important since the extrac-
tion of fish meal, even that made from wholesome fish using sanitary equipment and processes, is generally likely to be lower in
cost than extraction of whole fish. If this
is so, extraction of fish meal will be a
strong candidate for commercial acceptability
in areas where the product is acceptable when
used at reasonable levels in local foods.
    An alternative preparative step to reduce
moisture is use of the HTH (heat transfer
medium) method patented by Greenfield.[71]

Ground fish is suspended in fish or other oil
and dried by vacuum flash evaporation. The
suspended matter is then separated by centrifuge to form a sludge containing about 35
percent oil from which a form of FPC can be
separated by solvent extraction. Advantages
of this system are the low temperatures used,
the retention in the first stage of soluble
solids, the potential low cost, and the protection of the product from the atmosphere
during the drying stage.

Spinelli removes much of the oil and soluble protein by contacting ground fish with a
dilute acidic aqueous solution of a condensed phosphate, e.g., sodium hexametaphosphate,[72] which insolubilizes the soluble protein fraction. The protein is then washed
with water to remove undesired components.
The resulting cake can then be processed
using only two IPA extractions to less than
0.2 percent residual lipid. The oil can be
recovered from the aqueous washes. Spinelli
and Koury have shown that the phosphate complexes formed in this process retain their
nutritional value.[73]

A process preparative to IPA extraction
has been developed by Astra Nutrition Corporation of Sweden.[27] The fish are eviscerated, cooked in water, deboned, and then
separated by centrifuge, washed with hot water and centrifuged again. This process,
with subsequent IPA extraction, enables a
high quality FPC to be made from herring, a
relatively dark oily fish.

Enzymatic Processes. Autolytic digestion of
fish is extensively practiced in the orient
where fish sauces are made in many countries,
principally by the slow digestion of highly
salted fish.[74] Two biological approaches are
being considered for making FPC. The first
is the use of microorganisms, the second the

use of commercial enzymes.[75,76]

The use of microorganisms has not made
much practical progress as yet. Burkholder
et al. have described screening tests for
microorganisms which are highly proteolytic
or which are capable of removing fat from
fish by converting it to protein using a
supplementary nitrogen source.[77] However,
in practical trials, yields with these organisms were found to be poor and the products were not too promising. The use of
Aspergillus species followed by yeast to
ferment fish has been investigated by
Jeffreys and Krell.[78] Bertullo and
Hettich,[79] and Bertullo,[80] have prepared
hydrolysates using Saccharomyces; the bones
are removed from the digest before concentration and spray drying.

Fish proteins can be solubilized by autolytic action, but the speed and completeness of the hydrolysis are increased by the
addition of proteolytic enzymes. Hale has
compared the efficiency of commercially
available enzymes.[81] Proteolysis is carried
to a point at which a suspension of fish is
largely solubilized and forms three layers,
free oil, a sludge or emulsion of oil and
proteinanceous material, and a clean layer of
protein hydrolysate which is dried to form
the protein concentrate. The products are
water soluble and have tastes varying from
slight to definite, which have been described
as "cheesy", "slightly fishy", "malty",
"bitter", "fish meal", etc. Protein efficiency ratios are frequently lower than that
of casein, largely due to an imbalance of
amino acids in the soluble fraction recovered
as the end product. Tryptophan tends to concentrate differentially in the insoluble solids. The loss from the soluble fraction is
reduced as the yield of soluble product increased, i.e., as more of the insoluble

fraction is hydrolyzed. Thus the loss varies
inversely with pH. Histidine is also lost in
the process, especially at higher pH levels,
but this varied with the enzymes used.

Among others who have investigated the use
of proteolytic enzymes are Keys and Meinke[82]
and Nestle, who reduced bitter flavor by
treatment with activated charcoal.[83] Lum
used autolysis followed by a liquid-solvent
extraction to remove lipids followed by spray
drying. Such a process using solvents might
be more expensive than standard solvent extraction, but it gives soluble products.[84]

In summary it may be said that the enzyme
process appears to be potentially less expensive, but it presents problems of nutrition and product acceptance which have yet to
be overcome. Perhaps one of the best
approaches at present is to consider the use
of such processes as alternatives for converting by-products to animal feeds while
further development is being undertaken on
their application to human foods.

Future Developments in FPC Processing

At the present time, industry development in
FPC has been limited. Commercial operations
have been undertaken in South Africa, Peru,
and the United States, but none are presently
functioning on any significant scale. Astra
Corporation is continuing commercial development in part through Nabisco Astra Nutrition,
Inc. in the United States. The future development of commercial enterprises depends upon
the ability to manufacture FPC with characteristics attractive to the food industry at
a competitive cost.[85] This means that the
future aim of process development should be
reduction of cost and increase in functionality.

A major factor in the cost of FPC is that
of the raw material. Concentration should be

on preparing high quality FPC from menhaden,
anchovy, herring and other relatively low
cost raw materials and developing high value
by-products from these fish. Lowering cost
of preservation by such means as storage of
fish in solvent or processing to press cake
or other intermediate products at sea should
be investigated and developed intensively.
Reduction of residual odors and flavors in
FPC by inexpensive treatments such as reduction of soluble fractions, and treatment
with mild oxidizing or reducing agents should
be considered.

General process simplification, increase
in yield, and efficienty of operation is now
under study at the NMFS demonstration plant
to provide basic plant design and cost information. In looking at future operating procedures, the cost of alternative plant
configurations and operational modes should
be compared. Attention must be paid to mini-
mizing down time and maximizing operating
hours per year. In this connection, and for
cost sharing in common services such as power
supplies, management, etc., association with
other fishery operations may be useful.

Cost of operation is a function of the
plant size and the number of days of operation. Figure 2 shows some early estimates
made by the University of Maryland for the
cost of FPC made by a four-stage IPA counter-
current extraction process. The specific
figures may only be valid in a particular
case, but the relative figures for different
sizes and seasons will give essentially similar trends in a range of circumstances.
They show the expected advantages of greater
plant size and of increasing the number of
days operating per year. Keeping in mind
that seasons are limited, it is important to
conserve continued operation without bad
weather interruption and to extend the season

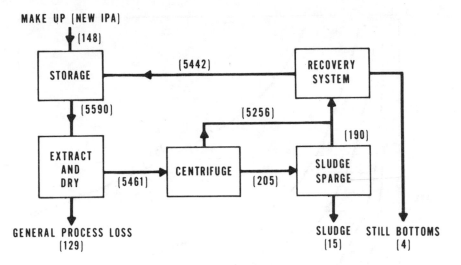

Figure 1. Material Balance of Isopropyl
Alcohol (IPA) for One Run of Red Hake 40.
(Figures in parentheses are 1 lb anhydrous
IPA/hr. measured on one run of 95.9 hours.

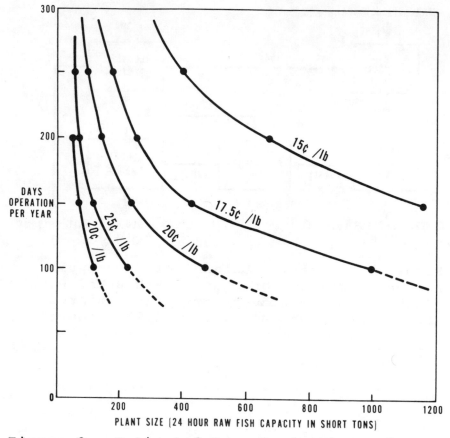

Figure 2.   Estimated Days Production and
Plant Sizes Required to Produce FPC at
Different Cost Levels.

by increased storage.

Finally, processes which preserve or enhance the functional nature of fish proteins offer products which can compete in higher value markets. Fish proteins are extremely sensitive to the effects of solvents and heat, and the best chance of success seems to be in some form of protein modification with alkali or enzyme treatment before drying, as being developed by Rutman,[64] and Spinelli.[62,63] Other interesting alternatives are the stabilization of low cost wet fibrillar protein and further chemical modification of fish protein by acylation* to give a new range of properties.[86] The intensive investigation of solvent extraction processes for fish is reaching an advanced stage. Although attention has been focussed primarily upon the nutritive value of fish proteins, it is fair to say that wider possibilities for using fish proteins and their products in human foods are now only beginning to be realized. In consequence, considerable advances in fish protein processes and products can be anticipated in the next few years.

References

1. Finch, R. 1970. Fish proteins for human foods. Critical Reviews in Food Technology 2: 519.

2. Fish protein concentrate - a comprehensive bibliography. 1970. Library of Congress, Washington, D. C.

----

*Acylation includes the reactions between proteins and various organic anhydrides.

3. PAG guideline for fish protein concentrates for human consumption. 1971. FAO/WHO/UNICEF Protein Advisory Group, United Nations, N. Y.

4. Whole fish protein concentrate. Federal Register, Washington, D. C., February 2, 1967, p. 1173.

5. Whole fish protein concentrate. Federal Register, Washington, D. C., August 4, 1970, p. 12390.

6. Schedule of Amendments No. 130, Canada Gazette, October 14, 1970.

7. Love, R. M., Lovern, J. A., and Jones, N. R. 1959. The chemical composition of fish tissues, D.S.I.R. Food Investigation Special Report No. 69, H.M.S.O., London.

8. Stansby, M. E. 1962. Proximate composition of fish. In Fish in Nutrition, eds. E. Heen, and R. Kreuzer, p. 55. London: Fishing News.

9. Brooke, R. O., E. M. Ravese, and M. A. Steinberg. 1962. The composition of commercially important fish taken from New England waters. II. Proximate analysis of butterfish, flounder, pollock and hake and their seasonal variation. J. Food Sci. 27: 73.

10. Lovern, J. A. 1962. The lipids of fish and changes occurring in them during processing and storage. In Fish in Nutrition, eds. E. Heen and R. Kreuzer, p. 85. London: Fishing News.

11. Horan, F. E. 1967. Proceedings of the International Conference on Soyabean Protein Foods. ARS-71-35. U. S. Department of Agri-

Agriculture, Peoria.

12.   Pariser, E. R., and Odlund, E.   1963.
MIT-UNICEF studies on the production of fish
protein concentrate for human consumption.
Comm. Fish. Rev. 25: 10.

13.   Dreosti, G. M.   1962.   Technological
developments in South Africa. Fish in Nutrition, eds. E. Heen, and R. Kreuzer, p. 425.
London: Fishing News.

14.   Dambergs, N.   1959.   Extracts of fish
muscle.   2. Solvent water ratio in extraction
of fat and water solubles. J. Fish. Res. Bd.
Can. 16: 63.

15.   Hallgren, B.   1966.   Nutritional value
and use of fish protein concentrate. Narings
Forskning 10: 37.

16.   Dubrow, D., Brown, N. L., Pariser, E. R.
and Miller, H.   1970.   FPC's quality virtually the same as its raw material's quality.
Comm. Fish. Rev. 32: 25.

17.   National Marine Fisheries Service, unpublished results, Washington, D. C.

18.   Goldmintz, D., and Hull, J. C.   1970.
Bacteriological aspects of fish protein concentrate production. Dev. Ind. Microbiol.
11: 335.

19.   Goldmintz, D.   1971.   Survival of
microorganisms in fish protein concentrate
stored under controlled conditions. Dev.
Ind. Microbiol. 12: 265.

20.   Dassow, J. A., Patashnik, M., and Koury,
B. J.   1970.   Characteristics of Pacific

hake (<u>Merlucius productus</u>) that affect its
suitability for food. In <u>Pacific Hake</u>
Circular 332, p. 127. Washington, D. C.:
U. S. Fish and Wildlife Service.

21. Dreosti, G. M. 1957. Mush in canned
pilchards. In <u>Progress Report No. 22</u>, p. 39.
Fishing Industry Research Institute, Cape-
town, S. A.

22. Koury, B., Spinelli, J. and Wieg, D.
1971. Protein autolysis rates at various
pH's and temperatures in hake, <u>Merluccius
productus</u>, and Pacific Herring, <u>Clupea
harengus pallasi</u>, and their effect on yield
in the preparation of fish protein concentrate. <u>Fishery Bulletin</u> 69: 241.

23. Nelson, R. W., and Barnett, H. J. 1971.
Fish preservation in refrigerated sea water
modified with carbon dioxide. 13th International Congress of Refrigeration, Washington,
D. C.

24. Dubrow, D. L., Brown, N. L., Pariser,
E. R., Sidwell, V. D. and Ambrose, M. E.
1971. Effect of ice storage on the chemical
and nutritive properties of solvent-extracted
whole fish - red hake, <u>Urophycis chuss</u>.
<u>Fishery Bulletin</u> 69: 145.

25. Guttmann, A., Dambergs, N. and Jangaard,
P. M. 1967. Preservation of raw material
for fish protein concentrate with isopropyl
alcohol. <u>J. Fish. Res. Bd. Can</u>. 24: 895.

26. Dubrow, D. and Hammerle, O. 1967.
Holding raw fish (red hake) in isopropyl alcohol for FPC (fish protein concentrate) production. <u>Food Tech</u>. 23: 120.

27.   Lawler, F. K.   1970.   Pure fish protein.
Food Eng. 42: 61.

28.   Marine Protein Concentrate.   1966.
Fishery Leaflet 584, U. S. Department of the
Interior, Washington, D. C.

29.   Idler, D. R.   1967.   The development and
scope of the Halifax process.   In Proceedings
Conference on Fish Protein Concentrate, Canadian Fisheries Report No. 10, Canadian Department of Fisheries.

30.   McPhee, A. D. and Brown, N. L.   1971.
Power consumption in solid-liquid slurries.
Ind. Eng. Chem. Process. Des. Dev. 10: 456.

31.   Levin, E.   1961.   U. S. Patent
2,972,542.

32.   Lahiry, N. L., Moorjani, M. N., Viswes-
wariah, K., Shurpalekar, S. R., Swaminathan,
M., Sreenivasan, A. and Subrahmanyan, V.
1962.   Preparation of edible fish flour from
oil sardine (Clupea longiceps). Food Sci.
(Mysore) 11: 2, 37.

33.   Yanez, E., Barja, I., Monckeberg, F.,
Maccioni, A. and Donoso, C.   1967.   The FPC
story.   6. Quintero fish protein concentrate:
Protein quality and use in foods.   Food
Technol. 21: 1604.

34.   Power, H. E.   1962.   An improved method
for the preparation of fish protein concentrate.   J. Fish. Res. Bd. Can. 19: 1039.

35.   Whaley, W. M., and Moshy, R. J.   1966.
U. S. Patent 3,252,962.

36. Cavanagh, J. C., and Inman, E. G. 1963.
German Patent 1,138,308.

37. Moshy, R. J. 1963. Canadian Patent
663,559.

38. Levin, E. and Worsham, E. M. 1951.
U. S. Patent 2,539,544

39. Ernst, R. C. 1971. FPC: The NMFS
experiment and demonstration plant process.
Comm. Fish. Rev. 33: 22.

40. Summary Report of Hake Run 1971. 1971.
Report on Contract No. 14-17-0007-980, Ocean
Harvesters, Inc.

41. Thijssen, H. A. C., and Rulkens, W. H.
1968. Retention of aromas in drying food
liquids. Chem. Tech. 5: De Ingenieur, 80
(47), 45.

42. Ash, C. S. 1933. U. S. Patent
1,934,677.

43. Blaw Knox Co. 1969. British Patent
1,167,673.

44. Hevia, P., Acavedo, F. and Kaiser, S.
1971. Isobutanol as a solvent for FPC production. J. Food Sci. 36: 708.

45. Thijssen, H. A. C. 1969. U. S. Patent
Appl. 874,214.

46. Brown, N. L. and Miller, H. 1969.
Experimental production of fish protein con-
centrate (FPC) from Mediterranean sardines.
Comm. Fish. Rev. 31: 10, 30.

47.   Dubrow, D. L. and Stillings, B. R.
1970.   Effect of heat on the chemical and
nutritive stability of FPC.   J. Food Sci. 35:
677.

48.   Dubrow, D. L.   1973.   Effect of drying
and desolventizing on the functional properties of fish protein concentrate (FPC).
Fish. Bull. 71:104.

49.   Ackman, R. G. and Odense, P. M.   1968.
Retention of isopropyl alcohol in fish protein concentrate.   J. Fish. Res. Bd. Can. 25:
804.

50.   Wills, J. H., Jameson, E. M., and
Coulston, F.   1969.   Effects on man of daily
ingestion of small doses of isopropyl alcohol.   J. Toxicol. Appl. Pharmacol. 15: 560.

51.   Drozdowski, B., and Ackman, R. G.   1969.
Isopropy- alcohol extraction of oils and
lipids in the production of fish protein
concentrate from herring.   J. Amer. Chem.
Soc. 46: 371.

52.   Hiltner, P. P., Metzner, H. and Peters,
H.   1943.   German Patent 733,896.

53.   Lorinez, F.   1957, 1971.   The manufacture of protein from home produced, so-called
"mass" fish.   Food Sci. Abs. 29: 33.   Elelmez
Ipar 5: 72.

54.   Libenson, C. M., and Pirosky, I.   1967.
French Patent 1,502,113.

55.   Moshy, R. J.   1963.   Canadian Patent
663,556.

56.   Ehrensvard, C. H. G., Lofquist, B. V., and Sjoberg, D. B. 1968. French Patent 1,533,966.

57.   Rogers, W. I.   1963.   U. S. Patent 3,099,562.

58.   Caiozzi, M., Arrieta, L., Villarroel, L., and Rauch, E. 1969. The fish protein concentrate story. 7. New method of FPC production for food use. Food Technol. 23: 206.

59.   Connell, J. J. 1969. The fish protein concentrate story. 8. On the use of detergents in FPC production. Food Technol. 23: 206.

60.   Pigott, G. M. and Chu, C-L. 1969. A new method of processing fish waste. I. The evolution of a process. In Proceedings of the 36th Annual Meeting of Pacific Northwest Pollution Control Association, Seattle.

61.   Hammonds, T. M., and Call, D. L. 1970. Utilization of protein ingredients in the U. S. food industry. Parts 1 and 2, The Future Market for Protein Ingredients. Ithaca: Cornell Univ.

62.   Spinelli, J., Koury, B. and Miller, R. 1972. Approaches to the utilization of fish for the preparation of protein isolates. Part 1. Isolation and properties of myofibrillar and sarcoplasmic fish proteins. J. Food Sci. 37:599.

63.   Ibid. 1972. Part 2. Enzymic modifications of myofibrillar fish proteins. J. Food Sci. 37:604.

64.   Rutman, M.   1971.   U. S. Patent 3,561,973.

65.   Tannenbaum, S. R., Ahern, M., and
Bates, R. P.   1970.   Solubilization of fish
protein concentrate.   I. An alkaline process.   Food Technol. 24: 96.

66.   Tannenbaum, S. R., Bates, R. P., and
Bradfield, L.   1970.   Solubilization of fish
protein concentrate.   II. Utilization of the
alkaline process product.   Food Technol. 24:
99.

67.   Anglemier, A.   1974.   In Economics,
Marketing, and Technology of FPC, eds.
N. Scrimshaw, B. Stillings, and S. Tannen-
baum.   Cambridge: M.I.T. Press.

68.   Dubrow, D. L., and Stillings, B. R.
1971.   Chemical and nutritional characteristics of fish protein concentrate processed
from heated whole red hake, Urophycis chuss.
Fishery Bulletin 69: 141.

69.   Allen, L. E.   1963.   Fish flour production in Chile.   Fishing News Int. 2: 106.

70.   Verrando, C.   1963.   U. S. Patent
3,064,018.

71.   Greenfield, C.   1953.   U. S. Patent
2,651,647.

72.   Spinelli, J.   1971.   U. S. Patent
3,598,606.

73.   Spinelli, J., and Koury, B.   1970.
Phosphate complexes of soluble fish proteins.
Their formation and possible uses.   Ag. and
Food Chem. 18: 284.

74.   Van Veen, A. G.   1965.   Seafood products
in Southeast Asia.   In Fish as Food, ed. G.
Borgstrom, vol. 3, R235.   New York: Academic
Press.

75.   Mackie, I. M., Hardy, R., and Hobbs, G.
1971.   Fermented fish products.   FAO Fisheries Report No. 100, FAO, Rome.

76.   Hale, M. B.   In press.   Making fish protein concentrate by enzymatic hydrolysis.
NOAA Technical Report (NMFS SSR-F 657).

77.   Bulkholder, L., Bulkholder, P. R., Chu,
A., Kostyk, N., and Roels, O. A.   1968.
Fish fermentation.   <u>Food Technol</u>. 22: 1278.

78.   Jeffreys, G. A., and Krell, A. J.   1965.
U. S. Patent 3,170,794.

79.   Bertullo, V. H., and Hettich, F. P.
1959.   U. S. Patent 3,000,789.

80.   Bertullo, V.   1970.   U. S. Patent
3,516,349.

81.   Hale, M. B.   1969.   Relative activities
of commercially available enzymes in the
hydrolysis of fish protein.   <u>Food Technol</u>.
23: 107.

82.   Keys, C. W. and Meinke, W. W.   1966.
U. S. Patent 3,249,442.

83.   Nestle, S. A.   1967.   Netherlands
Patent Appl. 6,612,977.

84.   Lum, K. C.   1969.   British Patent
1,157,415.

85.   Anon. 1970.   The economics of fish protein concentrate.   M.I.T., Cambridge, Mass.

86. Groninger, H. S.   1972. Preparation and
properties of succinylated protein from fish
muscle. Presented at the 32nd Annual Meeting, Institute of Food Technologists, Minnea-
polis, Minn.

VI
CANADIAN FPC RESEARCH AND DEVELOPMENT

L. W. Regier
Department of the Environment, Fisheries
Research Board of Canada, Halifax Laboratory,
Halifax, Nova Scotia, Canada

The Canadian interest in FPC (fish protein concentrate) arose from the need for more proteins and the possibilities of supplying them through underutilized species of fish. At the time when our studies first began, most species in the waters normally considered Canadian were still underutilized. Since the mid-50s, however, the fishing pressure has so increased that several species are being overfished. To meet our goal of an economically viable industry, the problems of raw material quality and supply, process variables, regulatory agency approval, and marketing must be brought to satisfactory solutions.

The first basis for product definition was the attainment of a highly nutritious protein with long shelf stability and a minimum of flavor and odor. In 1957, Guttman and Vandenheuval[1] arrived at a process which involved heating acidified fresh filleting waste from cod, haddock, and hake, followed by washing with water, pressing, and extraction with isopropanol (IPA). The work by Gunnarson showed that the IPA could be used on a pilot scale and in the first extraction.[2] Later studies by Dambergs on both low fat fish such as cod, and on fatty herring showed that direct isopropanol extraction was quite effective if the solvent concentration was controlled in the first extraction.[3,4] The optimum was shown to be in the 60 to 80 percent isopropanol range. Under these

conditions both the lipids and the water
solubles such as amines are extracted from
the proteins. These investigations resulted
in a process which is known as the Halifax
process.[5]

FPC prepared by this process in the Halifax pilot plant was subjected to detailed
analyses and animal feeding studies through
the cooperation and support of the Department
of Industry, Trade and Commerce of the Canadian government. These data formed a major
portion of the information used in the application to the Food and Drug Directorate of
the Department of Health and Welfare. The
cooperation of what is now the U. S. National
Marine Fisheries Service in allowing the use
of their extensive data was very helpful in
the submission which was made in 1969. Approval was granted in 1970, and the regulations of the production and composition of
fish protein was published in the Canada
Gazette of October 14, 1970. The details of
the regulations are given in the Appendix.
Approval was given for products made from
several families of whole edible fish or
their trimmings. No specific limitations
were placed upon the use of fish protein
meeting the required raw material, process,
and final composition requirements. The
produce can be incorporated in a variety of
food products to compete with proteins from
other raw material sources.

The internationally supported[6] limitation
on fluoride in FPC meant further work on
fluoride analysis methodology.[7] The results
of these studies showed that certain raw
materials must be deboned to lower the fluoride level to the 100 to 150 ppm levels in
the final product.[8] Although methodology for
determining bone levels in the final product
indicate the possibility of separation based
upon density as in an air classification

system, the wet raw material deboning
approach was used for this separation.[9] The
primary reason for this choice was the ready
availability of commercial units for this
purpose which can be used to provide raw
material for other potential processes as
well.

At this time, the process development and
the likelihood of regulatory agency approval
had reached a point where a commercial plant
based upon the isopropanol extraction process
was built at Canso, Nova Scotia. This plant
has a designed capacity of 200 tons of raw
material per day. Although the plant has
produced some material on a start-up basis,
it has not been put into production due to
financial, management, and raw material supply problems.

The food-use markets in the developed
countries need products which could supply
positive functional characteristics as well
as nutrition. It should be noted that a
large market potential based primarily on
nutritional quality exists in animal starter
rations which is not being filled primarily
by nonfat milk solids, and studies are under
way in this area by the Canada Department
of Agriculture and elsewhere.[10,11,12] In
1969 the studies at the Fisheries Research
Board Laboratory in Halifax were expanded to
put emphasis on the development of a functional FPC. Instead of trying to resurrect
the properties from the hot isopropanol extracted product, effort was made to retain
the functional properties of the original
fish proteins. This work led to a process
which gives a dry product that readily rehy-
drates taking up quite a bit of water, functions as an effective emulsifier, and
coagulates on heating. The process includes
water extraction of solubles, protein swelling and coagulation, isopropanol extraction,

and drying. It has been evaluated in a
"sausage test" in which the strength of a
cooked emulsion is measured. The protein
(FPC), fat, salt, and water concentrations in
this system are the same as those used in
some regular products such as weiners. A
patent application has been filed in Canada
and one is being filed in the United
States.[13]
     There are further laboratory and pilot
plant studies on functional FPC presently under way. The Research and Development
Directorate of the Fisheries Service, Department of the Environment, has recently author-
ized a one year expansion of efforts in the
Halifax Laboratory, Fisheries Research Board.
Studies are being made on the effects of species as well as raw material quality, and
process condition variables are being evaluated to get a more complete definition that
will allow pilot plant production and engineering for commercial production.

APPENDIX

CANADIAN FOOD & DRUG REGULATIONS FOR FISH
PROTEIN (Fish Protein Concentrate)

Schedule of Amendments No. 130, Passed by
Governor-in-Council Under P.C. 1970-1619 of
September 16, 1970, and published in the
Canada Gazette of October 14, 1970.

1. Section B.01.023 of the Food and Drug
Regulations is revoked and the following substituted therefor:
"B.01.023 (1) Notwithstanding subparagraph
(iv) of paragraph (b) of Section b.01.004, a
list of ingredients is not required on the
label of the following foods except as

provided in subsection (2)
(a) bakery products,
(b) black pudding,
(c) blood pudding,
(d) confectionery,
(e) flavouring preparations,
(f) gelatine desserts,
(g) non-nutritive seasoning sauces,
(h) pastry spice,
(i) pickling spice,
(j) poultry seasoning,
(k) preparations of synthetic colours listed
in paragraph (c) of section B.06.002,
(l) soft drinks, and
(m) white pudding.
    (2) A list of ingredients is required on
the label of any food referred to in subsection (1) where
(a) such food contains fish protein as an ingredient; or
(b) an advertisement for such a food mentions
an ingredient, not included in the common
name of the food, that is used to distinguish
the food or that is required by these Regulations to be declared on the label of the
food.
2. Part I of the Table to section B.15.002
of the said Regulations is amended by adding
thereto the following item:

	Arsenic ppm	Lead ppm	Copper ppm	Zinc ppm	Fluo-rine ppm
"Fish protein	3.5	0.5	-	-	150"

3. (1) Table VIII to section B16.100 of the
said Regulations is amended by adding thereto
immediately after item H.1 thereof, the
following item:

Item No.	Column I Additive	Column II Permitted In or Upon	Column III Purpose of Use	Column IV Maximum Level of Use
"I.1	Isopro-pyl Al-cohol	Fish Pro-tein	To Extract moisture, fat and other sol-uble com-ponents from fish	Good Manu-facturing Practice"

(2) Item P.1 of Table X to section
B.16.100 of the said Regulations is amended
by adding thereto in Column II and Column III
thereof the following subitems:

Column II Permitted in or Upon	Column II Maximum Level of Use
"(3) Fish Protein	(3) Good Manufacturing Practice"

4.   All that portion of section B.21.005 of
the said Regulations preceding paragraph (a)
thereof is revoked and the following substituted therefore:
"B.21.005. Fish except fish protein, and
meat products or preparations thereof are
adulterated if any of the following substances or any substance in one of the following classes is present therein or has been
added thereto:"
5.   The said Regulations are further amended
by adding thereto, immediately after section
B.21.025 thereof, the following section:
"B.21.027 (S) Fish Protein
(a) shall be the food prepared by
     (i) extracting water, fat and other sol-
uble components through the use of isopropyl
alcohol from fresh whole edible fish of the
order Clupeiformes, families Clupeidae and

Osmeridae and the order Gadiformes, family
Gadidae, or from trimmings resulting from the
filleting of such fish when eviscerated, and
    (ii) drying and grinding the protein
concentrate resulting from the operation described in subparagraph (i);
(b) may contain a pH adjusting agent; and
(c) shall not contain
    (i) less than 75 percent protein, which
shall be at least equivalent to casein in
protein quality,
    (ii) more than 10,000 bacteria per gram,
or
    (iii) Escherichia coli,
as determined by the official method."

References

1. Guttmann, A., and Vendenheuval, F. A.
1957. Fishery Reserve Board Canada, Progress
Report, Atlantic Coast Sta. No. 67, 29.

2. Gunnarsson, G. K. 1958. Unpublished
data.

3. Dambergs, N. 1959. Extracts of fish
muscle. 2. Solvent-water ratio in extraction
of fat and water-solubles. J. Fish. Res. Bd.
Canada 16: 63-71.

4. Dambergs, N. 1969. Isopropanol-water
mixtures for the production of fish protein
concentrate from Atlantic herring (Clupea
harengus). J. Fish. Res. Bd. Canada 26:
1919-1923.

5. Power, H. E. 1962. An improved method
for the preparation of fish protein concentrates from cod. J. Fish Res. Bd. Canada 19:
1039-1045.

6. Anonymous. 1970. Protein Advisory Group tentative suggestion for fish protein concentrates for human consumption. Document 2.8/26, 15 January 1970, FAO/WHO/UNICEF Protein Advisory Group, United Nations, N. Y. 10017, U. S. A.

7. Ke, P. J., Regier, L. W. and Power, H. E. 1969. Determination of fluoride in biological samples by a nonfusion distillation and ionselective membrane electrode method. Anal. Chem. 41: 1081-1083.

8. Ke, P. J., Power, H. E. and Regier, L. W. 1970. Fluoride content of fish protein concentrate and raw fish. J. Sci. Fd. Agric. 21: 108-109.

9. Dambergs, N., and Regier, L. W. 1970. Estimation of bone material in fish protein concentrates. J. Fish Res. Bd. Canada 27: 591-595.

10. Gorrill, A. D. L., Nicholson, J. W. G., and Power, H. E. 1972. Performance of dairy calves fed milk replacers containing milk, fish and soybean proteins for either 6 or 7 times per week, and early weaning based on starter intake. Can. J. Anim. Sci.

11. Makdani, D. D., Huber, J. T. and Michel, R. L. 1970. Fish protein concentrate as the only protein in liquid diets for calves. J. Dairy Sci. 53: 631-688.

12. Pond, W. C., Snyder, W., Walker, E. F., Stillings, B. R. and Sidwell, V. 1971. Comparative utilization of casein, fish protein concentrate and isolated soybean protein in liquid diets for growth of baby pigs. J. Anim. Sci. 33: 587-591.

13. Dingle, J. R., Kennedy, D. J., and Dyer,
W. J. Improved fish protein concentrate,
Case No. 4752, Canadian Patents and Develop-
ment Limited, Ottawa 4, Canada, Can. Pat.
Appl. No. 113,942, Filed 26 May 1971.

VII
AQUEOUS-SOLVENT PROCESSES

John Spinelli
Pacific Fishery Products Technology Center,
National Marine Fisheries Service, National
Oceanic & Atmospheric Administration, U. S.
Department of Commerce, Montlake Boulevard
East, Seattle, Washington 98102

Aqueous Processes

In these types of processing, only water or
water containing organic or inorganic reagents is used to facilitate the separation
of fish components into their lipid, protein, and nonprotein constituents. These reagents can include acids, bases, salts, and
surface-active compounds. Separation of fish
components is accomplished by extraction,
solubilization, or partial solubilization of
the tissue constituents followed by chemical
and/or mechanical partitioning.

Biological (involving the use of microorganisms) and enzyme hydrolysis methods
might rightfully be included in this category, but because these methods significantly
depart from the original FPC concept, they
have been considered in a separate review.

Aqueous-solvent Processes

This category includes those processes in
which a major portion of the oils and nonprotein constituents are removed with water
followed by an extraction with organic solvent to further remove residual lipids and
other nonprotein constituents. With this
type of processing, the fish proteins are
first coagulated by heat or a combination of
heat and chemical reagents. Oils, part of
the water, and the nonprotein constituents

are then mechanically separated by centrifuging or pressing. After coagulation, the proteins are generally water washed, and the
pressing or centrifuging is repeated. Following the washing, residual oils are then
removed by extraction with an organic solvent.

The aqueous processing as well as the various solvent extraction processes have been
described by Finch.[1] Briefly, however, it
can be said that the preparation of FPC by
complete solvent extraction systems has been
developed to the point where their virtues
and weak points are apparent. Although a
high quality FPC can be prepared by solvent
extraction systems, particularly when the
extractant is an alcohol such as isopropyl
alcohol (IPA) or ethanol, these methods of
preparation currently suffer from two distinct disadvantages. First, with solvent
extraction systems, insufficient consideration has been given to the problems of producing a high quality oil. For example, oil
produced by azeotropic distillation of ethylene dichloride produces a dark colored, partially polymerized oil that has little if any
utility. When fish is extracted with alcohols, a high quality oil can be produced,
but the engineering and economics of oil recovery due to the mutual solubilities of oil
and alcohol have not been completely established. Second, FPC produced by most solvent
extraction procedures with the exception of
hydrolyzed products is essentially inert.

The importance of these two points is
immediately realized when consideration is
given to the fact that a substantial FPC program cannot be based on low oil species such
as hake but must in reality be dependent on
underutilized fatty species of fish available
in both U. S. and foreign waters. It is
estimated that over six billion pounds of

these species are available in U. S. waters
alone, as compared to 1 billion pounds of
hake.   Economics would therefore dictate that
an efficient FPC process should produce both
a high quality protein and a utilizable oil.
    The inertness or loss of functionality of
the proteins that results when proteins are
extracted with polar organic solvents could
pose a distinct deterrent to their full utilization and potential usefulness.   This is
particularly true in the U. S. where food
manufacturers blend food ingredients that
complement one another to achieve the characteristics desired by the diet habits of the
consumer.   Hammonds and Call,[2] for example,
have pointed out that over two thirds of the
three billion pound potential market for ingredient proteins will be for those possessing functional properties.

Disadvantages of Aqueous Processing
The major disadvantage to aqueous processing
has been that yields are lower than on those
obtained with solvent extraction processes.
This can generally be attributed to a loss of
low molecular weight proteins that are soluble in the aqueous extracting medium.   In
addition to the problem of yield, it has been
found that obtaining and maintaining desirable organoleptic characteristics is more
difficult with aqueous processing. Problems
of organoleptic stability of FPC generally
reside with the quantity and type of residual
lipids that remain in the product. Methods
for stabilizing residual lipids have been
only partially successful, so that most investigators have still found it necessary to
lower the content of residual lipids in preparations where it was originally thought
that complete aqueous processing would
suffice.

Status of Aqueous Processes

To date, I know of no complete aqueous process method that has been developed to the
point of commercialization, i.e., preparation
for sale of an FPC that meets current U. S.
specifications for its use as a food additive. By definition, Rutman's product does
not meet the criteria for FPC because of its
high lipid content.[3] It has been reported
that Dreosti and Atkinson have developed an
all-aqueous process for producing FPC of high
acceptability and stability from headed and
gutted hake and factory trimmings.[4] In this
process, press cake is first produced, then
washed with boiling water, treated with BHT,
and dried in an air stream at 150° F to a
moisture content of less than 10 percent.
This product is reported to be almost equivalent in organoleptic properties to solvent-
extracted hake meal. As has been previously
pointed out, however, yields are lower due to
the loss of water soluble proteins that
accompanies the water washing steps.

Alkali or acid solubilization processes. In
a compilation of FPC methods several are described for dissolving fish in either alkali
or acids and reprecipitating the proteins at
their mean isoelectric point.[5] It would be
expected that yield would be lower with these
methods because of peptide and amino acid
losses. In addition, the precipitated proteins generally require extraction(s) with
organic solvents for purposes of deodorizing
and the removal of residual oils.

     There has been extensive reporting on me-
thods that utilize alkali or acid to solubilize fish proteins, but there has been no
comprehensive study made on the economics of
using this approach for making either FPC or
protein isolates. Low yields coupled with
rather extensive processing steps would

indicate that these methods might not be able
to compete with either straight solvent extraction or combination aqueous-solvent processes. In addition, complete nutritional
data is lacking with these processes so that
valid comparisons cannot be made for the purpose of overall evaluation. The merit of alkali or acid processing seems to lie with the
properties of the recovered proteins. Using
this type of processing, heat-coagulable proteins[6] and proteins with characteristics re-
sembling egg albumin[7] have been prepared.
Tannenbaum et al. have recently reported on
an investigative study in which FPC is used
as a starting material for preparing fish
protein isolates.[8] In this work, FPC was
partially hydrolyzed with NaOH and the proteins recovered by isoelectric precipitation.
Although working with the defatted FPC could
obviate the need for solvent cleanup, the
economics of using a once-processed product
as a raw material might lessen the economic
advantage that an unprocessed raw material
possesses. It seems quite possible, however, that these processes could be developed
to produce protein isolates with desirable
functional properties. These products would
therefore be competitive with protein isolates of animal origin and would probably be
valued more for their intrinsic physical and
chemical properties than for their nutritive
properties.

Aqueous-solvent processes. The idea of using
partially defatted fish, fish meal or press
cake as a raw material source for preparing
FPC has received considerable attention. The
major drawbacks in producing acceptable FPC
with these processes are related to the
difficulties of removing lipids, and color
and odor bodies that reside in the processed
starting meals. During processing (cooking

and drying), many chemical reactions occur
that make the subsequent solvent extraction
step difficult to accomplish efficiently.
Such reactions as lipid polymerization, the
formation of fatty acid protein complexes,
and the formation of Maillard-type products
all add to the difficulty of efficient solvent extraction.[9] Only recently has Astra
Nutrition solved most of these problems.
With the Astra process, fish is eviscerated,
washed, given a mild cook, deboned, centrifuged, and solvent extracted. FPC produced
by this method is reported to be excellent.
Yields, however, are about 33 percent lower
than those obtained by the alcohol extraction process.[10] Because of the deboning
step, however, the protein content is about
10 percent higher than in FPC made from
whole fish.

Utilization of condensed phosphate for the
preparation of FPC. It is well-known that
under acidic conditions condensed phosphates
will react with proteins to form insoluble
protein-phosphate complexes. Utilizing this
reaction, Spinelli et al. have developed a
combined aqueous-solvent process that produces FPC of quality and yield equivalent to
that obtained by alcohol extraction processes.[11] A schematic of this process is
shown in Figure 1, and the process has been
described as follows:
    Comminuted fish is mixed with an equal
part of water and sufficient sulfuric acid
is added to lower the pH to 5.7. The mixture is rapidly heated to 75°-80° C to inactivate endogenous proteolytic enzymes.
Immediately after heating, sodium hexametaphosphate (1 percent based on the weight of
wet fish) in aqueous solution is added to the
fish-water mixture, and the pH of the slurry
is lowered to 3.8-4.0 with 1 M H_2SO_4. The

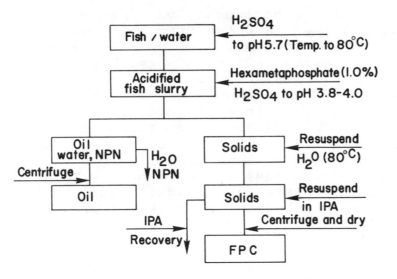

Figure 1.   Preparation of FPC by the Aqueous
Phosphate Process

slurry is then centrifuged, yielding an
aqueous-oil phase and the complexed protein-
bone (solids) fraction. The solids are generally resuspended twice in water to remove
additional oil and other nonproteinaceous
matter. Residual lipids are then removed by
resuspending twice in azeotropic IPA (at a
ratio of 1 part IPA to 1 part fish) and
dried. The oil is recovered from the aqueous
phase by conventional methods.

Yields of FPC made in the laboratory by
the above process are not significantly
different from those prepared by alcohol extraction procedures. PER values and the
proximate composition of FPC made by the
aqueous-phosphate procedure are equal to FPC
made by IPA extraction. The phosphate content of FPC made by the aqueous-phosphate
procedure is, as expected, higher than that
of IPA-produced FPC. A typical analysis is
given as follows:

Species	% phosphorous in FPC made by	
	IPA	API
Herring	1.12	2.10
Hake	2.70	3.75

The nutritional significance of the higher
phosphate content in the aqueous phosphate
FPC is yet to be determined.

Flexibility of aqueous-solvent processing.
Current emphasis on the preparation of FPC is
primarily oriented toward the preparation of
products with functional characteristics.
These range from rather simple properties
such as loss of wetting and dispersion to the
more complex ones of solubility and emulsion-
forming characteristics. With complete solvent systems, the flexibility of processing
parameters is largely limited to the choice

of solvent and processing temperatures.
Desolventizing and drying techniques employed
to meet current specifications for solvent
residues generally destroy most of the functional properties that may have been maintained by the proper choice of process parameters. Binary organic solvent systems have
been described in the literature but inherent
process parameters and desolventizing problems are similar to or possibly more difficult than those employing a single solvent.

Aqueous-solvent processes, however, offer
flexibility that would be difficult to
achieve with an all-solvent system. The Astra process presents a good example of this
flexibility where part of the processing can
be done at sea and subsequent solvent processing finished ashore. Recent work at the
author's laboratory (John Spinelli, unpublished data) shows that press cake made by
the aqueous-solvent process can be stabilized
against microbial and oxidative deterioration
for at least 30 days at 20° C.

Another example of the direction that
might be taken with aqueous solvent processing has been shown by Spinelli et al. where
functional protein isolates were prepared
from partially hydrolyzed fish protein.[12]
The partially hydrolyzed proteins were recovered as phosphate complexes, extracted
with isopropanol to remove residual lipids,
desolventized by aqueous extraction, and then
spray dried. The technique is also being
applied to produce a functional fish protein
concentrate.

Conclusions
The most advanced processes for producing FPC
are still those processes that are based on
complete solvent extraction procedures.
Aqueous processes, however, offer attractive
alternatives. At present, it would appear

that combined aqueous-solvent procedures
might actually be better suited for processing of fatty species of fish, because of reduced solvent requirements and simplified oil
recovery techniques. In addition, these processes have a degree of flexibility that is
not attainable with complete solvent extraction systems. With processes that utilize
solvents in the initial processing steps,
there is little if any recourse except to
finish the process with the use of additional
solvents. With aqueous methods, on the other
hand, the possibility of varying process
parameters is greatly enhanced. It would
seem quite probable, therefore, that aqueous-
solvent processes are better suited to
achieve full utilization of fish as a raw
material source of protein if various market
requirements are to be met.

References

1.   Finch, R.   1970.   Fish Proteins for Human
Foods.   CRC Crttical Reviews in Food Technology.

2.   Hammonds, T. M., and Call, D. L.   1970.
Utilization of protein ingredients in the
U. S. food industry. Part 2. The Future Market for Protein Ingredients.   Ithaca: Cornell Univ.

3.   Rutman, M.   1971.   Process for Preparing
High-energy Fish Protein Concentrate.   U. S.
Patent No. 3,561,973.

4.   Fish flour experiments in the Cape Town
Institute. 1969. Fishing News International, December.

5.   Library of Congress.   1970.   Fish Protein

Concentrate. A comprehensive Bibliography
Compiled by Special Bibliography Section,
Science and Technology Division, Washington,
D. C., Catalogue Card No. 79-606672.

6. Rogers, W. I. 1960. Preparation of Heat
Coagulable Protein. Canadian Patent No.
663,557.

7. Bonagura, A. G., and Moshy, R. J. 1960.
Preparation of Whipping Agent. Canadian
Patent No. 663,558.

8. Tannenbaum, S. R., Ahern, M., and Bates,
R. P. 1970. Solubilization of fish protein
concentrate. Food Technol. 24: 96.

9. Dreosti, D. M. Recent South African
advances regarding fish protein concentrate.
Paper presented at the 2nd International
Congress of Food Science and Technology, War-
saw, Poland.

10. Astra Nutrition. 1968. Edible Defatted
Fish Meal. British Patent No. 1,106,676.

11. Spinelli, J., Dyer, J., Lehman, L., and
Wieg, D. 1971. The fish protein concentrate
story. 13. Aqueous phosphate processing.
Food Technol. 25: 713.

12. Spinelli, J., Koury, B., and Miller, R.
In press. Approaches to the utilization of
fish for the preparation of fish protein
isolates. II. Enzymic modification of myofibrillar fish proteins. J. Food Sci.

VIII
FPC APPROACHES AND PROJECTS IN NORWAY

Eirik Heen
Norwegian Fisheries Research Institute,
P. O. Box 187, Bergen, Norway

Approaches

The present directions to research on FPC in
Norway are the result of several approaches
explored over the past 40 years. In prewar
years lean species of fish were in abundance,
and a commercial venture was attempted based
on processing eviscerated cod, which was put
through a conventional cooking, pressing, and
drying process. The resultant press cake was
converted into a fish meal with a pronounced
fibrous texture. Pilot scale operation was
extended to the production of whole meal from
deboned cod, a slightly more refined product,
but none of these efforts met with any success.

An attempt was made to produce a highly
purified fish protein through deproteinization used in analytical chemistry. A dehy-
dration-fractionization process was employed,
concentrating alcohol at increasing levels in
steps to separate the smaller molecules and
reactive substances from a more narrow spectrum of protein moieties. This technique
produced a pure protein mixture consisting
mainly of actomyosin and partly of albumins,
which were coagulable in the alcohol concentration. In 1955, a pilot plant was built to
evaluate the technical feasibilities of the
procedure. One of the purposes of the project was to see if the heat coagulability of
the fish protein could be retained in a cold
dehydration-extraction process with ethanol
in a concentration range of 40 to 80 percent.
It was found that the heat coagulability was
only partly retainable and that dehydration

with these solvents would denature the proteins.

Present Projects in Norway

We have now focused our attention on three
different products: the first is a good fish
meal, whole meal, or dried press cake meal;
the second is a defatted product; and the
third is a neutral, bland product similar to
other Type A FPCs presently being produced.

Fish meal type products are the cheapest
animal protein concentrates that can be made
available. Extensive feeding experiments
indicate that they are wholesome and nutritionally satisfactory, although they do not
meet the specifications for FPC proper due to
a fat content in the 7 to 9 percent range.
They have a pronounced fishy taste and develop a definite rancidity after comparatively
short storage. In trial tests, however, they
have met with acceptance in regions of the
Far East and Africa where they tally with the
local habits of preparing cereal dishes and
with the accepted condiment properties.
Stabilization and control over the degree of
rancidity is possible through antioxidants
and feasible forms of protection in packaging.

The second product is defatted through a
classical solvent extraction process. It has
a fishy taste, is gritty, and develops a
taste of its own. Provided that a well pro-
tected, good fish meal is used and the oil is
stabilized through antioxidants before the
extraction process, the recovered oil may be
used commercially, although it hardly compen-
sates for the extraction costs. It will,
therefore be more expensive than the first
products, but it still ranges in the lowest
price level.

The third product is produced by a modified wet extraction process which aims at a

neutral, bland product. Although there are
still many snags, a project is under way to
transform the individual production steps into an industrial process. The cost estimate
for the product is tentatively established at
about 50¢ per kilogram based on present raw
material prices. The species being used are
the same as those being used for conventional
oil and meal production with an anticipated
premium for special handling and transportation. The goal is to arrive at a product and
price which can compete favorably with milk
protein.

Finally, water soluble types of FPC or
lightly dispersible protein concentrate are
also being considered, and a joint study program is under way between several food processors and research establishments.

IX
LIQUEFIED FISH PROTEIN CONCENTRATE

Toyosuke Kinumaki
Tokai Regional Fisheries Research Laboratory,
Tokyo, Japan

Liquefied fish protein (LFP), developed by
Dr. Higashi, is produced by an enzymatic digestion method. It is a fish protein hydrolysate that forms a stable, light tan powder
containing about 85 percent crude protein
which is instantly soluble in water.[1,2]

Manufacturing Process
An outline of the process is shown in Fig. 1.
Whole fish is ground and used as a starting
material. When a high quality product is required, fish-meat emulsion is also available
as the starting material. After grinding,
the slurry is mixed with 0.8 to an equal
amount of water, and 0.3 to 0.5 percent of
a commercial proteolytic enzyme. During continuous stirring, the enzymatic digestion of
the fish protein is carried out for four
hours at 50 to 60° C. After digestion, the
temperature of the mixture is raised to about
90° C to inactivate the enzyme. The aqueous
fraction, the oil, and the insoluble part
consisting mainly of bones and other indi-
gestible fish tissues are separated in a
centrifuge or through a filter press. The
aqueous fraction is then deodorized with an
organic solvent such as cyclohexane. Although azeotropic distillation was proposed,[4,5] it was found that by blowing carbon
dioxide through the aqueous fraction, unacceptable odors are mostly removed along
with the solvent. The resulting aqueous
fraction is concentrated under reduced pressure at below 60° C in order to get a higher

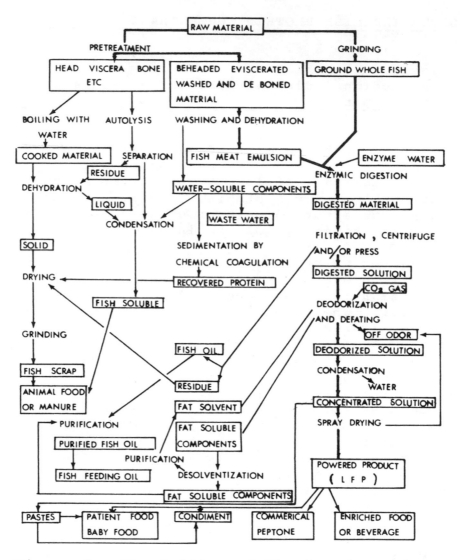

Figure 1. The Outline of the Manufacturing
Process of LFP. Thick arrows indicate main
flow.

yield during the spray drying procedure.
Finally, the powdered product is prepared by
spray drying; any remaining off-odor is completely removed during this operation.

An analysis of the composition of the
product obtained is shown in Table 1, and the
yield of each operating procedure is shown in
Table 2.

The yield of LFP is strongly influenced by
the type of enzyme used, the enzyme concentration, the amounts of enzyme inhibitors and
stabilizers, and the digestion conditions.[5,6]
Using pollack-meat emulsion as the starting
material, the yield was tested under the
least influence of autolytic. The yield was
obtained after a 4-hour digestion with 0.3
percent enzyme concentration to substrate at
optimum temperature and unadjusted pH. Three
different enzymes were compared with respect
to the recovery of the total nitrogen when
the starting material was turned into a
liquefied product. Pronase, a protease produced by Streptomyces griseus, solubilized 95
percent of the total nitrogen at an activity
of 35,000 unit per gram. Only 65 percent of
the nitrogen was recovered with the commercial bacterial protease from Bacillus polymyxa (100,000 units per gram) and 45 percent
with the commercial protease from B. spo-20
(10,000 units per gram).[6] When different
types of enzymes are standardized for activity using casein as a substrate, the yield of
LFP was found not to be proportional simply
to the proteolytic activity. These results
do not simply reflect the amount of proteolytic used in the experiments since standard-
ization of the enzymes using casein as a
substrate still gave different yields.

Inhibitors such as polyphosphate or even
NaCl added to the fish-meat emulsion decrease
the yield of LFP.[6] When the raw material is
precooked, the yield of LFP decreases, and

Table 1. Analyses of Products Obtained in Individual Operations

Product	Mackerel					Pollack					
	Mois-ture %	Pro-tein¹ %	Fat %	Ash %	VB-N mg %	pH	Mois-ture %	Pro-tein¹ %	Fat %	Ash %	VB-N mg %
Ground whole fish	70–75.5	16–18	4.5–8.0	2.5–3.0	18–18.5	6.3	77–77.5	15–18	1.7–3.8	2.5–3.0	12.5
Digested solution	91–92	6.5–8.5	0.08	0.6	28–45	6.0	88–92	6.4–8.5	0.09	0.4–0.6	32–52
Residue	65–70	22–22.5	9.5–10.5	1.2–2.0	28–33	6.0	72–75	13.5–18	–	7.8	22–53
Deodorized solution	91–92	6.4–8.5	0.07	0.6	–	–	92	7.0	0.06	0.3–0.6	37–55
Concentrated solution	80–83	15–18	–	1.2–1.4	–	–	–	–	–	–	–
Powdered product (LFP)	2.4–4.9	87–88	0.16	7.3–7.9	–	–	1.9–2.9	78–87	0.08	6.5	–
Fish flesh	69–77	19–29	1.3–15	1.5–2.0	8.2–16.2	5.6	79–82.5	16–20	0.7–0.8	1.1–1.6	7.6

1
Crude protein: N x 6.25

Table 2.   Yield in Each Operation of LFP
Manufacture on a 15-60 Kg Batch Scale.

Operation	Percent Yield Based on	
	Weight	Nitrogen
Grinding	92-99	-
Addition of enzyme	180-200	95-98
Digestion and filtration	65-89	55-92
Deodorization and defatting	96-98	86-98
Condensation	36-47	95-100
Spray drying	14-18	87-90
Overall process	5-15	37-90
(Average	(10)	(55)

Table 3.   Analysis of LFP Samples on Main
Constituents.

Starting material	Enzyme used	Mois- ture %	Pro- tein[1] %	Fat %	Sugar %	Ash %
Whole mackerel	Pronase[2]	4.2	90.7	0.07	1.7	4.0
Whole mackerel	BNP[3]	3.6	87.8	0.00	0.00	7.5
Whole horse mackerel	Pronase[2]	6.2	87.4	0.04	-	6.1
Whole horse mackerel	BNP[3]	8.6	78.5	0.0	0.0	5.8

[1]Crude protein: N x 6.25
[2]Fungal protease from Streptomyces griseus
[3]Bacterial neutral protease from Bacillus
polymyxa

Table 4. Analysis of LFP Samples on Minerals (mg %)

Starting material	Enzyme used	Ca	Mg	P	Na	Cl	Fe	As	Heavy metals[1]	Cu	Cd
Whole mackerel	BNP[2]	72.1	115.6	919.7	1005.7	-	0.14	0.15	4.01	1.3	Nil
Whole mackerel	BNP[2]	164.8	167.4	1034.6	1142.2	153.2	-	0.15	4.01	-	-
Whole pollack	BNP[2]	53.6	89.9	873.9	464.9	-	0.10	-	-	3.8	Nil

[1]Hazardous heavy metals except Cu were not detected
[2]Bacterial neutral protease from Bacillus polymyxa

Table 5. Amino Acid Composition of LFP Samples

Essential amino acid	Whole mackerel		Whole horse mackerel		Precooked whole horse mackerel		Pollack meal emulsion		
	Pronase[1]	BNP[1]	Pronase*	BNP*	Pronase[1]	Bioprase[2]	Pronase[1]	BNP[1]	OFP-10[3]
Isoleucine	247	330	286	293	239	190	278	233	201
Leucine	379	556	457	506	441	389	518	499	500
Lysine	711	549	516	550	510	549	674	726	792
Methionine	214	174	176	184	153	105	156	118	103
Cystine	—	56	—	—	50	45	55	25	44
Phenylalanine	219	255	221	243	177	131	201	146	133
Tyrosine	204	177	95	177	116	51	172	193	129
Threonine	345	254	307	294	268	226	278	246	260
Tryptophan	65	60	79	66	38	24	79	62	91
Valine	302	392	388	376	259	213	321	264	260
Total	2,686	2,803	2,515	2,689	2,251	1,923	2,932	2,485	2,489
Total amino acid	8,762	6,350	—	—	5,572	5,120	5,990	5,950	5,990
E/TA	30	44	—	—	40	37	49	42	42

1. Fungal protease from Streptomyces goiseus
2. Bacterial protease from B. polymyxa
3. Bacterial protease from Bacillus spo-20
*See above
**Bacterial protease from B. Subtilis

much of the protein is left in the insoluble
fraction.[4,5]

Bitterness in LFP depends on the kind of
starting material, the type of enzymes, and
the digestion condition.[1] When pronase is
used, edible but bitterish LFP is obtained.[8]
Bitterness can be reduced significantly when
beheaded, eviscerated, and deboned fish is
digested with Bacillus proteases. Enzymes
must be selected not only on the basis of
their capability to break down fish tissues
but also on the flavors left or generated in
liquefied products.

Properties and Nutritive Quality
The dissolving properties of LFP such as
solubility, wettability, dispersibility, and
speed of dissolution are excellent as compared with those of sugar or dried milk.
However, LFP prepared by short term digestion
is inferior in all the dissolving properties
except solubility.[5] LFP dissolves easily in
water and can be incorporated into soup,
bread, cereals, baby food, and the like without changing their physical properties.

The main constituents of LFP are shown in
Table 3. It contains more protein, but less
fat and ash than FPC prepared by the isopropanol extraction method.[5]

The mineral content of LFP is shown in
Table 4. It contains fewer inorganic substances such as calcium, fluoride, and others
than FPC because the bones are removed during
the manufacturing process.

Although their composition varies with the
type of enzyme, the kind of material, and the
digestion conditions, LFP consists of peptides, both large and small, and amino
acids.[4,7]

The essential amino acid composition of
LFP is almost the same as that of the raw
fish as shown in Table 5.[5] Rat-feeding tests

show that the biological value of LFP is
higher than that of milk casein.[2] Some LFP,
especially that from precooked material, is
lower in isoleucine, cystine, tyrosine, or
tryptophan. However, most LFP is rich in
methionine and phenylalanine. Therefore, the
low nutritive value due to the imbalance of
essential amino acids is mainly attributable
to lack of tryptophan. The tryptophan content
of LFP is lower in an earlier stage of the
digestion. This may be due to the fact that
tryptophan content is very low in a hot-water
extract of whole fish. When a material is
cooked to destroy its original enzymes prior
to digestion with a commercial enzyme, the resultant LFP often shows a poor content of
tryptophan and a low nutritive value in rat-
feeding tests.[2,3]

References

1. Higashi, H. 1966. Liquefied protein.
(In Japanese only) Nippon Shokuhin Kogyo
Gaku Kaishi 13: 37.

2. Higashi, H., Murayama, S., Onishi, T.,
Iseki, S., and Watanabe, T. 1965. Studies
on Liquefied Fish Protein. 1. Nutritive
value of liquefied fish protein. Bull. Jap.
Soc. Sci. Fish. 43: 77.

3. Yanase, M. 1965. Studies on Liquefied
Fish Protein. 2. Difference in tryptophan
content in enzymatic hydrolysate of fish by
different digestion methods. Bull. Jap. Soc.
Sci. Fish. 43: 87.

4. Onishi, T., and Higashi, H. 1968. Studies on Liquefied Fish Protein. 3. Odor and
peptide composition of Liquefied Fish Protein.
Bull. Tokai Reg. Fish Res. Lab. 55: 225.

5.   Iseki, S., Watanabe, T., and Kinumaki, T.
1969.   Studies on Liquefied Fish Protein.
4. Examination of processing conditions for
industrial production.   Bull. Tokai Reg. Fish.
Res. Lab. 59: 81.

6.   Iseki, S., Watanabe, T. and Kinumaki, T.
1973.   In preparation.   Studies on Liquefied
Fish Protein.   5. Yield of LFP in the digestion of fish meat emulsion.   Bull. Tokai Reg.
Fish. Res. Lab. 73: 85.

7.   Sugii, K., and Kinumaki, T.   1973.
Studies on Liquefied Fish Protein.   6.
Comparison of composition in different prod-
ucts by use of commercially available several
proteolytic enzymes.   Bull. Tokai Reg. Fish.
Res. Lab. 73: 103.

8.   Kitabayashi, K., Shado, K., Nakamura, K.,
and Ishikawa, S.   1963.   Proteolytic hydrolysis on digestion of aquatic animal meats.
On the bitterness in animal meat products.
Sci. Rept. Hokkaido Fish. Expl. Station 1:
88.

X
THE FISH PROTEIN HYDROLYZATE (FPH) PROCESS
A TARGET DESIGN APPROACH

Max Rutman and Wilhelm Heimlich
Centro Proteico Industrial, Casilla 1287,
Santiago, Chile

The development of food to feed the Chilean
infant population using fish as a protein
source has been the first priority of our
laboratories at the Industrial Protein Center
(Santiago, Chile). This protein could enrich
staple foods or could be used in the design of
new foods for nutritionally deficient social
groups.

   The methodology for achieving this nutritional purpose was selected after considering
the difficulties previously encountered in the
implementation of solvent-extracted FPC[1,2,3,4]

   The main question to be answered was, what
process could produce a protein good enough to
formulate a food to be consumed by the infant
target group?

   There has recently been an increasing concern about a general approach intended to
solve nutrition problems and about the need
for multidisciplinary work and multisectorial
action for achieving the desired success.[5,6,7]
This approach has not been used to design a
protein concentrate process. More emphasis
should be given, therefore, to design the food
within the constraints of a given system. In
other words, designing the food comes first,
then comes the process development. This new
approach is quite different from the previous
ones where the question was reversed; namely,
given a process for obtaining an FPC, how
could the FPC be used for nutritional purposes?

   In this article we will analyze the general

criteria for designing a food intended for the
target group, and then discuss its application, taking into account the particular constraints of Chilean natural resources and the
target population.

Criteria In Designing New Foods With A Nutritional Purpose

In the selection of foods designed for fight-
ing malnutrition, four aspects should be considered carefully and simultaneously:
1. Nutrition (N), 2. Economics (E), 3. Technology (T), and 4. Consumer Acceptability (A)
(Figure 1). The relationship between these
aspects will define the feasibility of reaching the target group with a given food. A
brief description of each aspect is given
below:

1. Nutrition (N). Circle N represents all
possible formulations with a given nutritional
value. They are obtained from our knowledge
of nutrition and from animal and clinical
experiments.

2. Economics (E). For any developing country
a program to nourish the target population
properly is very expensive. The consumer we
are interested in has little or no purchasing
power, and it is the country's obligation to
diversify, directly or indirectly, its resources towards nutrition. Circle E will represent, therefore, the family of foods which
a country will or can afford to produce for
the target group.

3. Technology (T). Circle T comprises all the
foods and their components which can be produced on an industrial scale. However, too
many laboratory products have been recommended
in the applied nutrition field, which up to
now remain at the same low scale of operation.
Many protein concentrates are a good example

of this situation.

4. Consumer Acceptability (A). Consumer reaction for a given food is of the utmost importance, and may be the key factor for a
successful program in applied nutrition. The
food should be not only nutritious, and
economically and technologically feasible, but
also acceptable to the target population.[7]
Circle A comprises those foods with textures,
flavors, and appearances which are associated
with existing food habits.

The Target Foods. The intersection of the
four areas, N, E, T and A, corresponds to the
family of foods which might reach the target
population to be called the target foods.

The intersection of N, E represents formulations having a good biological value which
are also economically feasible.

By linear programming we can select the
cheapest formulation within the intersecting
area. This approach, where protein concentrates from different sources were evaluated
for various formulas, was used by Devanney.[8]
However, when the technologies for obtaining
the foods or their components are added to the
picture, the solution area of our problem
shrinks, as shown by the intersection of N, E,
and T.

The consumer acceptability (A) of the food
makes the solution even harder, as shown by
the intersection of N, E, T, and A. Figure 1
shows an intersection and, therefore, a target
food family of solutions exists. However, we
will rarely find this intersection since there
are very few nutritious formulas given to
undernourished children with success.

In the area of FPC there have been serious
problems regarding technology, acceptability,
and economics, but no problems in connection
with nutrition.[1,2,3,4]

What is the potential for expanding each of

TARGET FOODS

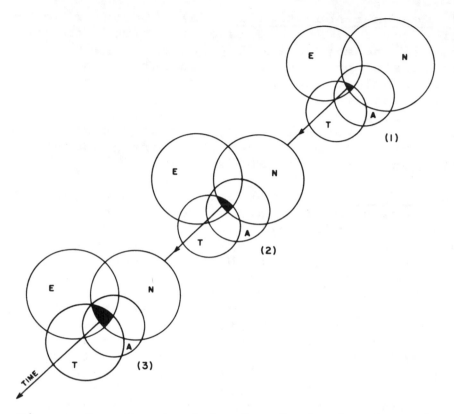

Figure 1. Constraints for designing target
foods, and how they might change with time.
N = Nutrition, E = Economics, T = Technology,
and A = Consumer Acceptability.

the circles and thus increasing the number of
available target foods? From our knowledge of
nutrition, it is difficult to think of expansion in this area. On the contrary, the more
we know about nutrition, the fewer number of
foods or components we can use safely. N actually becomes smaller with time. It is hard
to expand E because we are dealing with developing countries, although a change in priori-
ties within a country might increase E. The
Chilean government policy on nutrition programs sets a good example for an expanding E.

     We are left, then, with A and T. A could
be increased through marketing on a short
term basis and through education on a longer
term basis. T has a tremendous potential for
expansion which has not yet been properly exploited. For instance, in the area of FPC
only one type of technology has been tried in
more than 20 years.[1] It would seem proper to
emphasize new technological approaches, which
could provide a variety of components (lipids,
carbohydrates and proteins) formulated into
foods of different organoleptic and textural
characteristics.

Time. Malnutrition requires a quick solution,
and time is therefore of overwhelming importance since it will affect our target food
solution and the T, A, E, and N constraints.
For example, if we expect a 50 percent decrease in malnutrition over a period of five
years, the target food might be quite different than if we expand the period to ten
years. An example of the way time might affect the constraint areas is given below:
T: We will have to look for technologies
which can be easily implemented in developing
countries.
A: The food should be readily acceptable.
E: There should be a governmental policy.
N: To avoid long testing trials, no toxicity
doubt should exist about the foods or their

components.

Fish Protein Concentrate. From the three bulk
components of foods, proteins, lipids, and
carbohydrates, the first has received priority. Problems related to protein cost and
quality have been discussed else-
where.[1,2,3,4,8] Fish protein has been considered of great potential as a protein supplement because of its high nutritional quality
and probable low cost.
     There is a need for developing processes
which would yield different FPCs specially devised to obtain specific target foods. It
seems to be extremely difficult to develop a
universal type of protein which will work properly in any food. In this respect the definition of FPC should be extended to include
products with a fishy odor and a variable
lipid content. As stated above, the criteria
for designing a new FPC process should be
analyzed in the same way as the design of a
target food.

The Process
Constraints. In Chile, the government has
undertaken milk distribution for preschool and
school-age children at an enormous cost, importing over 30,000 tons of dried milk in
1971. There is great interest, therefore, in
developing milk analogs with built-in nutritional quality to suit the age of the respective target group.
     The large Chilean marine resources provide
the necessary raw material for preparing fish
protein as a source for a milk analog when
combined with carbohydrates and lipids.
     The constraints of the process are shown in
Table 1.

Process Description. The FPH process (Figure
2) can be divided into three steps:
1. Extraction of the purified fish pulp.

Table 1.   Process constraints

Economy (E)   Substitution of milk imports by
                     a cheaper analog for a govern-
                     mental milk distribution pro-
                     gram.

Nutrition (N)   High biological value fish pro-
                     tein concentrate, as supple-
                     mentary protein source.

Consumer   Milklike beverage with flavors
Acceptability   for enhancing acceptability.
(A)   Instant dry powder.

Technology (T) Quick technology.
                Maximum use of known technolo-
                gies, applied in Chile.
                Low investment.
                Raw material: Hake (<u>Merluccius</u>
                <u>gayi gayi</u>)
                Avoidance of any toxical and
                microbial hazard.
                Functional protein, soluble or
                suspendable in water.
                Storage stability: similar or
                better than milk.
                The final formula, protein,
                carbohydrate and lipids, should
                behave as milk.
                The process should be flexible
                for diminishing risks and in-
                creasing the variety of target
                foods.

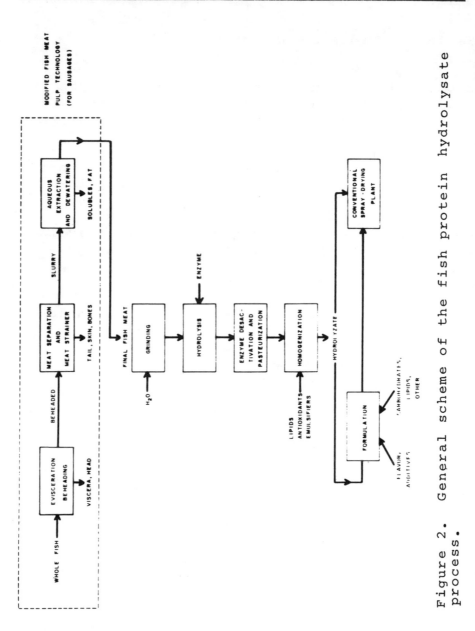

Figure 2.   General scheme of the fish protein hydrolysate process.

2. Fish pulp hydrolysis.
3. Concentration, formulation, and drying.

Step 1 is based on the pulp extraction met method used by the Japanese.[9]

Step 2 links both technologies by trans-forming a fishlike product into a milklike one.

Step 3 is known in dairy technology.

Purified fish pulp was obtained from hake (Merluccius gayi). The fish is beheaded, eviscerated, and the meat is separated and finally extracted using water.

This process splits the fish into 3 frac-tions (Figure 2): the purified pulp, the solubles, and the rest of the fish. Different processes have been developed for the utiliza-tion of each fraction. We will deal, however, only with the pulp which yields the FPH for human consumption. The yield of purified pulp on a nitrogen basis ranges from 30 to 40 per-cent according to the type and size of the fish.

The main purpose of extracting the purified pulp is to obtain a functional protein, fla-vorless, odorless, and free from unwanted components. The protein content increases from 80 percent on a dry basis in the evisce-rated hake to 95 percent in the purified pulp, the rest being 3 percent lipids and 2 percent ash. (Table 2)

The mechanical separation of skin, fish bones, and heads causes a loss of minerals (Figure 3). Part of the depot lipid attached to the skin is also removed. Water extraction is performed in two operations: mixing the pulp with water, and then dewatering by mesh and press. These operations are crucial for obtaining a high quality pulp. Water removes flavor compounds, pigments, blood, lipids, and enzymes, etc. (Figure 4). Some of these compounds strongly enhance lipid oxidation. There is a relatively low loss of proteins in the first extraction. The extraction

Table 2.   Protein Concentrate in the Stage of
Modified Fish Meat Pulp Technology of the FPH
Process.

	Percentage on a dry basis	
	Eviscerated hake	Purified pulp
Protein	80	95
Lipid	7	3
Ash	13	2

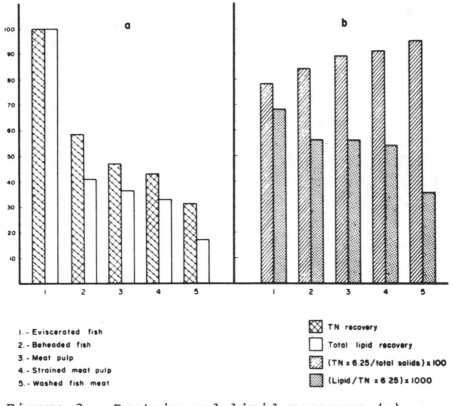

1.- Eviscerated fish
2.- Beheaded fish
3.- Meat pulp
4.- Strained meat pulp
5.- Washed fish meat

TN recovery

Total lipid recovery

(TN x 6.25/total solids) x 100

(Lipid/TN x 6.25) x 1000

Figure 3. Protein and lipid recovery (a),
and protein enrichment (b) at different
steps of the purified fish pulp process.
(TN = total nitrogen; TN x 6.25 = apparent
value of protein.)

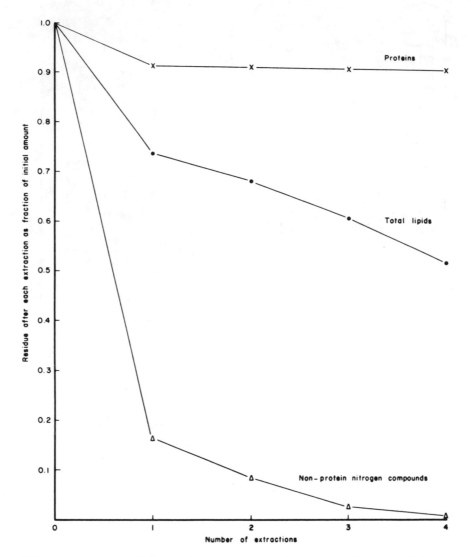

Figure 4. Effective removal of undesirable compounds (nonprotein nitrigen compounds) from fish pulp by successive water extractions.

conditions are: water/pulp, 5/1; pH 6.8;
temperature, 5° C; and time for each extraction, 5 minutes.

Water extraction at room temperature removes nonprotein-nitrogen (NPN) which is related to fishy flavor. Figure 4 shows how
several extractions, of 5 minutes each, drop
NPN to 1 percent of the original content. In
the unwashed pulp NPN is 12 percent of the
total nitrogen, composed mainly of pyrimi-
dines, creatine, etc., and a small fraction of
free amino acids.[10] Trimethylamine has been
measured as an index of the fish flavor. Figure 5 shows that under the described experimental conditions, equilibrium is reached
quickly. The model which might explain this
behavior shows how diffusion is nonlimiting in
the minced pulp matrix.

Ten percent of the total protein is also
lost during the extraction. This loss is
mainly sarcoplasma and heme proteins.[10]

Thirty to 50 percent of the lipids is also
removed in an emulsified form.[11] This lipid
extraction depends likewise on the pressing
operation.

Neutral as well as polar lipids are extracted in amounts related to the original
hake lipid composition.[11]

The lipid content of the purified fish pulp
runs from 2.5 to 3.5 percent on a dry basis.
These lipids are fairly unsaturated and well
above the percentage claimed to be safe for a
solvent-extracted FPC. The stability of the
remaining lipids should be measured in the
intermediate product or final food. Addition
of stabilized fat plus antioxidants has proved
to stabilize the unsaturated lipid.

Enzymatic Hydrolysis. The main purpose of
hydrolyzing the purified fish pulp is to get a
suspendable or soluble protein concentrate
with the required functional and organoleptic
properties to prepare beverages.

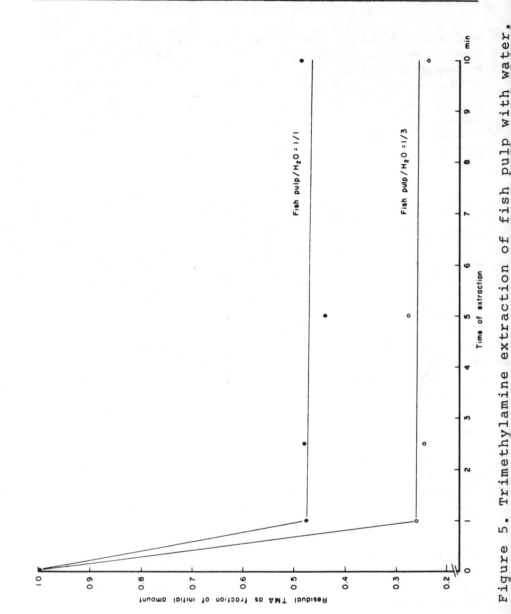

Figure 5. Trimethylamine extraction of fish pulp with water.

Fish protein hydrolysis has been used and tried before. The basic problems found by previous workers were: long time hydrolysis; flavor due to small molecules, peptides, and amino acids; microbiological hazards; engineering problems; and the disappearance of essential amino acids. Most of this work was carried out to separate lipids from proteins, or to obtain pure amino acids.[12,13,14,15,16]

Our approach was to try a short-time hydrolysis using different enzymes, at different conditions of pH and temperature.[16] It was possible to obtain the required hydrolysate with the desired functional properties and to avoid undesired flavor development.

The hydrolysis reaction is shown in Figure 6. A suspendable product with very little off-flavor was obtained by using 1 percent bromelain on a protein basis for 15 minutes in a programmed temperature reaction. The reaction conditions are as follows: pH 7.0 temperature profile as in Figure 7, and substrate 8.6 percent protein, plus 4.7 percent lipids and surfactants. The percentage of nonsedimented N was determined after 10 minutes of centrifugation at 3,000 rpm.

Some of the key factors of hydrolysis, such as viscosity and particle size, change rapidly in the first few minutes. (Figure 7).

It can be seen that the best particle size distribution is at 10 minutes of digestion: high nonheat coagulable nitrogen compounds, NCN, and low percentage of nonprotein nitrogen compounds NPN (the cause of off-flavors, small peptides, and free amino acids). Viscosity at this time is also low. The reaction conditions are as follows: Substrate 8.3 percent protein and bromelain, 12 mg/g protein, pH 7.0 and the reaction temperature profile as shown in this figure.

At about 38° C two simultaneous reactions will occur: enzymatic hydrolysis (due to the added enzyme), and the aggregation of protein

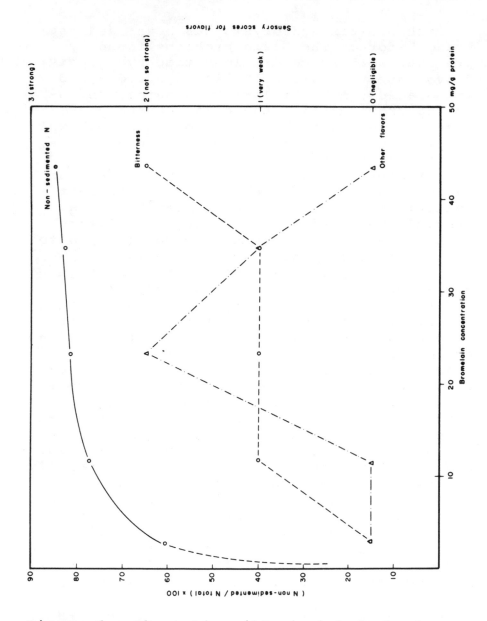

Figure 6. Short-time (15 min.) hydrolysis.
Effect of enzyme concentration on off-
flavor development and on the production of
suspendable hydrolysates.

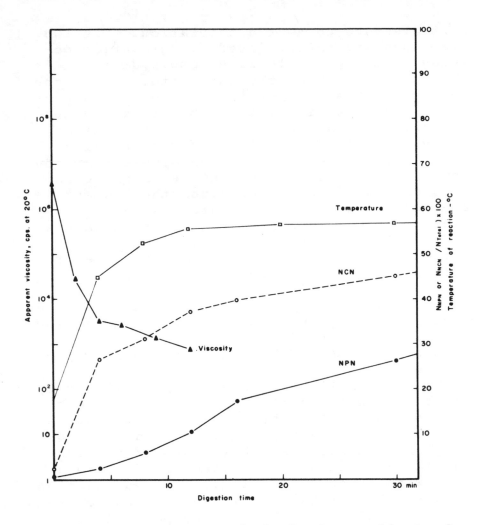

Figure 7.   Short-time hydrolysis.   Effect of
digestion time on some important properties
of the hydrolysate.

particles due to heat denaturation. The two
reactions are interrelated. Aggregation depends on the particle size, and hydrolysis on
the denaturation of the substrate. Since the
purpose of the process is to suspend the protein particles, it is desirable to avoid any
denaturation that causes strong aggregation
(coagulation) and the loss of waterholding
capacity. Therefore, the hydrolysis reaction
is carried out at a temperature as close as
possible to the one that gives the highest
enzyme activity without aggregation. The
hydrolysis should start at a low temperature
and should increase continuously with the reaction time (Figure 7). The temperature profile used is not necessarily the best.

The functionality of the hydrolysate has
been tested through the interaction with other
macromolecules, such as hydrolyzed wheat flour
and dextrines, to formulate the milk analog.
This mixture should be stable at boiling temperature without flocculation.

From the molecular point view, the hydrolysis should provide the right particle and
molecule size distribution. Small molecules
should be avoided if bitterness and astring-
ency are undesirable, while large particles
should be avoided if chalkiness and aggregation with other macromolecules are not wanted
(Figure 8). In Case A of Figure 8 the cause
of hydrolysis is such that the particle sizes
are distributed in the extremes, very large
(In) and very small (So) and, further, after a
certain reaction time, In remains almost constant and the main reaction is SC So. Because
of the particle size distribution, the final
product forms a relatively unstable suspension
and the off-flavors are rather strong. In
Case B it is digested to a low percentage and
the particle size distribution is more homo-
geneous towards small particles. This gives a
beverage with better functional properties and
flavor.[17]

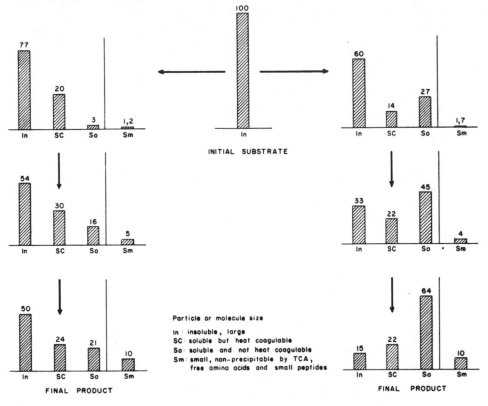

Figure 8.   Real causes of undesirable (A), and desirable (B) enzymatic hydrolysis obtained by using different enzymes and reaction conditions.

The molecular spectrum should be designed
for the specific target food. Ideally it
should be tailormade since there is a whole
family of possible hydrolysates to be used for
different products.[17]

With this short-time mild enzymatic hydrolysis we have avoided a loss of nutritive value, the formation of undesirable off flavors,
microbial hazards, and we have obtained the
right functional properties.

Lipid Addition. The addition of 10 to 30 percent on a dry basis of lipids to the FPH, such
as hydrogenated fish oil with antioxidants
(BHT, BHA, PG), will avoid the rapid lipid
oxidation of the remaining fat of the purified
pulp when the FPH is stored as a dry powder.
This approach was based on previous results.[18]
It seems that stabilized fat will dilute the
remaining unsaturated lipids and will allow a
better protection by the antioxidants. The
same results have been obtained with the addition of stabilized sunflower seed oil.

Microscopic studies of the emulsion formed
by FPH and stabilized fat show a substantial
diminishing of the clogging of protein particles, thus rendering more stable suspension.

The stabilized lipids are needed anyway in
the final milk analog as a source of energy
with a reduced bulk of liquid food.

An intermediate product called PH-65 has
therefore been produced for the formulation of
different milk analog. A typical composition
of PH-65 is given in Table 3.

Microbiology. The short-term programmed temperature hydrolysis avoids the growth of
microorganisms. The first stage, pulp production, as well as the third stage, water elimination, are based on standard sanitary procedures of the kamaboko and dairy industries.

The Product

The product studied is PH-65, an emulsion of FPH and lipids, containing 65 percent protein on a dry basis. (See Tables 3 and 4).

This product has been used for the formulation of milk analog, and for nutritional and toxicological evaluation.

Nutritional quality.

The process does not damage the essential amino acids and the high nutritional value of the pulp is unchanged after hydrolysis.[19] The amino acid composition is given in Table 3, showing a very high lysine content (11.3%), as well as a high available lysine value (10%). The product is therefore ideal for enrichment of cereals with a low lysine content.

Addition of 10 percent FPH to wheat flour increases the PER value from 0.66 to 2.5 and to rice, from 1.6 to 3.6.[19]

PH-65 was tried as the only source of protein for infants with results comparable to those of milk, as shown by Yanez et al.

Extensive toxicological studies were performed at the Laboratorio de Investigaciones Pediatricas, of the Universidad de Chile, and the product proved to be safe.[20]

Fisheries-Agriculture-Protein Complex

PH-65 has been used in the formulation of milk analog by mixing it with modified cereal flours.

The PH-65 process has been tried on a small pilot plant scale, and will be tried in 1972 on a larger scale. The industrial production is scheduled for 1974 within a fisheries-agriculture-protein complex (Figure 9), which will product 8,000 tons per year of dried milk analog for human consumption and 8,000 tons per year of calf milk replacer. The same plant can produce alternatively fish sausages and/or fish croquettes.

The stochiometry of the plant is such that

Table 3.   Composition and Nutritional Quality
of PH-65

PH-65 Composition (percentage)

Protein   66
Lipids
  Residual fish lipid   2.4
  Added lipid   22.6
Ash   1.5
Moisture   6.0

Biological Characteristics of PH-65

Amino acids composition (g/16 g N)

Alanine	5.49	Lysine	11.32
Aspartic acid	10.91	Metionine	3.26
Arginine	10.71	Phenylalanine	3.41
Cystine	0.35	Proline	2.84
Glutamic acid	18.42	Serine	4.43
Glycine	3.11	Threonine	4.59
Histidine	2.54	Tryrosine	3.41
Isoleucine	4.07	Tryptophane	1.46
Leucine	6.75	Valine	4.63

Available lysine (g/16 g N)   10.0
PER, Actual   Casein control   2.89
             Product   3.42
PER, corrected Casein control   2.50
             Product   2.98

Table 4.   Properties of PH-65

Color	White
Taste	Slightly astringent, easily masked by flavors
Odor	None
Texture	Smooth and homogenous
Suspension stability	No settling after 48 hr. at 4° C
Reconstitution	Similar to dry milk
Viscosity (10% solids)	Similar to milk
Higroscopicity	Slight

THE FPH INDUSTRIAL COMPLEX

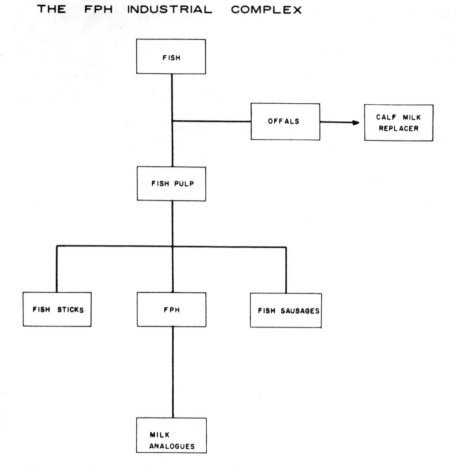

Figure 9.   Fish protein hydrolysate
industrial complex to be built in Chile.

20 thousand tons of hake will produce 16 thousand tons of dried milk analogs for human and animal consumption.

References

1. Rutman, M. 1972. Concentrados Proteicos de Pescado. Paper presented at the "Seminario Internacional de Desarrollo Pesquero-Industrial" April 1972, Lima, Peru.

2. Liston and Pigott. 1970. Fish Protein Concentrate. 3d. Int. Cong. of Food Sc. and Techn. August 1970.

3. Lovern, J. A. 1966. In World Protein Resources. Advances in Chemistry Series. ed. R. F. Gauld. American Chemical Society.

4. Lovern, J. A. 1969. Problems in the development of fish protein concentrates. Proc. Nutr. Soc. 28: 81.

5. Berg, A., and Muscat, R. 1972. Macronutrition. Proceedings Western Hemisphere Nutrition Congress III. New York: Futura Publishing.

6. PAG Bulletin. 1972. The potential of Fish Protein Concentrate for developing countries. (PAG Statement 16). Vol. 2, No. 3.

7. Meiss, A. N. and Cantor, S. M. 1971. Marketing considerations for improved protein food products. J. Am. Oil Chem. Soc., 48, 473.

8. Devanney, J. W. III. 1972. The economics of FPC. Proceedings Western Hemisphere Nutrition Congress III. New York: Futura Publishing.

9. Herrera, P. M. 1969. Studies on the effect of free fatty acid development on the fish paste forming ability of proteins of several species of fish. Master of Science Thesis. University of Washington.

10. Llanos, M. 1970. Estudio del proceso de lavado en la elaboracion de concentrado proteico de merluza. Efecto sobre nitrogeno total, proteico y no proteico. Thesis, Escuela de Quimica y Farmacia, Universidad de Chile, Santiago, Chile.

11. Munoz, P. 1970. Estudio del proceso de lavado en la elaboracion de concentrado proteico de merluza. Efecto sobre animas volatiles, lipidos totales, neutros y polares. Thesis, Escuela de Quimica y Farmacia, Universidad de Chile, Santiago, Chile.

12. Hale, M. M. 1969. Relative activities of commercially available enzymes in the hydrolysis of fish protein. Food Technology, 23: 107.

13. McBride, J. R., Idler, D. R., and MacLeod, R. A. 1961. The liquefaction of British Columbia herring by ensilage, proteolytic enzymes and acid hydrolysis. J. Fish. Res. Bd. Canada, 18 (1): 93.

14. Seripathy, N. V., Kadol, S. B., Sen, D. P., Swaminathan, M., and Lahiry, N. L. 1963. Fish hydrolysates. 3. Influence of degree of hydrolysis on nutritive value. J. of Food Science 28: 365.

15. Seripathy, N. V., Sen, D. P., and Lahiry, N. L. 1964. Preparation of protein hydrolysates from fish meat. Research and Industry, 9 (9): 258.

16.   Fujimaki, M., Kato, H., Arai, S., and
Tamaki, E.   1968.   Applying proteolytic enzymes on soybean.   1. Proteolytic enzyme
treatment of soybean protein and its effect
on the flavor.   Food Technology 22: 889.

17.   Rodriguez, C.   1972.   Determinacion de
esquemas de comportamiento de enzimas pro-
teoliticas sobre carne de merluza (Merluccius
Gayi, gayi).   In Press.   Comite Proteoco
Industrial, Santiago, Chile.

18.   Dreosti, G. M., and Atkinson, A.   1966.
Stabilized Fish Meal.   20th Annual Report p.
50.   Fishing Industry Research Institute.
University of Cape Town, Rondebosch, S.
Africa.

19.   Yanez, E., Ballester, D., Gattas, V.,
Araya, M., Monckeberg, F., and Rutman, M.
1972.   Chemical composition and nutritional
value of a fish protein hydrolysate.   Paper
presented at the IX International Congress
of Nutrition, Mexico.

20.   Ballester, D., Yanez, E., Brunser, O.,
Stekel, A., and Monckeberg, F.   1972.
Longterm effects of feeding a fish enzymatic hydrolysate to rats.   Paper presented
at the 9th International Congress of Nutrition, Mexico.

Part III

NUTRITION

XI
NUTRITIONAL AND SAFETY CHARACTERISTICS OF FPC

B. R. Stillings
Nabisco Research and Development Unit, Fair
Lawn, New Jersey 07410

Fish has long been recognized as having unique
nutritional characteristics and has been his-
torically an important component in the diet
of man. Because fish is an excellent source
of high-quality protein, increased efforts
have been made in recent years to preserve and
utilize this protein from fish that are not
currently being used for direct human consumption. Processes of various types have thus
been developed to convert fish into a broad
class of products called FPCs (fish protein
concentrates).

The literature contains numerous reports of
studies on the chemical, nutritional, and
safety characteristics of FPC. It has been
analyzed extensively for a variety of chemical
components; evaluated by rats, pigs, dogs, and
humans as a source of protein and minerals
either alone or as an ingredient in foods; and
it has been examined for wholesomeness and
safety.

The purpose of this paper, therefore, is to
review and highlight the results from some of
these studies on the composition, nutritional
characteristics, and safety of FPC. This review will not deal with studies conducted with
humans, since this area will be covered in a
subsequent paper by Scrimshaw. Also, because
of the extensive nature of the literature, it
is not possible to refer to all published reports. For a more extensive review, readers
are referred to a review paper by Finch[1] and

to a bibliography published by the Library of
Congress.[2] Further, this paper will deal almost exclusively with FPC prepared by solvent
extraction that is designed to be used for
nutritional purposes as an ingredient in
foods.

Composition

Proximate composition. The proximate (crude
protein, ash, lipids and volatiles) composition will only be dealt with in a general way,
since it is affected greatly by the source of
raw material and the process used. Crude protein may range from less than 75 to as high as
95 percent, ash from 2 to over 25 percent,
lipids from 0.1 to over 0.5 percent, and volatiles from 1 to over 10 percent.[1,3,4]
     The protein and ash contents vary inversely
and are affected by the species of fish processed. For example, when whole fish are
used, FPC made from menhaden is lower in protein and higher in ash than FPC made from herring. This variation can be largely eliminated by mechanically deboning the fish prior
to extraction, which results in FPC with protein and ash content of about 90 and 5 percent, respectively.
     The lipid content of FPC depends on the
efficiency of removal during solvent extraction. Efficient extraction usually results in
a residual amount of 0.5 percent or less.
Medwadowski et al.[5] have recently shown that
lipids in FPC were relatively stable when they
were present at levels of 0.1 percent of less.
When FPC contained more than 0.5 percent
lipids, changes occurred during storage at 37
and 50° C for 6 months that were reflected by
losses in extractibility and severe losses of
highly unsaturated fatty acids.
     As a point of interest, U. S. FDA regula-
tions specify that FPC shall not contain less
than 75 percent crude protein and not more

than 0.5 percent lipid and 10 percent moisture. For these components, Canadian FDD regulations specify only that "fish protein"
shall not contain less than 75 percent crude
protein.

Amino acids. The essential amino acid com-
positions of FPC and of egg and milk are
shown in Table 1. Values shown for FPC are
averages and ranges for several samples prepared by isopropyl alcohol extraction of whole
hake, menhaden, alewife, herring, anchovy, and
ocean pout. In general, the essential amino
acids are somewhat lower in FPC than in egg
protein, which has been used as an optimum reference standard. Lysine is an exception,
which is higher in FPC than in egg protein and
in milk protein. Additional data have been
published in the literature, but in general,
the amino acid values do not vary significantly from those reported here.

   The essential amino acid patterns of these
three proteins are shown in Table 2. Although
the total amounts of essential amino acids are
lower in FPC, data in this table show that the
pattern of amino acids in FPC compares more
favorably with those of egg and milk. Isoleucine, total aromatic amino acids and valine
are somewhat lower, and lysine is higher in
FPC protein.

   These data do not completely agree with the
results from studies on the limiting amino
acids in fish protein. Evidence available
from the literature, indicates that methionine
is usually the first limiting amino acid in
FPC and in fish meal. Miller[7] reported that
the supplementation of five commercial fish
meals with methionine increased the NPU (net
protein utilization) 13 to 58 percent. Likewise, Yanez et al.[8] showed that the NPU of FPC
prepared by ethanol extraction of hake increased significantly when supplemented with
methionine but did not increase when

Table 1. Essential amino acid contents of
protein in egg, milk and FPC (mg/gm of total
nitrogen)

	Hen's egg[1]	Cow's milk[1]	FPC[2] Aver.	Range
Isoleucine	415	407	265	(250-273)
Leucine	553	630	450	(415-476)
Lysine	403	496	509	(493-533)
Total aromatic AA's	627	634	442	(421-464)
Phenylalanine	365	311	246	(231-254)
Tyrosine	262	323	196	(188-210)
Total sulfur AA's	346	211	235	(221-256)
Cystine	149	57	44	(36- 54)
Methionine	197	154	191	(182-203)
Threonine	317	292	259	(248-271)
Tryptophan	100	90	73	(61- 82)
Valine	454	440	314	(282-341)
Total essential amino acids	3215	3200	2547	(2391-2696)

----

[1]Source: FAO[6]

[2]FPC made from red hake, Atlantic menhaden,
alewife, Atlantic herring, Pacific anchovy,
and ocean pout. Source: Sidwell et al.[3]

Table 2. Essential amino acid patterns of
protein in egg, milk and FPC (mg/gm of total
essential amino acids)

Amino acid	Hen's egg		Cow's milk		FPC	
Isoleucine	129		127		104	
Leucine	172		196		177	
Lysine	125		155		200	
Total aromatic AA's	195		197		174	
Phenylalanine		114		97		97
Tyrosine		81		100		77
Total sulfur AA's	107		65		92	
Cystine		46		17		17
Methionine		61		48		75
Threonine	99		91		102	
Tryptophan	31		28		28	
Valine	141		137		123	

supplemented with lysine. Stillings et al.[9]
studied the limiting amino acids in isopropyl
alcohol-extracted FPC prepared from red hake
and grouped the amino acids according to their
limitation from greatest to least as follows:
1. methionine, 2. histidine, tryptophan and
threonine, 3. valine, isoleucine, and phenylalanine, 4. leucine, lysine, and arginine.
Makdani et al.[10] reported that histidine and
methionine appeared to be equally first limiting in FPC prepared by either isopropyl alcohol extraction or by extraction with ethylene
dichloride.

Minerals. In considering the nutritional
characteristics of FPC, most emphasis and
attention has, quite logically, been given to
the protein component. Often overlooked, however, is that FPC is an excellent source of
several essential minerals. Table 3 shows the
mineral composition of FPC made from several
species of whole fish by isopropyl alcohol
extraction.[1] There is considerable variation
in the content of most minerals, which can be
attributed for the most part to the species of
fish used since all samples were processed by
the same general process. Values for fluoride, especially vary widely and have been
found to range up to 600 ppm in FPC made from
nondeboned Pacific hake (NMFS, unpublished).
FPC can contribute significantly, however, to
the requirements for several essential minerals. Based on the median of the ranges
shown in Table 3, as little as 10 grams of
FPC would furnish the following percentages of
the RDAs (recommended daily allowances) for an
8 to 10 year old child: calcium, 40 percent;
phosphorus, 25 percent; iron, 45 percent; and
magnesium, 10 percent. FPC is also a good
source of other essential trace elements such
as copper, zinc, chromium, fluoride, and
selenium. It has been suggested, however,
that FPC may not be an adequate source of

Table 3. Mineral composition of FPC made by
IPA extraction of 12 species of fish[1]

	%
Calcium	2.75 - 5.05
Phosphorus	1.87 - 3.39
Potassium	0.59 - 1.10
Sodium	0.34 - 0.44
Magnesium	0.16 - 0.28

	ppm
Iron	147 - 770
Copper	6 - 21
Zinc	112 - 163
Chromium	8 - 19
Fluorine	58 - 162
Selenium	1.8 - 3.8

----

[1]Source: Finch[1]

potassium for optimum protein metabolism.[11]
Also, it should be pointed out that the removal of bone during processing will have an
effect on the mineral content of FPC.

Another important aspect is the biological
availability of minerals in FPC. Studies
conducted in humans have shown that calcium
and phosphorus are highly available.[11,12] On
the other hand, the iron in FPC has been reported to be only 28 percent as available as
that in ferrous sulfate, but similar to that
in egg yolk.[13] Several studies on the availability of fluoride have indicated a high
availability when the intake is low and a low
availability at high intakes.[14]

Vitamins. FPC prepared by solvent extraction
is not a significant source of vitamins. Extraction of most of the lipids during processing removes fat-soluble vitamins. Water-
soluble vitamins are removed in the aqueous
fraction and have also been shown to be low in
FPC.[4,15]

Nutritional Quality

General. Fish flesh has long been known as an
excellent source of high quality protein. Although few published data are available, examples of the quality of protein in fish are
shown in Table 4.[16] As shown from these data,
the quality of protein in a variety of fish
was shown to be high and consistently above
that of beef protein. In processing fish into
FPC that is to be used as a protein supplement, one obvious objective is to retain to
the extent possible the quality of the original fish protein. Dubrow et al.[17] reported
that it is indeed possible to retain the quality of the protein during the processing of
fish into FPC. In this study, the protein
quality of freeze-dried, whole red hake caught
during different seasons was compared to that

Table 4.   Nutritive Quality of Fish Protein[1]

Source of dietary protein	Rate No	Sex	PER Actual	% of beef
Halibut	20	M	3.27	114
	20	F	2.98	104
Lingcod	15	M	3.60	126
Lemon sole	15	M	3.66	128
White spring salmon	15	M	3.68	129
Red snapper	15	M	3.86	135
Herring	15	F	3.18	111
Beef	20	M	2.86	100
	20	F	2.63	92

----

[1]Source: Beveridge[16]

of FPC made from the same starting material by
isopropyl alcohol extraction. With the exception of one sample, the PER value for the FPC
was virtually the same as that for the starting freeze-dried raw hake. There was, however, considerable difference in the PER
values of starting material caught during
different seasons of the year.

The raw material source, as well as the
processing procedures, may affect the quality
of protein in FPC. Since the quality of protein in FPC cannot be expected to be higher
than that in the raw material, it is important
that the protein in the starting material be
undamaged. Table 5 shows the quality of FPCs
prepared from several species of fish[3] (NMFS,
unpublished). In these studies, FPC was prepared by isopropyl alcohol extraction of
frozen whole raw fish except for hake
(merluccius productus) which was held in brine
and deboned prior to extraction. The data
show the quality of protein in FPC prepared
from these species of fish was reasonably consistent and equal to or slightly higher than
that of casein. Thus, one might expect that
if fish are adequately preserved after catching, the species of fish used in the production of FPC will have only a slight effect on
the quality of protein in the FPC prepared
therefrom. We have, however, noted that the
quality of protein in FPC prepared from some
whole fatty fish such as menhaden and sardines
tends to be slightly lower than that of FPC
prepared from lean fish such as hake.

The literature contains numerous references
to studies on the nutritional quality of FPCs
prepared from different species and by different processes. Table 6 summarizes data from
some of these studies. With the exception of
the sample prepared by ethylene dichloride
extraction, the PER values are high and
consistently above that for casein. Several
investigators have used methods other than

Table 5. Nutritive Quality of Fish Protein
Concentrates Prepared by Isopropyl Alcohol
Extraction of Various Species of Fish[1]

Species of fish	No. samples	PER % of casein
Hake, Urophycis chuss	58	107
Hake, Merluccius productus	10	112
Menhaden, Brevoortia tyrannus	6	102
Herring, Clupea harengus harengus	1	105
Anchovy, Engraulis mordax	1	108
Ocean pout, Macrozoarces americanus	1	102
Alewife, Alosa pseudoharengus	1	106
Moroccan sardine, Sardinia pilchardus	1	99

----

[1]Source: Sidwell et al.[3] and NMFS,
unpublished.

Table 6. Nutritive Quality of Fish Protein
Concentrates Prepared by Different Methods
from Various Species of Fish

Species of fish and processing method	No. samples	PER % of casein	Ref.
Hake, _Merluccius gayi_; dried, hexane or ethanol extraction; Chile	4	106	18, 19
Sardine, _Sardinella longiceps_; cooked and pressed, ethanol extraction; India	1	117	20
Bombay Duck, _Harpoden nehereus_; cooked and pressed, ethanol extraction; India	6	108	21
Krill, _Euphausia superba_ Dana; isopropyl alcohol extraction; Australia	1	103	22
Cod, _Gadus morhua_; isopropyl alcohol extraction, Canada	1	106	4
Herring, _Clupea harengus harengus_; isopropyl alcohol extraction; Canada	1	110	4
Hake, _Urophycis chuss_; ethylene dichloride extraction; U.S.A.	1	89	23

PER for determining the protein quality of
FPC, such as NPU[7,8,24,25] and RNV (relative
nutritive value).[26]   As with PER evaluations,
these methods have also generally shown the
protein quality of FPCs to be equal to or
higher than that of casein.   Thus, from the
data available it is evident that FPC with
protein of high quality can be produced from
several species and by several solvent extraction processes.   Compared to other protein supplements, the PER for isopropyl
alcohol-extracted FPC has been reported to be
about 60 percent higher than that for soy and
cottonseed flour.[3]

In addition to the effect of different
species of fish, the protein quality of FPC
is also affected by whether the whole fish is
used or only parts of the whole fish.   For
example, if fish are deboned prior to extraction, the protein quality of the final FPC is
slightly higher than that made from whole
fish.   Presumably, this slight difference in
quality can be attributed to the removal of
lower quality protein associated with the bone
fraction and the retention of the higher quality flesh protein in the final FPC.

Power[4] compared the nutritive value of FPC
prepared from whole fish, fillets, headed and
eviscerated fish, trimmings, and press cake.
As shown in Table 7, FPC prepared from fillets
was considerably higher in quality than that
made from the whole fish.   The use of headed
and eviscerated or the use of trimmings from
fish had little effect on the protein quality
of FPC compared to that made from whole fish.
When FPC was made from press cake prepared
from cod trimmings, however, the protein quality of the FPC was considerably lower than
that made from whole fish presumably due to
heat damage during processing.   Other work has
shown, however, that it is possible to produce
a high quality FPC from press cake or from

fish meal. As shown in Table 8, there was
little difference in protein quality of
menhaden-FPC prepared from whole fish, deboned
fish, press cake or fish meal. As mentioned
previously, there was a slight increase in the
quality of protein in FPC when made from deboned fish compared to that made from whole
fish. Also, FPC made by Astra Company is
prepared from a type of herring press cake and
the FPC is high in quality.[27]
    De et al.[28] reported that FPC made from de-
composed fish was higher in quality than that
made from fresh fish. In this study, fresh
water fish were allowed to decompose by storing in the laboratory for 24 hours and then
were processed into FPC. Although the yield
qualities were poorer, the PERs of FPC made
from decomposed fish were about 25 percent
higher than those of FPC made from fresh fish.
    Mention should also be made of the nutri-
tional quality of FPC produced by enzymatic
hydrolysis. This type of FPC is not always as
high in protein quality as FPC produced by
solvent extraction, because of a less favorable balance of amino acids.[29] As shown in
Table 9, however, enzymatically-produced FPCs
can be an effective protein supplement. When
evaluated as a sole source of protein, the
PERs ranged from 75 to 82 percent of that for
casein. When added to wheat flour, the PERs
were 91 to 99 percent of the values obtained
with comparable mixtures of casein and wheat
flour.
    Although the quality of protein in solvent-
extracted FPC has generally been reported to
be at least equal to that in casein, there
have been some exceptions. Morrison and
McLaughlan[30] found that the PER values for
various FPCs varied from 60 to 100 percent of
the PER for casein. In this study, FPC prepared by ethylene dichloride-extraction of cod
and haddock fillets had a PER 60 percent of

Table 7. Effect of raw material source on the protein quality of FPC prepared by isopropyl alcohol extraction[1]

Raw material source from Cod	PER % of casein
Whole	106
Fillets	119
Headed & eviscerated	103
Trimmings	103
Trimmings press cake[2]	88

----

[1]Source: Power[4]
[2]Trimmings cooked with indirect heat and pressed to 60 percent moisture.

Table 8. Protein quality of FPCs prepared by isopropyl alcohol extraction of Atlantic menhaden[1]

Raw material source	PER % of casein
Whole fish	101
Deboned fish	104
Whole fish-press cake	98
Whole fish-fish meal	99

----

[1]Source: Stillings, unpublished.

Table 9. Nutritive quality of FPCs prepared
by enzyme hydrolysis of whole red hake and
evaluated either as a sole source of dietary
protein or as a supplement to wheat flour[1]

	PER		
		Supplement to wheat flour	
Enzyme used to prepare FPC	Sole source of protein	2% protein	4% protein
	% of casein	% of casein	
Pancreatin	82	95	94
Alcalase	75	92	91
Autolysis	82	99	95

[1]Source: Knobl et al.[29]

[2]Diets contained 10 percent protein of which
either FPC or casein supplied 2 or 4 percent
and the remaining 8 or 6 percent was supplied
by wheat flour.

that for casein, FPC prepared by tertiary
butanol-extraction of whole menhaden had a PER
that was 104 percent of that for casein and
FPC prepared by isopropyl alcohol-extraction
of herring offal had a PER of 110 percent of
that for casein. Although the apparent protein digestibility for all FPCs was similar,
the availability of lysine and methionine was
found to be lower in the sample produced by
ethylene dichloride-extraction. In further
studies[31] it was found that FPC prepared from
ocean perch (whole fish, fillets or gurry) by
extraction with isopropyl alcohol was superior
to FPC prepared from the same batch of fish by
extraction with ethylene dichloride. Samples
produced by ethylene dichloride-extraction
were not toxic although they did contain high
levels of organic chloride. They also contained less lysine and methionine than those
produced with isopropyl alcohol. It was concluded that the process used can markedly influence the nutritional value of FPC.

Additional studies confirmed that ethylene
dichloride-extraction can reduce the total
amount and the availability of certain amino
acids.[32] Histidine and cystine were markedly
reduced in FPC produced by ethylene dichloride-extraction of freeze-dried cod fillets
for 16 hours. Of more importance, however,
the availability of amino acids as measured
by enzyme hydrolysis was markedly reduced in
FPC produced by ethylene dichloride. Extraction with either isopropyl alcohol or ethanol
had a minimum effect on the apparent availability of the amino acids. The destruction
of cystine by ethylene dichloride was found to
be pH dependent and occurred most readily
under slightly alkaline conditions. The evidence suggested that sulfhydryl groups of protein can be alkylated by ethylene dichloride
to produce thio-ether linkages with a resultant decrease in nutritional value.

Subsequently, it was shown that ethylene
dichloride can react with trimethylamine in
fish to yield chlorocholine chloride (CCC),
which is toxic and has an LD 50 of about 500
mg/kg of body weight. Animals fed ethylene
dichloride-extracted cod fillets at high levels had a high mortality rate. The amount of
CCC in ethylene dichloride-extracted fish,
however, was concluded to be insufficient to
cause death in rats, suggesting that other
toxic substances may have been present.[33]
Further work confirmed that cod fillets extracted for 24 hours with ethylene dichloride
and incorporated into diets at a level of 50
percent protein were toxic to the growing
rat. The toxicity did not appear explanable
on the basis of CCC content. Part of the
toxic material in the ethylene dichloride extracted fillets could be removed by methanol
extraction.[34]

Ershoff and Rucker[35] showed that the nu-
trient value of ethylene dichloride-extracted
cod fillets was dependent upon the temperature and length of time at which extraction
occurred. For example, rats responded normally when fed diets containing FPC that was
extracted at 65° C or 40° C for 24 hours or
at a temperature of 80° C for 6 or 3 hours,
and which was dried under vacuum without
steaming. In contrast, FPC was highly toxic
when prepared under similar conditions except
that it was extracted for 24 hours at a
temperature of 83° C and evaporated solvent
was not replaced during the last 6 hours of
extraction.

Although some of the above studies were
conducted with FPC prepared by prolonged
extraction in the laboratory, a recent study
showed that commercially prepared ethylene
dichloride-extracted FPC has a low nutritive
quality.[23] As shown in Table 10, FPC prepared by isopropyl alcohol extraction was

Table 10. Nutritive value of FPC as affected
by the method of processing[1]

Protein Source	Weight Gain g/day	PER % of casein
Casein	3.75	100
FPC:		
IPA extracted	5.41	118
EDC extracted	2.90	89
EDC & EtOH extracted	3.51	98
EDC & water extracted	3.81	102
EDC extracted plus dried EtOH extract	2.72	86
EDC & EtOH extracted plus dried EtOH extract	3.30	98

----

[1]Source: Makdani et al.[23]

higher in quality than casein, while ethylene
dichloride-extracted FPC was lower. Further
extraction of the ethylene dichloride-pre-
pared FPC with either ethanol or water raised
the protein quality to a level comparable to
that of casein. When the ethanol extract was
added back to the original ethylene dichloride-extracted FPC there was only a slight
depression in PER. When the ethanol extract
was added back to the FPC that had been extracted with both ethylene dichloride and
ethanol, there was no effect on nutritive
quality suggesting a beneficial effect from
ethanol refluxing other than solely removing
the substances soluble in ethanol. Although
these studies indicated that factors were
present that depressed the nutritive quality
of ethylene dichloride-FPC, the presence of
specific toxic factors and causative agents
could not be demonstrated. Isopropyl alcohol-
extracted FPC was higher in quality than
ethylene dichloride-extracted material and
further processing of the ethylene dichloride-
extracted FPC did not negate this nutritional
inferiority. These studies indicate that
alcohol washing of ethylene dichloride-
extracted FPC may increase nutritional quality
to a level comparable to that of casein. The
U. S. FDA regulations specify that ethylene
dichloride extraction will be followed by
isopropyl alcohol extraction. More recent
work, however, showed that the nutritional
quality of FPC prepared by ethylene dichloride
and isopropyl alcohol extraction was significantly poorer than that of either casein or
isopropyl alcohol extracted FPC[36]
(Frysztacki and Rasmussen, Unpublished).

Utilization of FPC when fed to malnourished
animals. With a few exceptions, studies with
normal animals have shown that the quality of
protein in FPC is high and comparable to

casein. Questions have been raised, however,
regarding the adequacy of fish protein when
fed to malnourished animals and humans. One
of the first studies with malnourished animals
was reported by Deuel et al.[37] The fish protein used in the study was prepared from the
edible muscle of mackerel by isoelectric precipitation followed by purification by means
of organic solvent extraction. Adult male
rats were placed on a low protein diet for a
period of 95 days. Thereafter, one group was
fed a diet containing 9 percent casein, while
a second group was fed a diet containing 9
percent mackerel protein. The results showed
that the extracted mackerel-protein was
superior to casein-protein in respect to
weight gain and stimulation of hemoglobin regeneration and that the two proteins were
equally effective in causing a regeneration
of plasma protein.

On the other hand, Barnes et al.[18] reported
that FPC was not as effective as casein in
rehabilitating malnourished baby pigs. With
normal weanling rats, the PERs of casein, soybean, cottonseed and FPC were similar. When
fed to malnourished baby pigs, however, casein
was definitely superior to the other proteins
in increasing the weight gain and in stimulating the regeneration of serum proteins. Thus,
this study indicated that the proteins in
casein and FPC (prepared in Quintero, Chile)
were similar in quality when fed to normal
weanling rats. When fed to malnourished baby
pigs, however, casein was superior to FPC in
increasing weight gain and in regenerating
serum proteins.

These studies were continued by Pond et
al.[38] who found somewhat different results.
In these studies the quality of FPC prepared
by isopropyl alcohol-extraction and of

isolated soy protein were compared to casein
when fed to malnourished baby pigs. As shown
in Table 11, the weight gains of protein-
depleted pigs fed FPC protein were at least
equal to those fed casein and were superior to
those fed isolated soy protein. Table 12
shows that the serum protein levels of protein
deficient pigs repleted for 6 weeks with FPC
protein were similar to those of animals fed
casein and were superior to those fed isolated
soy protein. Pond et al. concluded that the
FPC used in their studies was equal to casein
as a sole source protein for young animals
during repletion from protein-calorie malnutrition but that isolated soy protein was inferior to both FPC and casein in promoting
growth, feed intake and regeneration of serum
proteins. The difference in results obtained
by Barnes et al.[18] and by Pond et al.[38] may be
attributed to the different preparations of
FPC used.

The relative utilization of protein from
casein and FPC by malnourished weanling rats
was reported by Stillings and Hammerle.[39]
Rats that had been fed a protein depletion
diet for 8 weeks were repleted with diets containing either 10 or 20 percent protein from
either FPC prepared by isopropyl alcohol extraction or casein. As shown in Figure 1, the
growth response by animals repleted with 10
percent FPC protein was slightly greater than
those repleted with 10 percent casein protein. When both protein sources were included
in diets at a 20 percent level, the growth
response was similar. Figure 2 shows that the
regeneration of serum protein was similar but
that the regeneration by FPC protein was
slightly superior to that by casein protein.

The effect of protein repletion of protein-
depleted rats with diets containing 10 percent
protein from skim milk powder, peanut flour,
or FPC was also studied by Hariharan et al.[40]

Table 11. Weight gain and feed consumption of
protein deficient pi s during repletion on
casein, isolated soy protein (ISP), and fish
protein concentrate (FPC)[1]

	Control diet (25% casein)	Repletion diet (16% protein source)			
		Casein	FPC-A[2]	FPC-B[3]	ISP
No. of pigs	8	6	7	5	8
Average daily gain, kg.	0.42	0.30	0.31	0.37	0.22
Average daily feed, kg.	0.86	0.54	0.72	0.78	0.52
Gain/feed	0.49	0.56	0.43	0.47	0.42

[1]Source: Pond[38]
[2]NMFS-FPC
[3]Astra-protanimal

Table 12. Serum protein levels in protein-
deficient pigs before and after repletion with
casein, isolated soy, and FPC[1]

	Control	Casein	ISP	FPC-A[2]	FPC-B[3]
End of depletion					
Total protein	6.2		5.0		
Albumin	3.8		2.5		
Repleted 3 weeks					
Total protein	4.7	4.7	4.9	4.7	5.2
Albumin	3.9	3.3	2.8	3.4	3.0
Repleted 6 weeks					
Total protein	6.0	6.1	4.7	5.7	5.9
Albumin	3.8	3.6	3.4	3.8	3.7

----

[1]Source: Pond[38]
[2]NMFS-FPC
[3]Astra-protanimal

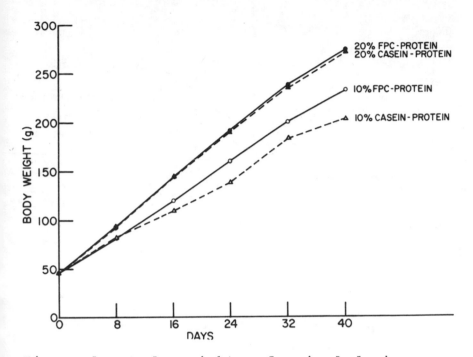

Figure 1. Body weights of animal during protein-repletion with either FPC or casein.[1]

----

[1]Source: Stillings and Hammerle.[39]

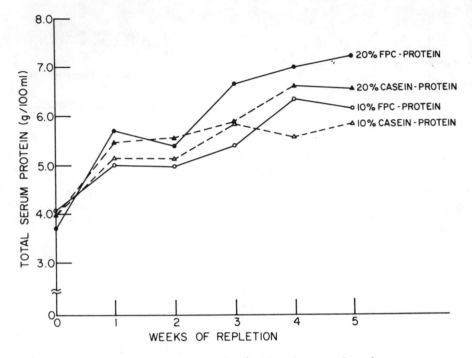

Figure 2.   Season Protein Values during
protein-repletion with either FPC or casein.[1]

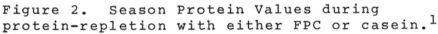

[1]Source: Stillings and Hammerle.[39]

The results showed that the rate of regeneration of serum proteins was similar for diets
containing skim milk and FPC but was definitely slower for diets containing peanut flour.
Likewise, FPC and skim milk were equally
effective in lowering the ratio in serum of
nonessential/essential amino acids and in increasing body weight gains of protein-depleted
rats. Both skim milk powder and FPC were
significantly superior to peanut flour in rehabilitating malnourished rats. A further
study showed, however, that a protein food
based on a blend (2:1:1) of peanut flour,
Bengalgram four, and FPC was as effective as
skim milk powder in meeting the protein requirements of protein-depleted animals when
diets contained 20 percent protein.[41]
    The overall results of these studies indi-
cate that FPC, when properly processed and
when little or no damage occurs to the protein during processing is equally effective
as casein in rehabilitating malnourished
animals. The reason for the inferiority of
the FPC studies by Barnes et al.[18] is not
clear. Studies reported by others have indicated that FPC prepared in Quintero, Chile
is high in quality and should be as effective
as milk protein in stimulating weight gains
and regenerating serum protein in malnourished
animals.

Supplementation of other proteins. As is well
known, FPC is intended to be used to supplement and enhance the quality of dietary protein rather than as a sole source of dietary
protein. Numerous studies have been reported
in which FPC was evaluated as a supplement to
other proteins. Again it is not feasible to
review each study in detail. We can, however,
attempt to draw a few general conclusions from
the information available in the literature.
    The addition of FPC to proteins that are

lower in quality will, of course, produce an
increase in overall protein quality. FPC is
particularly effective as a supplement to
rice, wheat, and corn. For example, the
addition of about 3.0 to 3.5 percent FPC to
either rice, wheat, or corn has been found to
increase the PER by 35, 100 and 300 percent,
respectively.[3] Sure[42,43] found that the addition of 1, 3, and 5 percent FPC to diets containing corn, wheat, rice, rye, grain sorghum,
and millet increased growth and PER, and the
greatest responses were obtained when FPC was
added to sorghum, millet, and corn. Several
other studies have been reported that showed
the enhancement of protein quality through the
addition of FPC to proteins of vegetable
origin[8,24,44,45] or to food mixtures.[46-51]

Few studies, however, have been designed to
determine the optimum level of FPC supplementation. Bressani[52] concluded that a minimum
of 3 percent FPC added to a diet based on
lime-treated corn produced the maximum PER,
although 8 percent was needed to produce maximum weight gains by rats.

Stillings et al.[25] used diets that contained 10 percent protein and reported that 6
percent FPC added to diets containing wheat
flour produced maximum weight gains, PER and
NPU. A similar optimum level was found when
FPC was added to semolina and processed into
pasta.[26]

Figure 3 shows that maximum weight gains of
rats were obtained when 10 percent of the
flour in bread was replaced by FPC and the
bread was added to diets at an 80 percent
level. Although 10 percent of the flour was
replaced by FPC, the diet contained only about
7 percent FPC since diets contained 80 percent
bread of which about 90 percent was the flour-
FPC mixture.[25]

The optimum level of FPC supplementation
will depend on several factors, especially the

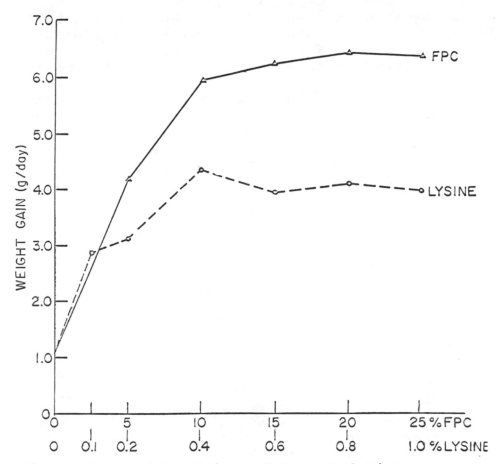

Figure 3.   Weight Gains of Rats Fed Diets
Containing 80 percent Bread Supplemented with
Varying Amounts of Either FPC or Lysine.[1]

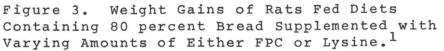

[1]Source: Stillings.[25]

combination and amounts of other proteins in
the diets. In general, however, the addition
of not more than 6 to 8 percent FPC to foods
containing protein mainly of vegetable origin
appears justified.

Some might argue that this level is in excess of the amount needed to meet amino acid
requirements. For example, based on a computer study of the amino acids supplied by diets
containing vegetable protein, it was concluded
that more than 3 percent FPC would rarely be
needed to meet 200 percent of the FAO reference amino acid pattern.[53] This assumes, however, that the total diet will be supplemented
with FPC, rather than individual food items,
and it does not account for differences in
amino acid availability or processing losses.

The combination of FPC with other protein
supplements and synthetic amino acids should
also be considered. It may be more effective
and economical to combine small amounts of FPC
with other supplements, such as oilseed proteins and lysine, rather than using only one
supplement. For example, in Figure 3, it is
evident that a greater response was obtained
by adding FPC to bread than by adding lysine.
Jansen,[54] however, showed that a combination
of 6 percent FPC and 0.25 percent lysine produced a greater response in PER when added to
bread than when only 6 percent FPC was added.
When either FPC or lysine were added separately to wheat flour, Hegsted[55] reported that the
cost per unit of utilizable protein was less
for FPC than for lysine.

Brief mention should be made to losses in
protein quality during processing of foods.
Adrian and Frange[56] found that during the baking of biscuits the PER of those enriched with
peanut flour declined 30 percent, those with
FPC declined 40 percent and those with skim
milk powder declined 100 percent. Others have
found somewhat different results. No loss in

protein quality was noted during the baking of
crackers supplemented with FPC.[57]   During processing of U. S.-type bread supplemented with
FPC, a 10 to 15 percent loss in protein quality was found.[25] With small loaves of bread,
however, Chilean investigators found a considerably larger loss during processing, presumably because of the higher proportion of
crust.[8] Processing of pasta supplemented with
FPC has been shown to have little effect on
protein quality.[8,26] Additional data on processing losses and on comparison with other
protein supplements are reported in a subsequent paper by Sidwell.

   From the data available, it appears that a
10 to 20 percent loss in protein quality can
be expected during processing of baked products. For pasta-type products the loss should
be less than 10 percent.

Toxicological studies. In contrast to the
voluminous reports on the nutritional quality
of FPC and on its use in foods, relatively few
studies on the wholesomeness and toxicological
safety of FPC have been published. A summary
of these studies is shown in Table 13. One of
the first was conducted by Allison et al.[58]
who investigated the safety of deodorized and
nondeodorized FPC prepared in Quintero, Chile.
The FPC was prepared from dried hake
(Merluccius gayi) by solvent extraction with
heptane and ethanol. The FPC was incorporated
into diets at levels ranging from 0 to 25 percent in 5 percent increments and the diets
were fed to male and female weanling rats for
periods ranging up to 12 months. Periodically, during the 12 months, animals were selected from each group, autopsied, and organs were
examined histopathologically. Over the entire
period, there was no evidence of any effect of
the FPC on blood cytology, body and organ
weights, and histopathology of tissues and

Table 13.   Summary of Toxicological Studies on
FPC

Investigator	Species of fish	Solvent used in process	Method
Allison et al.[58]	Hake	Heptane, ethanol	1 generation rats
Yanez et al.[8]	Hake	Hexane, ethanol	3 generations rats
Friedman et al.[59]	Hake	IPA	Highly concentrated fractions fed the rats
Newberne[63,64]	Hake	IPA	5 generations rats and mice
Stillings (unpublished)	Menhaden	IPA	1 generation rats
Schendel & Johnson[60]	-	Ethylene dichloride	4 generations rats
Hallgren[27]	Herring	IPA	3 generations rats
Jaffe[61]	Sardine meal	-	2 generations rats
	-	Ethylene dichloride	
Dreosti[62]	Fish meal extraction		2 generations rats

organs, and there was no other evidence of any
toxicity.

Yanez et al.[8] also reported a study in
which the toxicological safety of Quintero-FPC
was evaluated. The sample used was prepared
by extraction of hake with hexane and ethanol
and was incorporated into diets at a level of
30 percent. Diets were fed to rats for three
generations with each generation consisting of
three male and three female rats that received the FPC diet from weaning. Growth of
the rats was comparable to that shown by a
similar group of animals that received a
commercial rat diet. No pathological signs of
toxicity were evident, no abnormalities were
recorded in the microscopic postmortem examination, and in summary, the study revealed no
evidence of toxicity from the FPC.

A new approach to the evaluation of the
toxicological safety of foods was reported by
Friedman et al.[59] The approach consisted of
preparing extracts of isopropyl alcohol-extracted FPC and studying the toxicity of the
extracts. The FPC was extracted with solvents
of increasing polarity beginning with hexane
followed by chloroform then by ethanol and
finally by water. Each extraction was expected to concentrate substances of similar
solubility properties. The study was designed
so that the extracts could be fed at a level
equivalent to 10 times that obtainable by
feeding 50 percent of the diet as FPC. In
this study the original FPC sample, the extracts and the residue remaining after extraction were each included in diets at a level of
18 percent and were compared to a control diet
containing 18 percent casein. Diets were fed
to mice and rats for a period of four weeks
followed by exhaustive evaluation of tissues,
blood, excreta, etc. All perameters measured
failed to demonstrate any significant difference between test and control animals, and in

summary, the study failed to uncover any toxic
principles in FPC.

The studies conducted by Friedman et. al.[59]
using his new approach to toxicological safety
were continued using the conventional approach
to toxicological safety were continued using
the conventional approach (used in most
toxicological studies.[63,64] FPC prepared by
isopropyl alcohol extraction by the U. S.
National Marine Fisheries Service was included
in diets at a level of 25 percent and fed to
rats and mice over 5 generations. Control
groups were fed a diet containing casein or a
commercial rat chow. In a very exhaustive
evaluation of the results, no evidence of any
toxicity from the FPC diet was observed. Of
somewhat academic interest, however, it was
observed that after a continuous period of
time on a diet in which menadione was provided
to meet vitamin K requirements, many of the
rats fed FPC developed wide-spread hemorrhages characteristic of vitamin K deficiency.
It turned out that this was indeed a deficiency of vitamin K and that menadione could not
be utilized as a source of vitamin K when the
animals were fed FPC. When vitamin K was substituted for menadione, all animals fed FPC
responded normally and no hemorrhages were
observed.

A 12-week feeding study was conducted by
Stillings (unpublished) on FPC prepared by
isopropyl alcohol extraction of menhaden
(Brevoortia tyrannus). Diets contained 10,
20, and 40 percent protein from FPC, and control diets contained similar amounts of protein from casein. Seven male and seven
female weanling rats were assigned to each
diet. No significant differences were detected between experimental and control animals
in respect to growth, organ weights, and
histopathology of tissues and organs.

In addition to the previous reports on the
nutritional quality and possible toxicologi-

cal effects of extracting fish for long
periods of time with ethylene dichloride,
Schendel and Johnson[60] studied the effect of
feeding FPC prepared by ethylene dichloride
extraction to rats over several generations.
The FPC was prepared by the VioBin Corporation and was incorporated into diets at a
level of 25 percent. Diets containing the
FPC were superior to those containing casein
in respect to reproduction and general performance of rats through 3 matings of the
first generation, 7 matings of the second
generation, and 7 matings of the third generation. Histological examination of 12 organs
and tissues from animals of the first, second
and third generations showed no differences
between animals receiving FPC and those receiving casein. In this study, however, problems were encountered with animals on both the
control and the FPC diets, with respect to
poor reproductive performance. All animals
and especially animals consuming the casein
diet showed poorer reproductive performance
from the first to the third generation. Thus,
although there was no indication of toxicity
in rats consuming the FPC diet, the reproductive results of both the control and test
diets are in doubt because of an apparent
stress, of unknown origin, that affected all
animals.

Hallgren[27] reported the results of a reproductive study of rats fed FPC prepared by
Astra Company, presumably by isopropyl alcohol
extraction of cooked and pressed herring. The
fish protein was incorporated into diets at a
level of 20 percent and was compared to a diet
containing 20 percent casein. Rats were
raised for three generations on diets containing only fish protein as the source of protein
or, in the case of the control groups, with
protein from casein as the only protein
source. No differences were found between the

groups consuming fish protein and those
consuming casein in respect to the number of
pregnant females, number of litters born,
number of rats per litter, weight of young
when weaned, or the number of dead ones per
litter. Again, in these studies there was no
evidence of toxicity.

Jaffe[61] also reported on the results of a
toxicological study using Venezuelan whole
sardine meal or defatted and deodorized FPC
from the U. S. Two generations of pregnant
rats were fed a diet containing 80 percent
corn and 20 percent FPC while the control diet
was fed a Purina diet. Reproduction and
growth of litters were good and histological
examination of organs revealed no toxic effect
of the FPC. Presumably, the FPC from the
U. S. was prepared by the VioBin Company.

Dreosti[62] reported that no evidence of toxicity was found in studies on growth, breeding
performances, and histopathology of rats receiving a diet containing 28 percent FPC prepared in South Africa for 199-203 days.
Growth and histopathological studies on the
second generation of rats and raised on the
same diets for 87 days, also showed no evidence suggestive of toxicity.

In summary, several types of FPC prepared
from different species of fish have been
examined for evidence of toxicological properties. In all cases, no evidence of toxicity
has been revealed and the studies have indicated that the FPCs examined were indeed safe.

Summary and Conclusion

From the evidence available it is clear that
the balance of amino acids in fish protein and
its quality can be preserved during processing
into FPC. With few exceptions, FPCs prepared
by solvent extraction have been shown to be
high in protein with a quality at least equivalent to that of casein when evaluated by

laboratory animals. FPC prepared by extraction with ethylene dichloride has in some
cases been shown to be slightly lower in quality. When evaluated in protein-depleted animals, FPC has usually been shown to be as
effective as casein in stimulating weight
gains and regeneration of serum proteins.
Especially when prepared from whole fish, FPC
is also an excellent source of many essential
minerals. Numerous studies have amply demonstrated that FPC at levels up to 6 to 8 percent can effectively enhance the quantity and
quality of protein in foods that contain protein of vegetable origin. For nutritional
purposes, it may be more effective and economical to combine FPC with other supplements.
Several toxicological studies have shown that
FPC prepared by several processes from several species of fish is indeed safe and wholesome.
   FPC can be an effective protein supplement
and a significant source of dietary protein
providing other aspects related to relative
cost and organoleptic characteristics are also satisfactory.

References

1. Finch, Roland. 1970. Fish protein for
human foods. CRC Critical Reviews in Food
Technol. 2: 519.

2. Library of Congress. 1970. Fish protein
concentrate--a comprehensive bibliography.
Compiled by the Special Bibliographies Sec-
tion, Science and Technology Division for the
National Center for Fish Protein Concentrate,
Bureau of Commercial Fisheries, Fish and
Wildlife Service, U. S. Department of the
Interior.

3. Sidwell, V. C., Stillings, B. R. and
Knobl, G. M., Jr. 1970. The fish protein
concentrate story. 10. U. S. Bureau of
Commercial Fisheries FPC's: Nutritional quality and use in foods. Food Technol. 24: 40.

4. Power, H. E. 1964. Characteristics and
nutritional value of various fish protein concentrate. J. Fish. Res. Bd. Canada 21: 1489.

5. Medwadowski, Barbara, Haley, Alleah,
Van Der Veen, John and Olcott, H. S. 1971.
Effect of storage on lipids of fish protein
concentrate. J. Amer. Oil Chem. Soc. 48: 782.

6. Food and Agriculture Organization of the
United Nations, 1965. Protein requirements.
FAO Nutrition Meetings Report Series No. 37.

7. Miller, D. S. 1956. The nutritive value
of fish proteins. J. Sci. Food Agric. 7: 337.

8. Yanez, Enrique, Barja, Ita, Monckeberg,
Fernando, Maccioni, Alejandro, and Donoso,
Gonzalo. 1967. The fish protein concentrate
story. 6. Quintero fish protein concentrate:
Protein quality and use in foods. Food
Technol. 21: 1604.

9. Stillings, B. R., Hammerle, O. A. and
Snyder, D. G. 1969. Sequence of limiting
amino acids in fish protein concentrate produced by isopropyl alcohol extraction of red
hake (Urophycis chuss). J. Nutr. 97: 70.

10. Makdani, D. D., Huber, J. T. and Bergen,
W. G. 1970. Effect of histidine and methionine supplementation on the nutritional quality of commercially prepared fish protein
concentrate in rat diets. J. Nutr. 101: 367.

11.   Pretorius, P. J., and Wehmeyer, A. S.
1964. An assessment of nutritive value of
fish flour in the treatment of convalescent
Kwashiorkor patients. Amer. J. Clin. Nutr.
14: 147.

12.   Spencer, Herta, Samachson, Joseph,
Fowler, Josephine, and Kulka, Mary J. 1971.
Availability in man of protein and minerals
from fish protein concentrate. Amer. J. Clin.
Nutr. 24: 311.

13.   Fritz, James C., Pla, Gwendolyn W.,
Roberts, Talmadge, Boehne, J. William, and
Hove, Edwin L. 1970. Biological availability
in animals of iron from common dietary
sources. J. Agr. Food Chem. 18: 647.

14.   Stillings, B. R., Lagally, Herta R., and
Zook, Elizabeth. 1971. Further studies on
the availability of the fluoride in fish protein concentrate. Fed. Proc. 30.

15.   Wiechers, S. G. 1965. Vitamins in re-
fined and unrefined fish flour. 19th Annual
Report, Fishing Industry Research Institute,
Rondebosch, South Africa.

16.   Beveridge, J. M. 1947. The nutritive
value of marine products. XVI. The biological
value of fish flesh proteins. J. Fish. Res.
Bd. Can. 7: 35.

17.   Dubrow, D. L., Pariser, E. R., Brown,
N. L., and Miller, H., Jr. 1970. FPC's
quality virtually the same as its raw material's quality. Com. Fish. Rev. 32: 25.

18.   Barnes, R. H., Pond, W. G., Kwong, E.,
and Reid, I. 1966. Effect of severe protein-
calorie malnutrition in the baby pig upon
relative utilization of different dietary

proteins. J. Nutr. 89: 355.

19. Howe, E. E., Gilfillan, E. W., and Milner, Max. 1965. Amino acid supplementation of protein concentrates as related to the world protein supply. Amer. J. Clin. Nutr. 16: 321.

20. Moorjani, M. N., Nair, R. Balakrishman, and Lahiry, N. L. 1968. Quality of fish protein concentrate prepared by direct extraction of fish with various solvents. Food Technol. 22: 1557.

21. Sen, D. P., Rao, T. S. Sayanarayana, Kadkol, S. B., Krishnaswamy, M. A., Rao, S. Venkata, and Lahiry, N. L. 1969. Fish protein concentrate from Bombay-duck (Harpoden nehereus) fish: Effect of processing variables on the nutritional and organoleptic qualities. Food Technol. 23: 683.

22. Sidhu, G. S., Montgomery, W. A., Holloway, Gwenda L., Johnson, A. R., and Walker, D. M. 1970. . Biochemical composition and nutritive value of krill (Euphausia superba Dana). J. Sci. Food Agric. 21: 293.

23. Makdani, Dhirajlal, Bergen, Werner G., Michelsen, O., and Huber, John T. 1971. Factors influencing the nutritive value of 1, 2-dichloroethane-extracted fish protein concentrate in rat diets. Amer. J. Clin. Nutr. 24: 1384.

24. Shaikh, Iftikhar Ali, Arshad, M., Hug, M. Y. Ikram-Ul, and Ali, S. Magsood. 1967. Improvement of protein value of cottonseed protein isolate with fish flour and skim milk powder. Pakistan J. of Scientific and Industrial Research 10: 86.

25. Stillings, B. R., Sidwell, V. D., and
Hammerle, O. A. 1971. Nutritive quality of
wheat flour and bread supplemented with
either fish protein concentrate or lysine.
Cereal Chem. 48: 292.

26. Stillings, B. R., Sidwell, V. D., and
Hammerle, O. A. 1969. Supplemental value of
fish protein concentrate: The nutritional
quality of pasta made from wheat protein concentrate and semolina. The 54th Annual Meeting of the American Association of Cereal
Chemists, Chicago, Illinois, April 27-May 1,

27. Hallgren, B. 1966. Nutritional value
and uses of fish protein concentrates.
Naringsforskning 10: 37.

28. De, H. N., Mellah, Yasin, and Islam,
Aminul. 1965. Fish flour: Its biochemical
and nutritional studies. Part III. Protein
efficiency ratio values of some fish protein
concentrate (FPC) or fish flour and fish
vermicelli, and influence of decomposition of
fish on the above values. Scientific
Researchers 2: 27.

29. Knobl, George M., Jr., Stillings,
Bruce R., Fox, William E., and Hale,
Malcolm B. 1971. Fish protein concentrates.
Com. Fish. Rev. 33: 54.

30. Morrison, A. B., and McLaughlan, J. M.
1961. Variability in nutritional value of
fish flour. Can. J. Biochem. Physiol. 39:
511.

31. Morrison, A. B., Sabry, Z. I., and
Middleton, E. J. 1962. Factors influencing
the nutritional value of fish flour. I.
Effects of extraction with chloroform or ethylene dichloride. J. Nutr. 77: 97.

32. Morrison, A. B., and Munro, I. C. 1965.
Factors influencing the nutritional value of
fish flour. IV. Reaction between 1, 2- dichloroethane and protein. Can. J. Biochem.
43: 33.

33. Munro, I. C., and Morrison, A. B. 1967.
Factors influencing the nutritional value of
fish flour. V. Chlorocholine chloride, a
toxic material in samples extracted with 1, 2-
dichloroethane. Can. J. Biochem. 45: 1049.

34. Munro, I. C., and Morrison, A. B. 1967.
Toxicity of 1, 2-dichloroethane-extracted fish
protein concentrate. Can. J. Biochem. 45:
1779.

35. Ershoff, B. H., and Rucker, P. G. 1969.
Nutritive value of 1, 2-dichloroethane-
extracted fish protein concentrate. J. Food
Sci. 34: 355.

36. Frysztacki, C. A., and Rasmussen, A. I.
1972. Comparative nutritional quality of two
fish protein concentrates. Fed. Proc. 31:
696.

37. Deuel, Harry J., Jr., Hrubetz, M. C.,
Johnston, Cornelia H., Winzler, Richard J.,
Geiger, Ernest, and Schnakenberg, G. 1946.
J. Nutr. 31: 175.

38. Pond, Wilson G., Snyder, Wesley, Snook,
Jean Twombly, Walker, Earl F., Jr., McNeill,
Deborah A., and Stillings, Bruce R. 1971.
Relative utilization of casein, fish protein
concentrate and isolated soybean protein for
growth and pancreatic enzyme regeneration of
the protein-calorie malnourished baby pig. J.
Nutr. 101: 1193.

39. Stillings, B. R., and Hammerle, Olivia A.
1969. Relative utilization of the protein of
fish protein concentrate and of casein by
protein-depleted rats. Fed. Proc. 28: 812.

40. Hariharan, K., Desai, B. L. M., Rao, S.
Venkat, Swaminathan, M., and Parpia, H. A. B.
1966. The ratio between free serum non-
essential to essential amino acids in rats
depleted on protein free diet and repleted on
diets containing different proteins. J. Nutr.
& Dietet. 5: 52.

41. Shurpalekar, S. R., Joseph A. A., Lahiry,
N. L., Moorjani, M. N., Swaminathan, M.,
Nataraja, N., Sreenivasan, A., and Subrahmanyan, V. 1962. Relative value of a protein
food containing fish flour, groundnut flour
and bengalgram flour as compared with skim
milk powder in meeting the protein requirements of protein depleted rats. Food Sci. 11:
57.

42. Sure, Barnett. 1957. The addition of
small amounts of defatted fish flour to whole
yellow corn, whole wheat, whole and milled
rye, grain sorghum and millet. J. Nutr. 63:
409.

43. Sure, Barnett. 1957. The addition of
small amounts of defatted fish flour to milled
wheat flour, corn meal and rice. Influence on
growth and protein efficiency. J. Nutr. 61:
547.

44. De, H. N., Islam, Aminul, and Mollah,
Yasin. 1966. Fish flour--its biochemical and
nutritional studies. Part IV. Supplementary
effect of fish protein concentrate (FPC) on
the cereal proteins evaluated by determination
of PER values and measurement of liver protein
nitrogen, non-protein nitrogen and fat.

45. Desai, B. L. M., Hariharan, K., Jayaraj,
A. Paul, Rao, S. Venkat and Swaminathan, M.
1968. Studies on the protein efficiency ratio
of fish flour (from Bombay duck) and a protein
food based on fish, groundnut and bengalgram
flours and their supplementary value to low
protein diets. J. Nutr. & Diet. 5: 45.

46. D, H. N., Khan, S. A., Mullick, N. I. and
Islam, Aminul. 1969. Nutritive value of bengal gram (chick pea). Part 2. Assessment of
the nutritive value of formulated foods based
on bengal gram (chick pea) and fish protein
concentrate and egg powder by determination of
their protein efficiency and calorie efficiency ratio values and liver fat and protein-
nitrogen contents. Scientific Researches 5:
148.

47. Doraiswamy, T. R., Shurpalekar, S. R.,
Moorjani, M. N., Lahiry, N. L., Sankaran, A.
N., Swaminathan, M., Sreenivasan, A., and
Subrahmanyan, V. 1963. The effect of a
supplementary protein food containing fish
flour, groundnut flour and bengal gram flour
and fortified with vitamins on the growth and
nutritional status of children. Indian J.
Pediatrics 30: 266.

48. Shurpalekar, S. R., Moorjani, M. N.,
Lahiry, N. L., Indiramma, K., Swaminathan, M.,
Sreenivasan, A., and Subrahmanyan, V. 1962.
Supplementary value of proteins of fish flour
to those of groundnut flour and the protein
efficiency ratio of a protein food containing
groundnut, bengalgram and fish flours. Food
Sci. 11: 42.

49. Shurpalekar, S. R., Joseph, A. A.,
Lahiry, N. L., Moorjani, M. N., Sankaran, A.
N., Swaminathan, M., Sreenivasan, A., and
Subrahmanyan, V. 1962. Supplementary value

of fish flour and a protein food containing low fat groundnut flour, bengalgram flour and fish flour to poor rice diet. Food Sci. 11: 45.

50. Shurpalekar, S. R., Joseph, A. A., Moorjani, M. N., Lahiry, N. L., Indiramma, K., Swaminathan, M., Sreenivasan, A., and Subrahmanyan, V. 1962. Supplementary value of fish flour fortified with vitamins to poor indian diets based on different cereals and millets. Food Sci. 11: 49.

51. Shurpalekar, S. R., Jayaraj, A. Paul, Moorjani, M. N., Lahiry, N. L., Sankaran, A. N., Swaminathan, M., Sreenivasan, A., and Subrahmanyan, V. 1962. Supplementary value of fish flour and a protein food containing low-fat groundnut flour, bengalgram flour and fish flour to a maize-tapioca diet. Food Sci. 11: 52.

52. Bressani, Richardo. 1962. Enrichment of lime-treated corn flour with deodorized fish flour. In Fish in Nutrition, p. 266. London: Fishing News (Books).

53. Devanney, J. W. III, and Mahnken, G. 1970. Economics of fish protein concentrate. Report No. MITSG 71-3, Massachusetts Institute of Technology.

54. Jansen, G. R. 1969. Total protein value of protein and amino acid supplemented bread. Am. J. Clin. Nutr. 22: 38.

55. Hegsted, D. M. 1968. Amino acid fortification and the protein problem. Amer. J. Clin. Nutr. 21: 688.

56. Adrian, J., and Frangne, R. 1969. Nutritional advantage of biscuits enriched

with pure lysine or various protein additives:
Peanuts, fish, or milk. Ind. Aliment. Agr.
86: 801.

57. Sidwell, V. D., and Stillings, B. R.   In
press. Crackers, fortified with fish protein
concentrate: Nutrition quality, sensory and
physical characteristics. J. Amer. Diet.
Assoc.

58. Allison, J. B., Brush, M. K.,
Wannemacher, R. W. Jr., and McCoy, J. R.
1957. The determination of the nutritive
value and safety of fish flour. WHO/FAO/
UNICEF Nutrition Panel R.8/Add. 5.

59. Friedman, Leo, Glaser, Otto G., Brown,
Norman L., and Pariser, E. R. 1971. The
wholesomeness of fish protein concentrate: A
new approach to the evaluation of food safety.
Toxicol. & Appl. Pharmacol. 18: 239.

60. Schendel, Harold E., and Johnson, B.
Connor. 1962. Performance of rats fed fish
flour or casein as the sole source of dietary
protein through four generations. J. Nutr.
78: 457.

61. Jaffe, W. G. 1961. New studies of the
nutritive value of fish flour and its supplementary effect on wheat flour and bread, Arch.
venezol. Nutr. 11: 191.

62. Dreosti, G. M. 1962. Technological
developments in South Africa. In Fish in
Nutrition, p. 425. London: Fishing News
(Books).

63. Newberne, P. M., Glaser, O., and
Friedman, L. E. 1973. Biologic adequacy of
fish protein concentrate in five generations
of mice. Nutrition Reports Internal 7: 81.

64.   Newberne, P. M., Glaser, O., Friedman,
L. E., and Stillings, B. R.   1973.   Safety
evaluation of fish protein concentrate over
five generations of rats.   Toxicology and
Appl. Pharmacology 24: 133.

XII
EVALUATION OF FISH PROTEIN CONCENTRATE FOR
INFANT AND CHILD FEEDING

Nevin S. Scrimshaw
Department of Nutrition and Food Science,
Massachusetts Institute of Technology,
Cambridge, Massachusetts

There have been a considerable number of reports on successful feeding of various types
of fish protein concentrate (FPC) to infants
and young children. Unfortunately, the quality of the FPC has varied widely and the
studies have often been done without adequate
controls. In some cases, the source of the
FPC has not even been specified. This report
will attempt to evaluate each study and develop general conclusions regarding the value and
safety of properly processed and handled FPC
for child feeding.

   The first FPC to become widely available
for clinical trials was produced by the VioBin
process. Because of variations in processing
and differences in the length and conditions
of storage, this product was by no means uniform. Different batches at different places
and times gave inconsistent experimental and
clinical results. FPC products produced in
Morocco, India, Chile, and South Africa also
varied greatly in quality. The best standardized material for clinical testing was produced by the former Bureau of Commercial
Fisheries (BCF) of the U. S. Department of the
Interior. More recently, FPC has been available from the Astra process in Sweden, and the
Verrando process in Peru. All of these have
been solvent-extracted products. A non-
deodorized FPC from Norway has been fed to
Bangladesh refugees. In addition, an FPC

produced by microbiological digestion of fish
slurry in Uruguay has been fed to young children.

FPC Added to Predominantly Cereal Diets for Children

In the earliest studies and some later ones,
FPC was added to cereals. Gomez et al.[1] in
1958 fed undernourished children 15 g daily of
VioBin-FPC added to various foods such as
tortillas, beans, and soup. Recovery of the
children was reported to be good, but no controls or comparative data were presented. In
1959, Gruttner and Schafer[2] fed a protein
powder containing 97 percent protein prepared
from the muscle of Baltic cod to 92 premature
infants. When 1 percent of this material was
added to human milk instead of the 1 percent
casein usually used, the results were equally
satisfactory.

The Proceedings of the International Conference on Progress in Meeting Protein Needs
of Infants and Preschool Children, held in
Washington, D. C. in August, 1960,[3] contained
four papers referring to the clinical testing
of various types of FPC. Silvestre Frenk[4] fed
two different sources of deodorized, defatted
fish flour, in addition to beans and tortillas, to supply a total of 4 to 6.5 g protein
per day to six children with marasmic kwashiorkor. The net protein utilization of the
diet supplemented with fish flour was stated
to be significantly better and much less
variable than in the control group and in a
previous series in which corn and beans alone
were fed. Protein absorption as percent of
intake varied from 24.5 percent to 71.9 percent, but this is not unusual for severely
malnourished children even when fed milk.

John Hansen[5] compared nitrogen balance in
children on diets of 60 percent maize and 30
percent pea flour with and without

isonitrogenous supplements of either dried
skim milk (DSM) or fish flour. The protein
content was 18 and 20 percent, respectively,
and the protein intakes varied from 1.9 to
2.5 g protein/kg per day. Absorption and retention of nitrogen did not differ significantly, but the results with milk as the sole
source of protein were significantly better
and the maize-pea mixture alone was markedly
inferior.

Diets of maize meal plus other amino acid
or protein supplements were also compared.
The nitrogen retentions in mg/kg/day were:
maize meal, 33 ± 41; maize plus lysine and
tryptophan, 52 ± 52; maize meal plus pea
flour, 58 ± 29; maize meal plus pea flour plus
fish flour, 100 ± 40; maize meal plus pea
flour plus DSM, 110 ± 48; and DSM alone,
120 ± 45. From 11 to 24 children were studied
for each of six diets. There was no significant change in serum albumin concentration in
these children during the short periods on the
experimental diets.

Jean Senecal[6] chose fish flour of unspeci-
fied origin to supplement millet and peanut
flour for the treatment of malnourished children. The data are difficult to interpret because of the variety of dietary combinations
employed, the severity of the clinical malnutrition, and the relatively few individuals
on any single type of treatment. Formulas
containing 24 to 30 g of FPC per liter were
well accepted by 17 out of the 26 children included. Clinical improvement was also satisfactory, but much slower than that observed
when milk or protein hydrolysate was used. In
9 of the 17, clinical recovery was not satisfactory. For 3 of 4 healthy children a mixture containing 70 g of peanut, 20 g of
millet, and 10 g of FPC per liter was acceptable, and weight gain was satisfactory. A
mixture of 30 g peanut, 60 g millet, and 10 g

FPC per liter induced no weight gain during 2
months of feeding in 6 normal children 6 to 16
months of age, who had normal and regularly
rising weight curves in the months preceding
the trial.

All subjects were in positive nitrogen
balance and nitrogen retention ranged from 11
to 35 percent of intake. It is noteworthy
that treatment failure in the millet-peanut-
milk group was 22.5 percent, in the millet-
peanut-fish group, 26 percent, and in the
millet control diet, 70 percent. The authors
concluded that the value of peanut as a protein supplement was clearly demonstrated, but
that no clear advantage could be attained by
further addition of FPC.

DeMaeyer and Vanderborght[7] investigated the
digestibility, biological value, and net protein utilization of whole egg, cow's milk,
human milk, soy milk (Saridele Toffaroma from
Indonesia), fish flour, soybean flour, sesame
flour, cottonseed flour, peanut flour, and
biscuits made of fish, peanut and millet
flours by the nitrogen balance technique in 17
African children 3 to 7 years old. All were
hospitalized for minor parasitic infections,
infectious disease, or mild malnutrition. In
addition, a few children who had acute cases
of kwashiorkor when first admitted were involved in the experiment after satisfactory
recovery. The children were kept on each diet
for five days; the first two were described as
the adjustment period and the final three
days, the balance period.

The fish flour was prepared by OVAPIRU in
Usumbura, Ruanda-Urundi from two fish species,
Limnothrissamoidon and Stolothrissa tangani-
cae, both abundant in Lake Tanganyika. The
six children receiving 25 g of "fish flour"
had an average protein consumption of 16.6 g
per day, representing 4.4 percent of their
daily caloric intake. Absorption was 82.4

percent ± 4.7 percent. The biological value
averaged 82.9 ± 7.57 and the NPU 68.5 ± 8.6.
Reference cow's milk, consumed at 23 g per day
as 6.2 percent of the daily caloric intake,
gave an absorption of 88.4 ± 2.93, with a
biological value of 91.4 ± 4.5 and an NPU of
80.9 ± 5.62. All three values were better
than for any of the vegetable proteins tested
but somewhat less than the corresponding
values for whole egg, cow's milk, or human
milk.

Graham et al.[8] reported in 1962 the feeding
of wheat flour enriched with 10 percent VioBin
-FPC to infants who had reached the convalescent phase of severe protein-calorie malnutrition of either the marasmic or marasmic-
kwashiorkor type, after treatment with modified cow's milk. When wheat flour enriched
with 10 percent VioBin was fed isocalorically
and isonitrogenously in comparison with either
modified cow's milk or a vegetable mixture of
good biological value, serum albumin, hematocrit, and nitrogen balance results were similar. When FPC was used as the sole source of
protein in one infant, the results were
equally satisfactory.

For one infant it was necessary to replace
the cottonseed oil with a fat emulsion because
of large bulky stools and poor nitrogen retention. These same conclusions, with some additional data, are given in the authors' 1963
paper.[9]

In 1962, Thomson and Merry[10] gave, for 1
month, a laboratory-produced deodorized fish
meal made from Clupea pilchardus, not otherwise described, in the form of biscuits to
children 2 to 4 years old, attending five
different maternal and child health centers.
Twenty-one children who received the biscuits
containing 12 to 14 percent FPC, 20 to 24
percent peanut meal, 12 percent millet flour,
and 25 percent sugar with lysine content

standardized at 3.5 percent, as supplements
to their usual home diets, were compared with
13 receiving DSM and with 13 controls. The
protein supplement amounted to 70 g for the
FPC biscuit groups and 80 g for the DSM group
per week. Analysis of variance showed significantly greater weight gain (712 g) for the
FPC group than for the children receiving DSM
(386 g), while the controls gained only 266 g.

In a second trial, these authors gave
boarding school children 6 to 8 years of age a
supplementary FPC biscuit in the morning and
evening, supplying 10 g of protein in addition
to 15 g of protein from DSM. They concluded
that adding the fish biscuit resulted in much
greater than expected weight gain, but the
study included no controls.

In 1963, Doraiswamy and co-workers[11] in
India fed 40 g of a protein food based on a
2:1:1 blend of peanut flour, chick pea, and a
fish flour prepared by the Central Food Technological Research Institute, Mysore, from
sardines and fortified with vitamins A and D,
thiamine, and riboflavin. When 29 boys 6 to
12 years of age, in a local orphanage, were
fed the mixture for 6 months, 80 percent were
said to have gained significantly in height
and weight compared to growth in 17 percent in
a matched control group. In a companion
paper,[12] the same Institute reported that 7
pairs of boys 9 to 10 years of age were fed
this same mixture or their usual rice-based
diet. Their daily nitrogen intakes were 10.42
g and 7.51 g, and their nitrogen retentions
2.68 g and 1.36 g, respectively.

In 1963 a study, Lee et al.[13] fed 24 Korean
children 10 percent VioBin-FPC as a weaning
food for two months, incorporated into wheat
flour noodles. Total serum protein, hemoglobin, hematocrit, and red blood cell count increased, but serum albumin decreased. Hwang[14]
reported in 1963 that 10 percent FPC added to

Korean diets improved nitrogen balance more
than did the addition of 10 percent liver.

A 1964 paper of Pretorius and Wehmeyer[15]
compared the effects of maize meal diets
supplemented approximately isonitrogenously
with VioBin-FPC or FPC from the Fishing Industry Research Institute of South Africa (FIRI)
with DSM for six weeks in a total of 45 convalescent kwashiorkor patients. The diets
provided about 3.5 g protein/kg/day, of which
approximately 2 g came from the supplement.
All three diets were well tolerated and no
significant differences in weight, plasma
protein, plasma amino acid, or nitrogen levels
were noted, although weight gain was less in
the group receiving the FIRI flour. Three-day
balance studies were carried out in the
seventh week after admission on 10 patients
from each group. The differences in absorption and retention of nitrogen, phosphorus,
and magnesium were not significant. The two
FPC groups ingested and retained significantly
more calcium than did the DSM group.

Wikramanayake's 1966 paper[16] describes two
groups of convalescent children fed for four
weeks either a mixed diet with multiple
sources of animal protein or one in which all
of the animal protein was replaced by FPC
cooked in coconut milk with curry powder.
This provided about 20 g of FPC protein with
lunch and dinner. The diets were made iso-
caloric with added rice, bread, and vegetables. All diets were accepted after about a
week, although the mixed animal protein diet
was preferred. Height, weight, plasma protein, and hemoglobin increased comparably on
either diet.

In 1967, Spada et al.[17] fed 39 children
from 2 to 7 years of age a vegetable mixture
containing 3 percent Quintero-FPC for an average of 170 days. Acceptability and weight
gain were good, but no control group was

reported.

Comparative data on both Quintero- and VioBin-FPC for human consumption were provided in 1967 by Yanez et al.,[18] who fed 5 infants 3 to 5 months old with FPC as the sole source of protein in a formula made up of 15 percent FPC, 12 percent butter, 17 percent corn starch, 18 percent sucrose, and 35 percent lactose, supplemented with 3 percent of a vitamin and mineral mixture. The average weight gain of 25 g per day did not differ between the groups fed the two kinds of FPC and was considered satisfactory. Similar results were subsequently reported for 9 additional infants given the Quintero-FPC formula and for 3 who received the VioBin-FPC formula for 30 to 90 days.

Yanez et al.,[19] in 1969, described 12 infants 2 1/2 to 4 1/2 months of age fed a formula providing 340 calories and 31.8 g protein from a mixture of Quintero FPC and sunflower seed meal per 100 ml ad libitum for 11 weeks. Growth results were excellent. A similar mixture was given for 6 months in the form of a mid-morning and mid-afternoon beverage and as a component of lunch to 80 preschool children who consumed breakfast and supper at home. Increases in height and the hemoglobin, hematocrit, and serum albumin values were within normal limits.

Fernando Monckeberg and co-workers of the University of Chile (unpublished data, 1966), fed FPC produced at the Quintero plant in 1963 and 1964 to 21 infants, varying in age from 2 to 6 months, for periods of 3 to 6 months. The diet consisted of fish protein concentrate, sunflower oil, dextrose, and vitamin supplements fed in a liquid formula whose protein concentration was roughly equivalent to that of milk--approximately 3 to 4 percent. Children were brought into the metabolic ward and maintained for approximately three weeks

on a milk/dextrose formula in order to
establish a baseline, and were then changed to
the fish protein concentrate formula. All
were maintained for approximately an additional month on the milk formula at the end of
the FPC feeding period to establish a second
baseline. Milk and FPC formulas were fed on
an ad libitum basis.
      No unusual problems were encountered.
Specifically, no rejection of the FPC formula
was experienced with any of the children, no
digestive upsets were encountered, and, in
fact, children had less of a problem with
diarrhea from the FPC formula than they did
with milk. Weight gains were above the
Chilean norms. Changes in electrophoretic
pattern and radiologically determined bone age
were considered normal. They concluded that
the FPC formula could be fed on a long-term
basis to infants as the sole source of protein
with no adverse reactions when substituted
isonitrogenously for milk. The value of the
formula for children with severe protein-
calorie malnutrition was not tested.
      Spencer et al.,[20] in 1968, found that re-
placing 37 percent of the protein of a good
mixed diet with an FPC protein (produced by
the U. S. Bur. Com. Fish) did not change
nitrogen utilization. They interpreted this
as an indication that the FPC protein was
readily available for absorption.
      Moroccan-produced FPC was fed by Tavill and
Gonik[21] in 1969 for 6 months to 50 healthy
weanlings and to 90 randomly selected infants
from lower socioeconomic groups in Casablanca.
The larger number of infants selected to receive FPC was in anticipation of a higher
drop-out rate, but there were only two drop-
outs, both in the control group. Infants in
the test group received meals that supplied
just over 10 g of FPC, twice daily, in a
neighborhood feeding center. This was the

maximum amount acceptable to the mothers.
The vegetable protein component of the diet
supplied the equivalent of a total of 12.6 g
of reference protein per day, an amount exceeding the estimated protein requirements.
The estimated average additional protein
contribution from food consumed at home was
4.4 g. Mothers were provided with a daily
ration for the control children of 70 g of
half cream and half DSM as part of the regular
nutritional program of the health center. No
statistically significant differences in
weight and height gains or in disease morbid-
ity occurred between the groups.

A 1970 feeding trial by Brinkman et al.[22]
in an orphanage in Trinidad was extended for
9 weeks in 2- to 5-year-old children receiving mixed diets providing an average of 3 g
of protein/kg/day. Half of the total protein
(22.5 g) was provided by either 28 g of
VioBin-FPC to 37 children or 65 g of DSM to
35 children. After the first three days, all
diets were well accepted, well tolerated, and
totally consumed, with no differences in
growth performance or hemoglobin levels between the two groups.

Type B FPC produced in Norway was used on a
large scale among Bangladesh refugees in the
Calcutta area from October to December, 1971,
and subsequently given to thousands of Bangladesh refugees, both children and adults, in
other areas (Cato Aall, personal communication, 1973). Approximately 10 g/day were
added to the diet of rice and vegetables in a
variety of different ways with high acceptability. Nutritional results were said to have
been good, but circumstances did not permit
quantitative observations. In these trials,
the taste and odor of fish proved to be an
advantage.

The well controlled studies at the Institute of Nutrition of Central America and
Panama (INCAP) of FPC as a protein source for

malnourished children are still unpublished
(F. Viteri, personal communication, 1969).
Using 9 children fully recovered from
kwashiorkor, ranging in age from 3 to 6 years,
the INCAP workers found that the amount of
BCF-FPC protein required to maintain nitrogen
equilibrium did not differ from that found for
egg or milk protein, and was less than that
required from good vegetable mixtures. Each
of these protein sources was evaluated at four
intake levels, ranging from 0.5 g/kg to 1.5 g/
kg. Unexpectedly, in view of the above result, the slope of the FPC regression line for
nitrogen retention was slightly less than that
for milk or egg, although greater than for the
Incaparina formulas tested in the same way.
The approximate digestibility of FPC averaged
80 ± 4 percent.

On the basis of results in 5 children with
kwashiorkor given FPC 20, 10, 10, 5, 5 days
after initial milk therapy, the therapeutic
effects of FPC could not be distinguished
from those obtained with milk, as judged by
weight gain, recovery of lean body mass
(measured by the creatinine/height index), and
rise of serum protein to normal levels. Information on the suitability of FPC for the
initial treatment of kwashiorkor was not
given.

With this record of favorable experience,
it would seem reasonable to conclude that properly processed FPC can be a valuable protein
source for human feeding, including the supplementary and mixed feeding of both healthy
and malnourished young children. FPC, when
properly used, is comparable in protein value
to milk and other proteins of animal origin.
However, several published papers have been
interpreted in a manner that, to some extent,
unjustifiably confuses this conclusion, and
they require particularly careful review and
analysis. These come from three different

laboratories: The National Institute of
Nutrition in Hyderabad, India, the Christian
Medical College in Vellore, South India, and
the British American Hospital in Lima, Peru.

Srikantia and Gopalan,[23] in 1966, fed 6 g
of protein per kg and 200 calories per kg to
57 children hospitalized for kwashiorkor.
Thirty-three of the children received a diet
in which 80 percent of the protein came from
Viobin-FPC and 20 percent from wheat bread,
while 24 were given a diet of 80 percent DSM
and 20 percent wheat gluten. The FPC had a
fishy odor and was rejected by 10 of the 33
and poorly tolerated by another 5. For the 18
children who accepted the FPC, the results in
terms of clinical recovery, including rise in
serum albumin, were as satisfactory as for
those receiving DSM. Weight gain was less for
those receiving the FPC, presumably because of
poorer acceptability and hence lesser intake,
but actual food consumption data were not
given. The authors' general conclusion that
"Fish flour does not appear to be a satisfactory substitute for DSM in the treatment of
kwashiorkor", should be qualified because the
particular FPC employed had obviously deteriorated and the problem was one of palatability
rather than nutritional properties. In fact,
the result demonstrated that even an unpalat-
able FPC had the protein value necessary for
the successful treatment of at least some
cases of PCM.

In 1964, Moorjani et al.[24] described
"Fricola", a fish-enriched farinaceous product
prepared from eviscerated, freshly caught
fish, cooked and blended with cooked rice in a
ratio of 3:1, with 4 percent of dry shredded
coconut added to the product. The complete
mixture was dried in the form of thin flakes
on a roller dryer. Its PER was given as 3.5
compared with 2.9 for casein. This product
was fed in 1965 by Pereira et al.[25] to 15

Indian children in Vellore with typical
kwashiorkor. In the first trial, after two
weeks of skim milk protein at 3 g/kg/body
weight per day, Fricola was given to provide
5 g of protein/kg/day. The clinical response
was satisfactory compared to that of 7 control
children kept on the skim milk formula.
There were no significant differences between
the two groups in loss of edema, gain in
weight, or in increase in serum protein and
albumin.

In a second trial, however, 6 children with
kwashiorkor were given Fricola from the time
of admission, but only 3 showed a satisfactory
response. For the other 3, feeding with Fricola was stopped and recovery became satisfactory after the change to skim milk protein.
The authors concluded that the processed fish
was promising as a food for convalescent infants and for healthy children, but could not
be recommended for children seriously ill with
kwashiorkor. These results are not conclu-
sive, however, because heat damage was sus-
pected in the roller drying of some batches of
the product.

A later paper by Pereira and co-workers[26]
has created controversy because the method of
evaluation was the ratio of non-essential to
essential amino acids determined in a simple
one-dimensional chromatogram by a slight modification of Whitehead's method (see Lancet 1:
250, 1964). In children with PCM, the ratio
is originally high and decreases gradually
during recovery when they are given a diet
providing 3 g of skim milk protein and 150
kilocalories/kg body weight/day.[27]

Pereira and her group fed test diets to 19
orphanage children 2 to 5 years of age, and,
in a second study, 3 boys and 3 girls of 4 1/2
years. These diets supplied 2 g of the test
protein/kg/day in addition to the protein
contained in a low protein basal diet, for a

total of 42 g of protein per child per day.
Skim milk, fresh fish (oil sardines), mutton,
fish flour (prepared from oil sardines), and
legumes (Phaseolus radiata) were tested in
this manner. The ratios decreased significantly with either DSM or mutton, but not with
either fresh fish or legumes. The effect of
FPC was intermediate.

Based on their interpretation of the report
by Srikantia and Gopalan, and their own experience with Fricola, the authors accepted
these results as further evidence that fish
protein is not completely satisfactory in the
treatment of children with PCM. Because the
significance of the E/T ratio under these conditions is not clear, and because the conclusion is applied to both "fresh fish" and FPC,
the interpretation of this observation remains
uncertain. Supporting clinical data were not
obtained.

In 1965, Graham et al.[28] reported comparisons of 10 percent of either VioBin- or
Quintero-FPC added to wheat flour. Results
were generally satisfactory in 10 infants who
had been treated initially for marasmus or
kwashiorkor with milk. When used for the initial treatment of 3 cases of marasmus and 1
case of marasmic kwashiorkor, the recovery of
serum albumin values and growth lagged, although the children made a satisfactory.
clinical recovery. Similar results were obtained with FPC as the sole source of protein
in the initial treatment of marasmus and two
marasmic kwashiorkor cases.

These observations were followed by a 1966
paper[29] in which data were computed on 17 infants 5 to 54 months of age with at least one
6-day period of feeding in which FPC was the
sole source of protein in comparison with a
good vegetable mixture (40 percent cottonseed,
30 percent broad bean, and 20 percent quinua
flours), or wheat flour enriched with 10

percent FPC. The pooled results with all
three diets showed weight changes comparable
to those obtained previously with milk.

At all calorie and protein levels, increases in serum albumin were less than previously observed with milk, a result also
reported by Scrimshaw et al.[30] for the vegetable mixture Incaparina (29 percent cottonseed flour, 67 percent corn flour, 3 percent
torula yeast, and 1 percent calcium carbon-
ate). There is little doubt of this phenomenon even with good vegetable protein mixtures,
although its significance is uncertain.
Presumably, it indicates that an amino acid
pattern adequate for overall protein needs
can be less than optimum for albumin synthesis. The indication that this is also true
of fish protein, whether FPC or fresh fish,
is of interest, but hardly justifies classi-
fying this protein as inferior. More knowledge is required on the relative effects of
other proteins of animal origin and of varying amino acid patterns on albumin synthesis
and other biochemical parameters.

Any new protein source for the initial
treatment of kwashiorkor is hard to evaluate
because of the complication of superimposed
infections and the ethical need to change to
milk feeding in any child showing poor recovery. The problem is that there is no
assurance that a given child would have recovered faster if fed with milk. Recovery
from kwashiorkor, even under standard milk
therapy, is a highly variable process at best
because of individual differences in degree
of malnutrition and, especially, in superimposed infections. However, it must be pre-
sumed that DSM, when available, is to be
preferred over either FPC or good vegetable
protein mixtures for the initial treatment of
kwashiorkor, although either will support
satisfactory recovery in most cases. After

this period, the three are equally satisfactory for convalescence as well as for subsequent maintenance and prevention of
malnutrition.

Related Observation
In a different category is the paper by
Delfino et al.[31] in 1968, describing the feeding of a fish protein concentrate made by using the proteolytic yeast, Hansenula
montevideo. Seventy premature infants who
weighed between 1,100 and 2,500 grams at birth
were fed the material at levels of a half to
one g/kg/day, and 15 malnourished infants,
initially between 2 and 5 months of age, were
fed the mixture for 30 days at a level of 1 g
protein/kg/day. In addition, the yeast was
fed to 60 adults, half of whom were in the
geriatric age range. No cases of diarrhea
were encountered and the product was acceptable in the form presented. Its digestibility
varied between 97 and 99 percent, higher
values than observed for ordinary fish flour
or meat flour. In the 30-day study, hematocrit, total serum protein, albumin, and
globulin fractions all increased significantly. Considerable additional data are given,
indicating that this product has a high
nutritional value.
     The residual fluoride content of FPC has
also received attention. The Committee on
Aquatic Food Resources of the U. S. NAS/NRC
does not consider the levels likely to be encountered in use to constitute a health hazard
for any segment of the population. On the
contrary, the addition of fluoride to the diet
from this source would have the advantage of
its anti-caries activity. It is conceivable
that some child consuming abnormally large
amounts of ordinary FPC on a daily basis
could experience some mild mottling of the
enamel, but this is benign and associated with

high resistance to dental caries. The amount
of fluoride in FPC varies somewhat with the
type of fish, the area from which the fish are
obtained, and other factors, and should be
routinely monitored. If there is any reason
to do so, fluoride levels can be easily
lowered by partial removal of bones through
sieving or air classification. However, the
100 ppm limit to fluoride content of FPC imposed by the FDA is unnecessarily restrictive
and burdensome to the cost of the final product. This is based on a level that would
cause no dental fluorosis even at the maximum
possible use of the concentrate in all potential foods. A limit of 250 ppm would seem to
be reasonable. Such a level would not have
any toxic effect and only rarely a cosmetic
one.

Summary

There is very extensive evidence that properly
prepared FPC is an effective source of protein
for human consumption and that it can be used
interchangeably with milk and vegetable protein mixtures of good quality to meet the protein needs of infants and young children. For
the prevention of protein-calorie malnutrition
in infants and young children and the feeding
of patients convalescing from malnutrition,
this interchangeability is also well demonstrated. The slightly lower serum albumin
levels in children fed either FPC or vegetable
mixtures of good quality compared to levels in
children fed milk have no proven clinical
significance.
    Because the initial treatment of kwashior-
kor yields variable and uncertain results
even under optimum circumstances, physicians
are understandably reluctant to continue feeding sources of protein less accepted than milk
to children who are recovering poorly. Thus,
although there is evidence that either FPC or

good vegetable protein mixtures can be used
successfully in the treatment of cases of
kwashiorkor, milk is still the protein source
of choice for this purpose. Except for the
initial treatment of kwashiorkor, properly
processed FPC should be considered fully
interchangeable with all other good sources of
protein for all nutritional purposes. The
fluoride content of FPC in the quantities
likely to be consumed is an asset in the prevention of dental caries and does not constitute a health hazard.

References

1. Gomez, F., Ramos-Galvan, R., Cravioto, J.,
Frenk, S., and Labardini, I. 1958. Studies
on the use of deodorized fish flour in malnutrition. Preliminary report. Bol. Med.
Hosp. Infantil (Mexico) 15: 485.

2. Gruttner, R., and Schafer, K. H. 1959.
Die biologische Wertigkeit des Fischproteins
im Ernahrungsversuch an Fruhgeborenen und im
Tierexperiment. Klin Wochensch. 37: 255.

3. Progress in Meeting Protein Needs of
Infants and Preschool Children. 1961. Pro-
ceedings of an International Conference held
in Washington, D. C. August 21-24, 1960.
Publication 843, National Academy of Sciences-
National Research Council. Washington, D. C.

4. Frenk, S. Biological value of some new
sources of protein in Mexican malnourished
children. In Progress in Meeting Protein
Needs of Infants and Preschool Children, op.
cit., p. 21.

5. Hansen, J. D. L. The effects of various
forms of supplementation on the nutritive

value of maize in children. In Progress in
Meeting Protein Needs of Infants and Preschool
Children, op. cit., p. 89.

6. Senecal, J. Studies on the use of peanut
flour in infant feeding. In Progress in Meeting Protein Needs of Infants and Preschool
Children, op. cit., p. 119.

7. DeMaeyer, E. M., and Vanderborght, H. L.
Determination of the nutritive value of
different protein foods in the feeding of
African children. In Progress in Meeting
Protein Needs of Infants and Preschool Child-
ren, op. cit., p. 143.

8. Graham, G. G., Baertl, J. M., and
Cordano, A. 1962. Evaluation of fish flour
in the treatment of infantile malnutrition.
In FAO International Conference on Fish in
Nutrition. 19-27 September, 1961. Washing-
ton, D. C. In Fish in Nutrition. p. 271.
London: Fish. News (Books) Ltd.

9. Graham, G. G., Cordano, A., and Baertl,
J. M. 1963. Studies in infantile malnutrition. 2. Effect of protein and calorie intake
on weight gain. J. Nutr. 81: 249.

10. Thomson, F. A., and Merry, E. 1962.
Weight increase in toddler children in the
Federation of Malaya: a comparison of dietary supplements of skim milk and fish biscuits. Brit. J. Nutr. 16: 175.

11. Doraiswamy, T. R., Shurpalekar, S. R.,
Moorjani, M. N., Lahiry, N. L., Sankaran, A.
N., Swaminathan, M., Sreenivasan, A., and
Subrahmanyan, V. 1963. The effect of a
supplementary protein food containing fish
flour, groundnut flour and Bengal gram flour
and fortified with vitamins on the growth and

nutritional status of children. Indian J.
Pediat. 30: 266.

12.   Shurpalekar, S. R., Daniel, V. A.,
Doraiswamy, T. R., Lahiry, N. L., Moorjani,
M. N., and Swaminathan, M. 1963. The effect
of a supplementary protein food containing
fish flour (from oil sardine) on the metabolism of nitrogen, calcium and phosphorus in
children. Indian J. Pediat. 30: 272.

13.   Lee, K. Y., Shin, M. S., Kim, M. H.,
Lee, E. S., Cho, B. K., and Lewis, J. A.
1964. Effect of protein supplementation by
fish flour at weaning period. Yonsi Med. J.
(Korea) 5:.

14.   Hwang, W. I. 1963. Digestion and absorption rate of protein from some Korean
diets in human subjects. Korean Med. J. 8:
59.

15.   Pretorius, P. J., and Wehmeyer, A. S.
1964. An assessment of nutritive value of
fish flour in the treatment of convalescent
kwashiorkor patients. Amer. J. Clin. Nutr.
14: 147.

16.   Wikramanayake, T. W., de S. Wijesundra,
C., de Silva, C. C., and de Silva, N. N.
1966. Supplementation with fish flour of a
rice diet fed to convalescent children. J.
Trop. Pediat. 12: 7.

17.   Spada, R., Maccioni, A., Vega, L.,
Oxman, S., Monckeberg, F., Gattas, V.,
Barja, I., and Donoso, G. 1967. Ensayo de
mezclas a base de harina de pescado, torta de
maravilla y leche descremada en preescolares.
Nutr. Bromatol. Toxicol. 6: 107.

18.   Yanez, E., Barja, I., Monckeberg, F.,

Maccioni, A., and Donoso, G. 1967. The fish
protein concentrate story. 6. Quintero fish
protein concentrate: protein quality and use
in foods. Food Technol. 21: 60.

19. Yanez, E., Ballester, D., Maccioni, A.,
Spada, R., Barja, I., Pak, N., Chichester,
C. O., Donoso, G., and Monckeberg, F. 1969.
Fish-protein concentrate and sunflower press-
cake meal as protein sources for human con-
sumption. Amer. J. Clin. Nutr. 22: 878.

20. Spencer, H., Lewin, I., Fowler, J., and
Samachson, J. 1968. Utilization of fish
protein concentrate in man. Fed. Proc. 27: 423.

21. Tavill, F., and Gonik, A. 1969. Use of
fish protein concentrate in the diets of weanling infants. Amer. J. Clin. Nutr. 22: 1571.

22. Brinkman, G. L., Sharadambal, B., and
Madhave, V. 1970. A feeding trial of fish
protein concentrate with preschool children.
Amer. J. Clin. Nutr. 23: 395.

23. Srikantia, S. G., and Gopalan, C. 1966.
Fish protein concentrates in the treatment of
kwashiorkor. Amer. J. Clin. Nutr. 18: 34.

24. Moorjani, M. N., Upadhye, A. N. Lahiry,
N. L., Parpia, H. A. B., Dumm, M. E., and
Pereira, S. M. 1964. "Fricola" A fish-
enriched farinaceous product. Feeding tests
with kwashiorkor children. FAO Symposium on
the Significance of Fundamental Research in
the Utilization of Fish. 26-30 May, 1964.
Husum, Germany. 2p.; World Fish Abstr. 15:
41.

25. Pereira, S. M., Isaac, T., Tewarson, B.,
and Dumm, M. E. 1965. Processed fish protein
in the treatment of kwashiorkor. Indian J.

Med. Res. 53: 651.

26. Pereira, S. M., Begum, A., Sundararaj, R., and Dumm, M. E. 1968. Effect of dietary protein on serum amino acids. Amer. J. Clin. Nutr. 21: 167.

27. Ittyerah, T. R., Pereira, S. M., and Dumm, M. E. 1965. Serum amino acids of children on high and low protein intakes. Amer. J. Clin. Nutr. 17: 11.

28. Graham, G. G., Baertl, J. M., and Cordano, A. 1965. Dietary protein quality in infants and children. I. Evaluation in rapidly growing infants and children of fish protein concentrate alone and in combination with wheat. Amer. J. Dis. Child. 110: 248.

29. Graham, G. G., Baertl, J. M., and Cordano, A. 1966. Studies in infantile malnutrition. 5. The effect of dietary protein source on serum proteins. Amer. J. Clin. Nutr. 18: 16.

30. Scrimshaw, N. S., Behar, M., Wilson, D. Viteri, F., Arroyave, G., and Bressani, R. 1961. All-vegetable protein mixtures for human feeding. 5. Clinical trials with INCAP mixtures 8 and 9 and with corn and beans. Amer. J. Clin. Nutr. 9: 196.

31. Delfino, A. H., Caillabet, E., Bidegain, S., Ricon, M. G., Bertullo, V. H., Alvarez, C., Moris, A., and Corbo, M. 1968. El bio-proteo-catenolizado (B.P.C.) de pescado en la recuperacion del nino desnutrido. Rev. Instit. Invest. Pesqueras 2: 173.

XIII
EVALUATION OF THE PROTEIN QUALITY OF FISH
PROTEIN CONCENTRATE FOR MAINTENANCE OF ADULTS*

Vernon R. Young
and
Nevin S. Scrimshaw
Department of Nutrition and Food Science,
Massachusetts Institute of Technology,
Cambridge, Massachusetts 02139

In our laboratories at M.I.T. we have studied
the protein quality of fish protein concentrate (FPC) in young men. The FPC was prepared from red hake and obtained from the
Bureau of Commercial Fisheries, College Park,
Maryland.
    Our studies, to date, have been concerned
with the evaluation of the nutritive value of
FPC per se, where the test protein provided
about 90 percent of the dietary protein intake. Two different and complementary approaches were followed in these experiments.
In the first, we examined the extent to which
FPC provides an excess of essential amino
acids per g protein nitrogen required for
adult maintenance and compared the results
with those obtained in similar studies using
other high quality animal protein sources.
Because this approach is not a standard one,

----

*Supported by a grant from the U. S. Bureau of
Commercial Fisheries. The facilities of the
MIT Clinical Research Center were utilized in
these studies and are supported by a grant
(RR-88) from the General Clinical Research
Centers Program of the Division of Research
Resources, National Institutes of Health.

we have also extended our studies to the
determination of the biological value (VB) and
net protein utilization (NPU) of FPC in young
adults.

Studies on the Effects of FPC Replacement with Nonspecific Nitrogen

The quality of a dietary protein is a measure
of its capacity to meet the nutritional requirement for protein, which is comprised of
two components. The first is the requirement
for the individual essential amino acids and
the second is the requirement for nonspecific
nitrogen, used also for the synthesis of body
proteins and other functionally important
nitrogen-containing compounds. These two components may be related on the basis of the
ratio of weight of the total of essential
amino acids per unit weight of nitrogen, and
Table 1 shows this ratio for whole hen's egg
and fish compared with the 1957 FAO reference
protein.
    Whole egg protein contains a higher E/T_N
ratio (3.08) than the 1957 FAO reference protein (2.02), but protein scores based on this
reference amino acid pattern agreed reasonably
well with results obtained by biological
assay.[1] Expressed in another way, the essential amino acids in whole egg supply about 36
percent of total amino nitrogen compared with
24 percent for the 1957 FAO reference protein.
Furthermore, the nitrogen balance data of Rose
and Wixom[2] in two adult subjects suggest that
only from 14 to 23 percent of the total dietary nitrogen need be supplied through essential amino acids in order to maintain nitrogen
balance.
    For these reasons a series of investiga-
tions have been conducted in our laboratories
to determine the extent to which the relatively high E/T_N ratios of various high quality,[3-5] including FPC, can be reduced by

isonitrogenous substitution of the protein
with a nonspecific nitrogen source without influencing the nutritional value of the protein. Using diets in which whole egg protein
furnished 90 percent of the total dietary protein, we found that the E/T_N ratio of the
basal diet could re reduced from 2.18 to 1.85
without influencing the efficiency of dietary
nitrogen utilization.[3] At these ratios essential amino acids furnish between 21 to 25 percent of the total dietary nitrogen.

The basic experimental procedures followed
in our studies with FPC have been previously
described in detail[3-5] and are further illustrated in Figure 1 for a subject consuming the
egg protein diet. The subjects were given an
experimental diet supplying approximately 0.4
g test protein/kg body weight/day during a
two-week control (0 dilution) period, and
urinary nitrogen excretion was monitored
daily. After stabilization of urinary N output, the test protein was isonitrogenously replaced to a variable extent with a mixture of
glycine and diammonium citrate in which each
provided equal amounts of N.

An increase in urinary N output occurred,
as shown in Figure 1, when 40 percent of the
egg protein N, provided by the control diet,
was replaced by the nonspecific nitrogen
source, indicating that the replacement or
dilution of the test protein caused a decrease
in the efficiency of N retention and thus a
reduction in protein quality. However, a 30
percent and in some cases a 40 percent dilution of egg protein did not influence protein
quality as judged by this criterion, and we
concluded, therefore, that the concentration
of essential amino acids in egg protein is
about 30 to 40 percent higher than minimally
required for maintenance in adult human subjects.[3]

From the concentration of essential amino
acids in FPC shown in Table 1, and from our

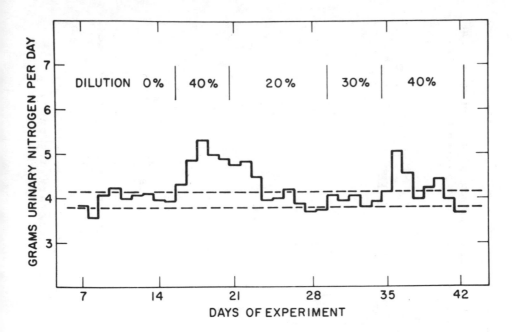

Figure 1. Urinary nitrogen excretion per day in a young adult male subject fed an egg protein diet with zero, 40, 20, 30 and 40% replacement of egg protein nitrogen with glycine and diammonium citrate. Broken lines represent mean baseline nitrogen excretion ± one standard deviation. Experimental details given in reference 3.

Table 1. Proportions of essential amino acids to total nitrogen in the experimental FPC diets, whole egg protein, and the 1957 FAO Reference Protein

Amino Acid	Basal egg formula	Basal FPC formula mg/g N	% Diluted FPC formula[1]			1957 FAO Reference Protein
			20	25	30	
Isoleucine	398	281	225	211	197	270
Leucine	530	472	378	354	330	306
Lysine	384	496	397	372	247	270
Total S Amino Acids	321	241	193	181	169	270
Total Aromatic Amino Acids	608	466	373	350	326	360
Threonine	300	271	217	203	189	180
Tryptophan	99	63	50	47	44	90
Valine	444	322	258	242	225	277
Total Essential Amino Acids	3084	2612	2090	1960	1827	2016
% EAAN[2]	35.7	33.2	26.6	24.9	23.2	23.6
E/T$_N$ ratio[3]	3.08	2.61	2.09	1.96	1.83	2.02

1. % isonitrogenous replacement of dietary nitrogen with glycine and diammonium citrate mixture with each supplying equal amounts of nitrogen.
2. % of total nitrogen contributed by essential amino acids.
3. G total essential amino acid per g total dietary nitrogen.

earlier results obtained with whole egg protein diets, it was predicted that the total
dietary nitrogen of an FPC diet could be
isonitrogenously replaced with nonspecific
nitrogen to the extent of about 25 percent
without a change in its nutritive value for
most young adults. Two studies, involving a
total of 12 young men, were conducted to test
the hypothesis. Urinary nitrogen excretion
was used as an index of changes in dietary
nitrogen utilization, and the results of the
first experiment with seven subjects are shown
in Table 2.

Comparison of urinary N output levels during the dilution periods with those obtained
with undiluted diet indicates that most subjects tolerated a 30 percent dilution. This
level of replacement would be predicted to be
tolerated from previous results obtained in
similar experiments with whole egg[3] and beef[4]
and milk proteins.[5] However, we also observed
that when some subjects were again given the
basal FPC diet following a period of FPC dilution, there was a marked decrease in urinary
nitrogen excretion, indicating an increased
rate of dietary N retention, because the total
N intake was constant during the experimental
diet period. The results for one subject who
responded in this manner are shown graphically
in Figure 2.

The reason for this marked retention of
nitrogen could be the depletion of one or more
essential amino acids so that more efficient
use was made of the dietary FPC when refed in
undiluted form. The total S-amino acids and
tryptophan are in relatively low concentrations in the FPC diets[6-8] when compared with
the whole egg as used in our previous studies,
and this may explain the lack of completely
satisfactory results at the predicted minimum
E/T_N ratio. Plasma-free tryptophan concentrations in samples taken after an overnight fast

Table 2. Effects of Isonitrogenous
Substitution of FPC with Glycine and
Diammonium Citrate on Urinary Nitrogen
Excretion in Young Men (Exp. 1)

Subject	N Intake (g/day)	% Dilution of Dietary Protein			
		0	25	30	0
			g/day		
HN	4.31	4.40±0.45[1]	4.28[2]	4.26	--
BF	4.83	4.32±0.41	4.37	--	3.58
WH	3.55	3.70±0.20	3.40	3.77	--
RS	3.48	3.55±0.20	3.96	3.96	--
GC	3.95	4.47±0.25	4.17	4.17	3.31
WS	3.92	4.13±0.27	3.85	4.35	3.41
JG	4.29	4.31±0.22	4.57	--	3.85

1. Mean ± for last 8 days of a 15-day period
with FPC at 0.38 g protein/kg/day.
2. Mean values, after stabilization, for
periods lasting 6-17 days.

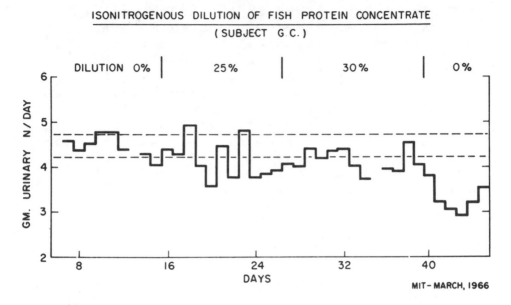

ISONITROGENOUS DILUTION OF FISH PROTEIN CONCENTRATE
(SUBJECT G.C.)

Figure 2. Urinary nitrogen excretion per
day in a young adult male subject fed a diet
in which FPC provided 90% of total dietary
protein and at various levels of FPC nitrogen replacement with glycine and diammonium
citrate. Further details are given in Table
2.

(Table 3) were lower in two additional subjects who also showed increased N retention
upon return to the basal FPC diet; there did
not appear to be a correlation with changes in
plasma tryptophan levels. However, it is
possible that postprandial plasma tryptophan
levels may have revealed more useful information in helping to explain the metabolic basis
for the N balance response following dilution
of FPC with the nonspecific N source.

A second metabolic balance study with five
young men was conducted to determine whether a
20 percent dilution would also result in the
development of an apparent amino acid depletion, and the levels of urinary nitrogen excretion are summarized in Table 4. A 20 percent replacement of the FPC with glycine and
diammonium citrate did not reduce the overall
utilization of dietary nitrogen, as indicated
by the lack of differences in urinary N output
between the 0 and 20 percent dilution periods.
Also, a consistent and marked decrease in
urinary N excretion (i.e., a marked increase
in dietary N retention) during the first several days of return to the basal FPC diet after
the dilution period was not observed in this
experiment.

These results contrast with those of
Kofranyi and Jekat,[9] who described experiments
seemingly comparable to ours. They reported
that tuna fish protein could not be diluted at
all. The fish protein used in their study
may, however, have undergone damage during
processing and storage.

From the results of our two studies, it
appears that FPC can be diluted to the extent
of 20 percent without an apparent change in
the nutritional quality of this food protein
source. Similar studies on the dilution of
beef[4] and cow's milk proteins[5] also show that
these proteins could be isonitrogenously replaced to the extent of 20 to 25 percent

Table 3.   Serum Albumin[1] and Free Tryptophan[2]
Concentrations in Young Men Studied for the
Effects of Dilution of FPC with Glycine and
Diammonium Citrate (Exp. 1)

Subject	% Dilution of Protein							
	0		25		30		0	
	Alb	Try	Alb	Try	Alb	Try	Alb	Try
HN	4.3	13.9	4.3	14.7	4.7	16.2	--	--
BF	4.2	12.5	4.4	11.6	--	--	5.4	12.4
WH	3.9	14.1	4.2	14.0	4.4	14.6	--	--
RS	3.5	11.0	3.9	14.3	4.0	13.7	--	--
GC	4.1	14.0	4.2	12.0	4.2	9.0	4.2	10.9
WS	3.9	15.3	4.4	8.2	4.0	6.5	3.8	10.0
JG	4.2	11.3	4.7	10.5	--	--	3.9	9.2

1.   grams per 100 ml
2.   µg per ml
Blood samples were taken after an 10-hour
overnight fast.

Table 4. Effects of a 20% Replacement of FPC[1] with Glycine-Diammonium Citrate on Urinary Nitrogen in Young Men (Exp. 2)

Subject	N Intake	% Dilution of Protein		
		0	20	0
		grams per day		
ND	3.90	3.16±0.34(10)	3.27±0.17(12)	3.04±0.24(5)
KE	4.89	4.98±0.41(5)	4.88±0.30(10)	4.25±0.23(5)
BI	4.08	3.24±0.46(5)	3.43±0.39(9)	3.55±0.21(5)
MS	4.72	4.32±0.11(4)	4.93±0.35(10)	4.27±0.11(5)
WT	5.65	6.03±0.59(4)	5.08±0.55(8)	5.18±0.53(5)

Figure in ( ) indicates number of observations. The 0, 20 and 0% dilution periods were 20, 20 and 7 days, respectively.

1. Total protein intake (90% from FPC) was 0.38 per kg per day.

without a change in their nutritional value.
Thus, based on these comparative findings, it
is concluded that the protein of FPC is of
relatively high quality for human adult
maintenance.

Estimation of the BV of Fish Protein Concentrate

In the second approach followed in our
studies we determine the digestibility and
biological value (BV) of FPC at a level of
protein intake that was significantly below
that necessary to achieve N equilibrium in
the young adult subject. This level was
equivalent to 0.3 g protein (N x 6.25) per kg
body weight per day. The results for N
balance are summarized in Table 5. At this
protein intake all subjects were in negative
N balance. The biological value (BV) was
calculated according to the conventional procedure, as previously described.[10] Mean values for obligatory urinary and fecal N losses
were based on those for similar subjects
studied earlier.[11]

The mean "true" digestibility was 97 percent and the mean BV was determined to be 75
for the six subjects who participated in the
experiment (Table 5). These values may be
compared to those obtained with other protein
sources as studied in our laboratory under
similar dietary and experimental conditions
(Table 6). The comparisons made in Table 6
indicate, for the level of test protein intake used, that when FPC is essentially the
sole dietary protein source, its protein
nutritional quality is somewhat lower than
that for dried skim milk, but similar to
National Research Council reference casein.

Recently Calloway and Margen[12] have
questioned the soundness of the theory behind
the conventional measurements of BV and their
application in estimating the minimum amount

Table 5.   Nitrogen Balance and Biological Value
(BV) with Fish Protein Concentrate Studied in
Young Men

Subject	N Intake[2] g/day	N Balance g/day	BV	Digestibility (%)
GD	3.28	-0.78	76	96
MT	4.10	-0.88	78	95
DD	3.34	-0.90	67	100
SR	3.53	-0.83	71	94
MB	3.93	-0.55	82	100
SD	2.87	-0.54	77	98
Mean ± SD	3.5±0.45	-0.75±0.16	75±5	97±3

----

1.   FPC given at a level of 0.3 g protein
(N x 6.25) per kg body wt. per day.   Experimental period was 15 days and results based on last
7 days.
2.   FPC furnished 90% of total N and oatmeal and
tomatoe juice the remainder.   NPU of FPC by rat
assay was 72 (casein control, 63).

Table 6. Comparison of the Biological Value of
FPC with Various Protein Sources Studied in
Young Men

Protein Source[1]   Biological Value[2]

Hen's Egg   95±3 (8)
Lactalbumin   94±6 (6)
Dried Skim Milk   87±6 (8)
Casein   79±4 (6)
FPC   75±5 (6)

Yeast   71±10 (6)
Opaque-2 Corn   80±9 (8)

----

1. Test proteins given at a level of 0.27 -
0.30 g protein/kg body weight/day.
2. Mean ± SD for number of subjects shown in
parenthesis.

Table 7. Calculated biological value (BV) and
net protein utilization (NPU) for egg protein
at maintenance and submaintenance levels of N
intake in young men

Level of protein	BV		NPU
(g/kg/day)			
0.2	107 ± 21*	(11)	103 ± 19
0.3	93 ± 16*	(11)	89 ± 14
0.4	65 ± 19*	(8)	61 ± 18
0.5	72 ± 14*	(11)	71 ± 13

----

*Mean ± standard deviation for number of
subjects shown in parentheses.

of a protein to meet the needs for N maintenance in adult subjects. We also have data,
summarized in Table 7, that support their
conclusions. At levels of egg intake of 0.3 g
protein/kg body weight and below, utilization
of the protein N was high, but this efficiency
decreased markedly when the level of N intake
approached or just exceeded the amount equivalent to the sum of obligatory urinary and
metabolic fecal N losses. From these observations, it is possible that at levels of FPC
intake about 0.3 g protein/kg, the nutritive
value of the protein might compare rather more
favorably with that of other high quality animal protein sources than at the limiting level
of intake (i.e., 0.3 g/kg) used in our studies
so far. Only further direct experiments will
resolve this uncertainty.

Conclusion
The protein quality of FPC has been studied in
a series of experiments with young men given
the test protein as the principal source of
dietary N and at submaintenance levels of
total protein intake. The results of experiments on the isonitrogenous replacement of
FPC with a nonspecific nitrogen source consisting of a mixture of glycine and diammonium
citrate, and estimations of the biological
value of FPC, reveal that the nutritional
quality of FPC for human maintenance needs
compares favorably with that of other good
quality protein sources.

References

1. FAO/WHO Protein Requirements. 1965.
Report of a Joint FAO/WHO Expert Group. FAO
Nutrition Meetings Report Series No. 37.
Food and Agriculture Organization of the
United Nations. Rome.

2.   Rose, W. C., and Wixom, R. L.   1955.   The
amino acid requirements of man.   XVL. The role
of the nitrogen intake.   J. Biol. Chem. 217:
997.

3.   Scrimshaw, N. S., Young, V. R., Schwartz,
R., Piche, M. L., and Das, J. B.   1966.
Minimum dietary essential amino acid-to-total
nitrogen ratio for whole egg protein fed to
young men.   J. Nutr. 89: 9.

4.   Huang, P. C., Young, V. R., Cholakos, B.,
and Scrimshaw, N. S.   1966.   Determination of
the minimum dietary essential amino acid-to-
total nitrogen ratio for beef protein fed to
young men.   J. Nutr. 90: 416.

5.   Scrimshaw, N. S., Young, V. R., Huang,
P. C., Thanangkul, O., and Cholakos, B. V.
1969.   Partial dietary replacement of milk
protein by nonspecific nitrogen in young men.
J. Nutr. 98: 9.

6.   Yanez, E., Barja, I., Monckeberg, F.,
Macioni, A., and Donoso, G.   1967.   The fish
protein concentrate story.   6. Quintero fish
protein concentrate: protein quality and use
in foods.   Food Technol. 21: 60.

7.   Miller, D. S.   1956.   The nutritive value
of fish proteins.   J. Sci. Food Agric. 7: 337.

8.   Stillings, B. R., Hammerle, O. A., and
Snyder, D. G.   1969.   Sequence of limiting
amino acids in fish protein concentrate by
isopropyl alcohol extraction of red hake
(Urophycis chuss).   J. Nutr. 97: 70.

9.   Kofranyi, E., and Jekat, F.   1964.   Zur
Bestimmung der Biologischen Wertigkeit von
Nahrungsproteinen.   9. Der Ersatz von
lockvertigen Eiweiss durch nichtessentiellen

Stickstoff. Hoppe-Seyler's Z. Physiol. Chem.
338: 154.

10. Young, V. R., Ozalp, I., Cholakos, B. V.,
and Scrimshaw, N. S. 1971. Protein value of
Colombian Opaque-2 corn for young adult men.
J. Nutr. 101: 1475.

11. Young, V. R., and Scrimshaw, N. S. 1968.
Endogenous nitrogen metabolism and plasma free
amino acids in young adults given a "protein-
free" diet. Brit. J. Nutr. 22: 9.

12. Calloway, D. H., and Margen, S. 1971.
Variations in endogenous nitrogen excretion
and dietary nitrogen utilization as determi-
nants of human protein requirement. J. Nutr.
101: 205.

Part IV

UTILIZATION

XIV
UTILIZATION OF FPC AND ACCEPTABILITY

V. D. Sidwell
College Park Fishery Products Technology Lab.,
National Marine Fisheries Service, National
Oceanic & Atmospheric Administration, U. S.
Department of Commerce, College Park,
Maryland 20740

Introduction
FPC (fish protein concentrate) may be defined
as a product made from fish in which the protein is more concentrated than in the original
raw product. It may range from a light-
colored bland powder to a dark powder having
an intensely fishy flavor. Hake-FPC, produced
by solvent extraction of hake, is nearly odorless, light-colored, insoluble in water, and
not easily wettable. In general, when a fatty
fish is used to make FPC, the color will be
darker and the flavor somewhat stronger. It
also is not water soluble or easily wettable.
    Although most of the work in our laboratory
was done on foods that are quite American, our
main objective was not to develop protein-rich
foods per se, but to observe how FPC func-
tioned in a media of other ingredients. Also,
we wanted to observe how machinable the doughs
were that contained 10 percent FPC. Last, but
not the least important, we wanted to obtain
some measure of acceptability.
    Generally, we do not add any more FPC than
10 percent of the dry ingredients in the food
products, especially the baked products or
pasta. At this level the changes that occur
in flavor, texture, or appearance can easily
be remedied by minimal changes in formulation
or in processing. The flavor can be easily
masked with flavoring compounds. Also, at
this level we have been able to produce quite

acceptable food items.

Use of FPCs with Varying Intensities of Flavor and Odor

The utilization of FPC in a food is determined
primarily by the flavor and odor of the FPC
per se, rather than by the flavor and odor it
will impart to the fortified food. The question arises, must FPC be nearly flavorless and
odorless to fortify all food products? To obtain some information on this problem, we took
six FPCs that varied in intensity of flavor
and odor. One FPC was made from deboned fresh
fish, and two were made from whole fish. The
difference between the last two FPCs is the
number of extractions, one was four stages and
the other five stages. The other three FPCs
were made from menhaden press cake, fresh menhaden fish meal, or cured fish meal.

The menhaden-FPCs were incorporated into
grits, bread, plain cookies, and chocolate
chip cookies at the 10 percent level of fortification.

To evaluate the sensory characteristics of
FPCs, we use the grit test using as basic ingredient (90 percent), Quaker Instant Corn
Grits, and 10 percent FPC. Enough hot water
was added so the consistency was comparable to
a thickish gruel.

The panelists evaluated the experimental
FPC against a standard FPC aroma, flavor by
mouth, aftertaste, color, and mouth feel. The
standard in this case was a hake-FPC with desirable characteristics. If the characteristics of the test sample were worse than the
standard, it would have a value of 2 or 1;
better than the standard 4 or 5. If they were
equal to the standard, then it would have a
value of 3. To avoid confounding the various
characteristics with color, the test was conducted in a darkened room under red light.
The color was evaluated in another room under

daylight.

This is a critical test for all characteristics, except aroma. Many times, as soon as
the hot water hits the FPC-grit mixture,
there is an expulsion of an odor and as soon
as it has disseminated, the aroma is much
milder.

The results of the flavor evaluation of the
six FPCs used in grits, bread, plain cookies,
and chocolate chip cookies are listed in Table
1. In the grit test the menhaden-FPC with the
mildest flavor was made from iced whole fish
but extracted with a five-stage counter-
current process. The FPCs made from press
cake or fish meal had the strongest flavor;
the others were intermediate.

The flavor of the FPCs was slightly better
in bread than it was in the grits. There was
a decided improvement in the flavor of the
cured fish meal-FPC when incorporated in
bread. The flavor of the plain cookies with
deboned fish FPC and the five-stage extraction
was similar to those made with the hake-FPC.
The others were stronger than the standard,
especially the cookies with FPC made from
press cake. The menhaden-FPCs that imparted
the strongest or the mildest flavor in the
plain cookies were used to make chocolate chip
cookies. The chocolate flavor masked the
strong flavor of the press cake and cured fish
meal-FPCs so that the flavor was comparable to
that of the FPCs that were quite mild in the
plain cookies.

Since the standard hake-FPC was very finely
ground in the fluid energy mill and the experimental sample in the Rietz grinder, the
difference in particle size was reflected in
the grit test, as seen in Table 2. Deboning
the fish did not change the texture of the FPC
FPC; it was similar to the texture of the FPCs
made from iced whole fish. The texture of the
bread was approximately like the control made

Table 1. Flavor[1] of grits, bread, plain
cookies and chocolate chip cookies fortified
with 10% fish protein concentrate (FPC) made
by isopropyl alcohol extraction of fresh hake
or menhaden, menhaden press cake or menhaden
fish meal.

Raw Material	Grits	Bread	Plain Cookies	Chocolate Chip Cookies
Hake-FPC (control)	3.0	3.0	3.0	3.0
Menhaden-FPC made from:				
Iced fish deboned	2.2	2.6	2.8	3.0
Iced whole[2]	2.2	2.5	2.4	-
Iced whole[3]	3.0	2.5	2.9	2.6
Press cake	1.4	1.8	1.8	2.7
Fish meal (fresh)	1.5	2.1	2.4	-
Fish meal (cured)	1.0	2.0	2.1	2.7

----

1. Equal to the standard 3; milder than
standard, greater than 3; stronger, less than
3.
2. Four-stage counter-current extraction.
3. Five-stage counter-current extraction.

Table 2. Texture[1] of grits, bread, plain cookies and chocolate chip cookies fortified with 10% fish protein concentrate (FPC) made by isopropyl alcohol extraction of fresh hake or menhaden, menhaden press cake or menhaden fish meal

Raw Material	Grits[1]	Bread[2]	Plain Cookies[3]	Chocolate Chip Cookies[3]
Hake-FPC (control)	3.0	3.0	3.0	3.0
Menhaden-FPC made from:				
Iced fish deboned	2.2	2.3	3.2	3.0
Iced whole[4]	2.3	2.9	2.9	-
Iced whole[5]	2.6	2.9	3.4	2.7
Press cake	2.4	2.3	3.2	3.0
Fish meal (fresh)	2.5	2.9	3.2	-
Fish meal (cured)	2.1	2.6	3.2	2.6

----

1. Equal to standard 3; more desirable than standard, greater than 3; less desirable, less than 3.
2. Equal to standard 3; spongier than the standard, more than 3; doughier than the standard, less than 3.
3. Equal to standard 3; crisper than standard, greater than 3; softer, less than 3.
4. Four-stage counter-current extraction.
5. Five-stage counter-current extraction.

with hake-FPC, except the breads with FPCs
made from iced deboned fish and press cake
were doughier than the control. The texture
of the cookies with the various experimental
menhaden-FPCs were comparable to the control
with hake-FPC.

The menhaden-FPCs were much darker than the
control. Naturally this is going to be reflected in the products fortified with these
FPCs. The appearances were somewhat lighter
when they were incorporated into bread and
cookies. The appearance of the cookies made
with FPCs from deboned fresh fish, five-stage
extracted iced whole fish, and the fresh fish
meal were comparable to the hake-FPC cookies.
The others were darker. All color differences
disappeared when the various FPCs were incorporated into a chocolate chip cookie.[1]

FPCs made from fatty fish tend to be
stronger in flavor and odor, as well as darker
in color. Moroccan-FPC, made from sardines,
is quite dark, but rather mild in flavor. It
was used by the investigators at the Department of Food Science and Technology, University of California, Davis, to fortify brown
sugar cookies with 0, 3, 5, and 10 percent
FPC. The panelists were not told they contained FPC, but were instructed to sample the
cookies and comment on their impressions. All
the panelists found the 10 percent formulation
to be less palatable than the cookies with
less FPC. Most of the comments were directed
to the heavier and chewier texture of the
cookies, rather than the flavor. There was no
substantial difference between 0, 3, or 5 percent FPC fortified cookies.[2]

The utilization of an FPC, therefore,
should not be considered primarily by the flavor and odor of the FPC per se, but also by
the flavor and odor it will impart to the fortified food.

Another interesting observation was noted

in our experiment, which was the differences
in the loaf volumes of the bread that contained the various FPCs. There was no variation in the handling of the dough. The bread
was prepared by the sponge method with no
emulsifiers or stabilizers. The bread that
contained FPC made from press cake or fish
meal had a significantly larger loaf volume
than the bread with FPC made from deboned or
whole fish, which were very much like the control loaf in size. This phenomenon was not
explained. We can only postulate. The FPC
made from press cake or fish meal is somewhat
more wettable; also, there may be some residual fat that may act as a surfactant.

Baked Products Fortified with FPC and Their Acceptability

Bread and breadlike products are probably
among the best vehicles for the use of FPC,
since some form of bread appears in most
diets. It is not always like the bread that
is familiar to Americans. It may be a tortil-
la, roti, chapati, baladi, or the water bread
available in Italy and France. In the United
States most of the work on fortification of
bread with FPC has been limited to bread that
is typically American where nine out of every
ten loaves are made in large bakeries and distributed to the consumer through a distributor, rather than directly to the consumer, as
it is done in many other countries. Bread
sold in America has to have an extended shelf
life of four to five days; therefore, much research has been done by scientists to find
ways to keep the bread fresh; consequently, we
have a typical American bread. In most countries the bakers either bake and sell the
fresh bread daily to the consumer or, in turn,
the consumer makes the bread at home to meet
the needs of the family.[3]

Bread. In breadmaking, the first thing we
needed to know was what effect the addition of
varying amounts of FPC has on dough characteristics. The Farinograph studies showed that
more water and mixing time were needed to
bring the dough to the same stage of development. There was a tendency to level off after
the 15 percent FPC level of fortification.
The Extensigraph studies showed us that the
dough lost the characteristics of stretching
and of springing back. In other words, the
dough became short.

These findings were further substantiated
when the bread was prepared by the Straight-
Dough method.[4] The only variation from the
published method was the amount of water added
and the length of time needed for the development of the dough. The dough became shorter
with each increment of FPC. This reduced the
capacity of the dough to retain the gas formed
during fermentation. Also, it reduced the
amount of handling the dough could withstand;
consequently, there was a decrease in loaf
volume with each increment.[5]

Pomeranz et al. found that fat is an important ingredient in the bread formulation.
Eight percent fish meallike FPC replaced the 4
percent dried skim milk in the standard formulation. They were able to increase the volume
of the bread by 19 percent over the bread with
no shortening, if 3 percent shortening was included in the formulation. Then, if they replaced the shortening with 1 percent sucrose
tallowate, they obtained a 21 percent volume
increase over the bread with no shortening.
It can be assumed that the shortening in the
bread can be replaced by a glycolipid.[6]

Next, we were faced with the problem of
making a loaf of bread that was equal in size
and weight to the bread that is commonly sold
as a high-protein bread on the American market, which runs from 2300 to 2400 ml per pound

loaf.

We found that the sponge method and the formulation listed in Table 3 made a pound loaf of FPC-bread with an average volume of 2500 ml. A sponge is made with part of the flour and water and all the fat, yeast, and yeast food. After a four-hour fermentation period, the remaining ingredients including the FPC are blended; the sponge is added and mixed until the dough is at the peak of development. Thereafter, the dough must be handled delicately, for the dough with the FPC has become somewhat short.

Tsen et al. at Kansas State University reported a formulation and procedure that was not too different than the one used by us. The greatest difference was that no fat was included in the basic formulation. In its place they used 0.25 percent, 0.5 percent, and 1.0 percent surfactant--sodium stearyol-2-lactylate.

The loaf volume they obtained with 0.5 percent sodium stearyol-2-lactylate was comparable to the ones we obtained with 3 percent lard in the formulation, 2574 and 2500 ml, respectively.[7,1]

While working in Chile, Vergara presented fifteen panelists with three bread samples: the first contained no FPC; the second contained 10 percent FPC and the third contained 10 percent FPC and butter. They were asked to record if the bread met their standards in odor, color, flavor, and texture. The bread with the FPC compared poorly with the control sample in the areas of odor and consistency. When butter was added, however, the odor became as satisfactory as the control sample, and the consistency almost doubled in acceptance.[8]

At the Department of Food Science and Technology of the Univers ty of California, Davis, FPC made from Moroccan sardines was incorpo-

Table 3.   Formulation for the preparation of
hake-FPC bread

                           gm
                           700
Flour   % of the flour

FPC   10.0
Yeast (dry)   2.5
Yeast food[1]   0.5
Sugar   8.0
Salt   2.0
Fat (lard)   3.0
Water   66.0

----

[1]Formulation for the yeast food taken from
AACC (1970).[4]

rated into bread at levels of 3, 5, and 10
percent. The bread was presented to two
groups of 25 panelists who were asked to sample the bread and comment upon its flavor.
They were not told that the bread contained
FPC. The panelists found the 10 percent FPC-
bread less palatable than the 3 or 5 percent
FPC-bread. Most of the comments were confined
to color and texture. Less than 1 percent of
the panelists identified the off-flavor as
"fishy." Fifty percent of the people preferred the bread with 3 percent FPC over the
nonfortified bread because it seemed "richer"
or more "bakerylike." The investigators
queried the people and found that they normally purchased specialty breads.[2]
In South Africa, the Nutrition Department
of Council for Scientific and Industrial Research conducted an extensive consumer acceptance study on the FPC-fortified bread developed by the food scientists at Western Cape
Province. A 90 percent extraction flour was
used to make the bread so it could be classi-
fied as a whole wheat bread. The acceptability test started in November 1956. By the
end of February 1959, nearly 40 million loaves
had been fortified with 2 percent FPC. No reaction of the public to indicate unaccept-
ability of these quantities of fish flour was
observed and it is fairly safe to say that
additions up to 4 percent of FPC do not impart an unacceptable flavor and odor to the
bread and that the loaf obtained with such as
addition would be acceptable to the bread
consumer in South Africa.[9] While this study
has been extremely useful, it stopped too
soon. In time the bread might have attained a
social status, and eventually the people who
needed the more nutritional bread would have
purchased it as a social status symbol. If
the enriched product is made for the social
strata above the poor, the benefits of the

product will soon filter down to the lower
strata.

Chapati. Chapati is a flat unleavened pan-
cakelike bread that is commonly used in India.
Sen et al. processed Bombay duck to make FPC
in seven different ways. Among the seven resulting FPCs, three were quite bland; the
others had a mild fish flavor and odor. The
investigators incorporated 5 and 10 percent of
each FPC into chapatis. The chapatis with 5
percent FPC were acceptable. Texture and
appearance were normal--no fishy flavor or
odor. At the 10 percent level of FPC fortification, at least 75 percent of the panel found
some of the chapatis slightly fishy. Although
they had slight reservations, they did not
find the chapatis unacceptable. The texture
of the chapatis with 10 percent FPC was normal; also, the appearance was acceptable and
normal to 88 percent of the panelists.[10]
These findings are quite contrary to those
reported by Bass and Caul,[11] probably because
they used the same formulation throughout the
study, regardless of the amount of FPC supplementation. Since the chapatis were made without regulating the amount of water needed to
make the doughs of comparable consistencies,
the changes in the physical and sensory
characteristics were probably more pronounced.

Tortillas. Tortillas, commonly eaten in
Mexico and other Central and South American
countries, are made from ground lime-treated
corn. Gomez et al.[12] fed a group of malnourished children for 60 days tortillas,
bread, noodles, beans, biscuits, donuts, and
pastries that were fortified with 5 to 10 percent FPC without any noticeable rejections of
the fortified foods over the experimental
period.
At our laboratory, a study was conducted to

determine the acceptability of tortillas
fortified with 5 percent, 10 percent, and 15
percent FPC. The tortillas with 5 percent and
10 percent FPC were as acceptable as the control with no FPC. The color of the tortillas
became darker as the amount of FPC increased
in the formulation, otherwise there was very
little difference in texture and flavor.[13]

Biscuits. A protein-rich biscuit containing
FPC processed from Boal fish and hammerhead
shark was prepared by Nath. The fish flesh
was boiled, extracted, and dried, producing a
product that was flavorless and odorless until
it came in contact with water. The fishy flavor and odor also reappeared when it was mixed
with wheat flour and water, made into a soft
dough, and fried. Lastly, a biscuit was made
with sugar, wheat flour, fat, ammonium carbo-
nate, and water. It was found that an acceptable tasting biscuit fortified with 25 to 40
percent FPC could be made this way. After
storage in a container for four months, there
was no reversion.[14,15]
    In Malaysia, Thomson and Merry found the
need to seek another source of protein, since
skim milk powder was going to be supplied only
temporarily to UNICEF. Legumes are not
commonly grown in Malaysia; therefore, they
had no good source of a vegetable protein,
but there was a large fish supply. They conducted acceptability studies on a deodorized
fish meallike FPC and on FPC-biscuits.
    The trials were held at seven Malaysian
Maternal and Child Health Clinics where
mothers, as well as children, tasted the FPC.
The mothers encouraged the children by telling
them that it tasted like a dried fish which is
commonly eaten at home. A similar trial was
conducted on the biscuit. The adults did not
like them as well as the children because they
were too sweet The children on the fish

biscuit gained more weight than the ones in
the control group on the skim milk, banana, or
sweet potato dietary regime.[16]

Pasta Fortified with FPC and Its Acceptability

Pasta is another type of food that is commonly
eaten by all groups of people regardless of
economic status. Like bread, it can be an excellent vehicle for introducing FPC into the
diets of individuals who need more animal protein in their diets.

Sidwell et al. made macaroni products from
semolina and varying amounts of hake-FPC (0,
3, 6, 9, and 12 percent). Sufficient water
was incorporated into the semolina-FPC mixture
to keep it free-flowing yet cohesive under
pressure. The mixture was extruded and the
resulting pasta was air dried overnight.[17]

The dried pasta became darker with each
increment of the hake-FPC. The color changed
from a bright yellow for the control (0 percent FPC) to a dark gray yellow for the pasta
with 12 percent FPC. During cooking much of
the dark color washed into the cooking water,
which lightened the cooked pasta considerably.

1. Panelists were asked to rate the degree
of odor difference between the experimental
samples and the control. 2. The cooked pasta
was placed in warm, mildly salted distilled
water and served in small tightly covered
containers. 3. No differences were detected
between the pasta containing 0 percent and 3
percent FPC. A few panelists were able to
detect a slight odor difference between the 0
percent and the 6 percent or 9 percent FPC
pasta. There was a distinct odor difference
detected for the 12 percent FPC pasta. The
panelists liked the flavor of the 0, 3, and 6
percent FPC pasta, but had a definite dislike
for the 12 percent FPC pasta. While the addition of 3 percent FPC to semolina did not
change the texture, levels of 6 percent and 9

percent tended to harden the pasta.[13,17,18]

Crisan reported that in Brazil, investigators made macaroni with a mixture of white wheat flour (distributed under Title II P.L. 480) and 6 percent FPC. The addition of FPC improved the texture of the product, and the pasta was firmer and more in keeping with the Italian description of al dento, a highly desirable attribute.

In Brazil the school lunch menu generally contains a thick stewlike soup. The macaroni is included as one of the ingredients. The soup with the FPC-macaroni was readily accepted, since the differences between the fortified and nonfortified macaroni was not distinguishable.[19]

Baertl et al. found that the FPC-fortified noodles, which in Peru may be considered a prestige food for the lower economic strata of society, were well accepted and tended to displace foods of lesser nutritional value. It was rather interesting to note that he stressed the importance of adding the fortification to a food with prestige value commonly used by that segment of the population that one hopes to reach.[20,21]

Woo and Erdman found that noodles made with all-purpose flour and fortified with 10 percent and 15 percent FPC had a nutritive value greater than casein, and PER values of 3.35, 3.83, and 3.21, respectively. The taste panel scored the cooked noodles with 10 percent FPC significantly higher in overall acceptability than those with 15 percent FPC. The 10 percent FPC-noodles were rated nearly as well as the ones with no FPC. Some adult judges had objections to the dark color of the FPC-fortified noodles. This characteristic may not be objectionable to Orientals, however, since many are used to even darker noodles made of rye flour. All the children in the panel liked the experimental noodles. When three Korean adult judges received the FPC-

fortified noodles, as commonly served in a
soup, they judged them as highly acceptable.[22]

Comparison of Physical and Sensory Characteristics of Bread and Pasta Fortified with Varying Amounts of FPC, Dried Skim Milk, and Soy Flour

So many times we speak of the lack of functional qualities of FPC compared to other protein supplements. Practically no data are
available, however, where there is a direct
comparison of the final food product that contains equal amounts of the high protein
supplements, like FPC, soy, and dried skim
milk.

We added varying amounts (0, 3, 6, 9, 12,
and 15 percent) of FPC, soy flour, and dried
skim milk to the bread formulation listed in
Table 3. The doughs were prepared under the
same conditions in all respects except the
amount of water. The doughs that contained
higher levels of FPC were less sticky and
easier to handle than the doughs with comparable amounts of soy flour or dried skim milk.

It may be noted that 3 percent supplementation of soy and dried skim milk had a marked
effect on the loaf volume, a decrease of 9
percent and 8 percent, respectively, against 2
percent for FPC. Nine percent FPC can be
added before the reduction in loaf volume is
comparable to ones that contain 3 percent soy
or dried skim milk. At the 9 percent level,
the loaf volume with FPC was significantly
larger than the ones with the same percent of
soy or dried skim milk.[1] Some of the volume
of the loaf of bread can be restored by including a surfactant or a glycolipid in the
formulation.[6,7]

In another study, 3 and 6 percent protein
from either FPC, soy, or dried skim milk or
0.2 and 0.4 percent lysine was added to the
pasta. The objective of this study was to

compare the nutritive values, as well as the
sensory and physical characteristics of pasta
supplemented with various types of protein.[1]

The nutritive value of both the cooked and
uncooked pasta was determined. The PER value
slightly improves after cooking in all experimental batches except the ones supplemented
with dried skim milk and lysine. In fact,
there was a notable decrease in the pasta
fortified with lysine. The PER values can be
more than doubled if 6 percent protein from
FPC is added to the semolina, and the dimen-
sion of improvement is nearly the same for the
pasta containing dried skim milk. The soy
pasta does not make as great an improvement as
the pasta with the other two protein supplements. There was a slight improvement over
the control with the lysine-fortified pasta,
but it was quite small in comparison to the
other protein supplements; in fact, the results indicated that the lysine leaches out
upon cooking.

When 3.5 or 7 percent FPC is added to the
pasta formulation, the amount of material
that leaches into the cooking water is practically the same as it is for the control,
which contained only semolina. As may be seen
in Table 4, there was a marked increase when
the pasta was supplemented with 8.4 or 16.8
percent dried skim milk. Some of this increase may be due to the amount used, as well
as the solubility of the supplement. The
leaching from the soy-fortified pasta was
slightly greater than the control. The solids
leached from the pasta enriched with lysine
was no greater than it was for the control.

The amount of protein that leached into the
cooking water was least in the pasta fortified
with dried skim milk and lysine. The amount
of protein that leached out increased with
cooking time. The largest amount was lost at
the 10-minute cooking time; after that it

Table 4. Percent solids that leached from
pasta fortified with either 3 or 6% protein
from various high-protein supplements or with
.2 and .4% lysine and cooked for varying times

Composition	Amount of Protein Added %	Cooking time (mins.)			
		5 %	10 %	15 %	20 %
Semolina		4.1	5.8	6.2	6.6
Semolina with:					
3.5% FPC[1]	3	5.0	6.4	7.0	7.1
7.5% FPC	6	4.9	6.6	6.6	6.6
8.4% DSM[2]	3	6.7	9.7	12.8	12.8
16.8% DSM	6	10.8	12.4	12.1	12.8
5.7% soy[3]	3	5.9	6.6	7.8	8.5
11.4% soy	6	5.9	7.4	8.0	8.2
.2% lysine		5.2	6.6	7.1	7.0
.4% lysine		5.0	6.7	7.0	7.0

[1]Fish protein concentrate.
[2]Dried skim milk.
[3]Soy flour.

seemed to level off.

Kapsiotis reported that due to the lack of the binding quality of FPC, it had limited use in pasta products. He found that 20 to 30 percent of the FPC in the fortified pasta leached into the cooking water. By changing the cooking procedure he was able to reduce the losses to 5 percent.[23] Sidwell and co-workers found that the binding quality of the semolina was not visibly modified by the addition of 10 percent FPC or less.[1]

The addition of the protein supplements has a definite bearing on the texture of the cooked pasta. The addition of the dried skim milk caused the cooking time for the pasta to shorten while the addition of soy caused it to lengthen, based on the more or less standard time of 10 minutes. The cooked characteristics of pasta with FPC were very much like the ones for the control.

All the pastas were cooked in unsalted tap water for 10 minutes. They were drained and served warm to the panelists. The results of the evaluation are listed in Table 5. The panelists observed the color difference: the FPC-pasta was grayish and the soy-pasta was a bright yellow. They did not pick up the texture differences between the milk pasta and the control, but they were aware of the hardness of the soy-pasta. The flavor of the FPC-pasta was as favorable as that of the control. They did not like the pasta with 6 percent protein from dried skim milk. Why the panelists did not like the pasta with 3 percent protein from soy is difficult to explain.

Snacks Fortified with FPC

Snacks are widely eaten in the United States; in fact, it is a $3 billion business which may offer another way to incorporate high protein supplements into a diet.

Table 5. Sensory evaluation of pasta
fortified with either 3 or 6% protein from
various high-protein supplements or with .2
and .4% lysine and cooked for 10 minutes

Composition	Amount Protein Added %	Appearance[1]	Texture[2]	Flavor[3]
Semolina		3.00	3.13	2.93
Semolina with:				
3.5% FPC[4]	3	2.71	3.00	3.04
7.5% FPC	6	1.25	3.00	3.04
8.4% DSM[5]	3	3.17	3.00	3.17
16.8% DSM	6	3.00	3.00	2.54
5.7% soy[6]	3	2.21	3.75	2.67
11.4% soy	6	2.04	3.75	3.29
.2% lysine		2.83	3.80	2.71
,4% lysine		3.00	3.12	3.25

----

[1]Equal to standard 3; lighter than standard,
greater than 3; darker, less than 3.

[2]Equal to the standard 3; firmer than
standard, greater than 3; softer, less than 3.

[3]Equal to standard 3; milder than standard,
greater than 3; stronger, less than 3.

[4]Fish protein concentrate.

[5]Dried skim milk.

[6]Soy flour.

Crackers. Sidwell and Stillings investigated
the possibility of adding FPC to saltines.
Crackers were made in Nabisco's pilot plant in
Fairlawn, New Jersey, according to their formulation, to which FPC was added.

In the one experiment, 10 percent of the
flour was replaced with FPC. The main objective was to note the effect of processing on
the nutritive value of the protein-rich
cracker. Baking did not affect its nutritive
value.

In a second study, the saltines contained
varying amounts (0, 4, 8, 12, and 16 percent)
of FPC. The objective was to study not only
the nutritive quality, but also the physical
and sensory characteristics. The supplementation of 4 percent almost tripled the nutritive quality; 8 percent almost quadrupled it.

The panelists found no significant differences in texture until 16 percent FPC was
added to the formulation when they also per-
ceived a flavor and color difference.

The cracker became harder with each increment, until 16 percent FPC was added. This
asset may be advantageously used in a biscuit
or cracker-type product.

No rancidity or other storage changes were
observed in crackers containing 0, 4, and 8
percent FPC after storage in an air-tight
container for 161 days at temperatures of 72,
90, 108, and 126° F. [24]

Donuts. Rusoff et al. added a number of high-
protein supplements to donut mixes. The most
successful supplements were toasted soy,
whole fish FPC, fish fillet FPC, and peanut
and cottonseed proteins. Other protein supplements like wheat gluten, and soy albumin
casein derivatives made a poor high-protein
donut. Many protein supplements cannot be
used in preparing mixes because the water
absorption is so high that it interferes with

the mechanical extrusion for automated production of donuts or donutlike products.[25] Rusoff reported that the donuts with FPC were highly acceptable.[26]

At our laboratory we did some work on yeast-raised donuts and found that with each addition of FPC the delicate texture of the donut decreased and it became more breadlike. The fat absorption was low. The flavor and appearance were quite acceptable. We felt that this fortified donut could be a basis for a high-protein breakfast snack.[1]

We have tried to extrude doughs fortified with 10 percent FPC by several methods. We found that doughs can be portioned, rolled, and formed into a pretzel with no change in the operation. The dough was a little short at the beginning, but upon standing about 10 minutes it lost the shortness and the operation proceeded without difficulty. The only modification in the processing suggested by the author is a reduction of heat during the baking so the color would be lighter.[1]

A mixture of corn meal and FPC was cooked under pressure, then extruded to make a puffed snack called corn curls. The physical characteristics were alike for the curl with FPC and without FPC. The change in color due to the FPC was the biggest difference.[1]

Beverage. It is possible to include FPC as the source of protein in a beverage using the following formulation: 4 percent FPC; 3 percent fat; 10 percent carbohydrates; 0.2 percent sodium citrate; 0.3 percent carrageenan; and 82.5 percent water. A variety of emulsifiers-stabilizers can be used in this formulation. They all will keep the materials in suspension for at least twelve hours.

The dry ingredients were mixed and added to hot water to which the fat has been added. Also a small amount of hydrogen peroxide added

to the mixture removed traces of undesirable
flavors. The mixture was heated to 175° F and
held for 20 minutes, homogenized, cooled
rapidly, and then spray dried. The dried
product could be easily reconstituted in water
to form a stable beverage.
   The composition of the beverage is comparable to cow's milk in respect to protein and
fat, but it contains twice as many carbohydrates. To this the necessary vitamins and
minerals can be added which would help to make
it a more complete nutritional beverage. The
flavor of the basic formulation is quite
bland, so it can be readily used for infant
feeding. It can be colored and flavored to
appeal to the older age groups.[16,21]
   Soups can be made from FPC in combination
with spices and flavorings, or it can be combined with legumes and/or vegetables. Since
legumes play an important role in diets of
many population groups, it may be advantageous
to make soup mixes with legumes and FPC. A
sensory evaluation of pea soup containing
varying amounts of FPC on the dry weight basis
showed that the panelists accepted the soup
with 5 percent or 10 percent FPC as well as
the soup with no FPC.
   Contasso reported that in Peru, Verrando
developed a soup mixture that contains 30 percent FPC, 8 percent dried skim milk, 25 percent rice flour, 6 percent semolina, 12 percent green pea flour, 4 percent potato starch,
7 percent salt, and 8 percent condiments and
seasonings. In 1965 Verrando was selling this
soup mixture, 130 grams per package for 5.90
soles. I was not able to find information on
the success of this market test.[27]

Conclusions and Comments
FPCs that vary in flavor, color, and odor
should be available to food manufactures.
Which one the user will choose depends upon

the food product and the level of fortification.

FPC can be used in a wide range of food
products. The suggested fortification level
is 6 to 8 percent of the dry ingredients, for
then the problems of handling and of changes
in formulation and of flavor are minimal.

The limited information available indicates
that when comparable amounts of FPC, dried
skim milk, and soy flour are incorporated into
a food product, FPC poses less problems in the
modification of an established formulation.

By no means are all the problems in the use
of FPC solved. So far most of the work on
fortification has been done with the cereals,
wheat, and corn. Additional questions still
remain. For example, how does the flavor of
FPC blend with other cereals such as oats and
rye? Can a more flavorable FPC be blended
with soy to make an acceptable high-protein
supplement. In what foods can the FPCs with
varying degrees of flavor be utilized? In
this case the combination of flavors becomes
especially important. We found, quite by
accident, that artificial smoke and ham flavor
cannot be used in a navy bean soup fortified
with FPC. Upon standing, a smoked herring
flavor developed. The same was true when the
oil of orange was used to flavor a sponge cake
fortified with FPC--a definite fish flavor
developed.

Last, but not least, we need a long term
acceptability study. We need to know if the
FPC-enriched products can be eaten over and
over again. This factor becomes especially
important if the more flavorful FPC are used
to fortify foods.

References

1.   Sidwell, V. D., unpublished data.

2. Chichester, C. O., Monckeberg, F., and
Yanez, E. 1969. The determination of nutri-
tional effectiveness and acceptability of fish
protein concentrate. Joint UNIDO/FAO Expert
Group Meeting on Production of Fish Protein
Concentrate, Rabat, Morocco, December 8-12.

3. Schaus, R. L. 1971. Bread the staff of
life is getting stronger. Cereal Science
Today 16: 178.

4. American Association of Cereal Chemists.
1970. Chemists Cereal Laboratory Methods,
Section 10-50. St. Paul: The American
Association of Cereal Chemists.

5. Sidwell, V. D., and Hammerle, O. A. 1971.
Changes in physical and sensory characteristics of doughs and of bread containing various
amounts of fish protein concentrate and
lysine. Cereal Chem. 47: 739.

6. Pomeranz, Y., Shogren, M. D., and Fenney,
K. F. 1969. Improving breadmaking properties
with glycolipids. 2. Improving various protein enriched products. Cereal Chem. 46: 512.

7. Tsen, C. C., Hoover, W. J., and Phillips,
D. 1971. High-protein breads. Use of
sodium stearoyl-2 lactylate in their production. Bakers Digest 45: 20.

8. Vergara Uribe, A. 1954. Harina de
pescado para consumo humano, pruebas de
aceptabilidad al gusto. Arch. Venezolanos
Nutr. 5: 365.

9. South African Council for Scientific and
Industrial Research, National Nutrition
Research Institute, Pretoria, 1959. A study
of principles of food enrichment and their
application to foods policy in South Africa

with reference to the use of fish flour for
the protein enrichment of bread. C.S.I.R.
Res. Rpt. 172.

10. Sen, D. P., Sayanarayana Rao, T. S.,
Kadkol, S. B., Krishnaswamy, M. A.,
Venkata Rao, S., and Lahiry, N. L. 1969.
Fish protein concentrate from Bombay-Duck
(Harpoden nehereus) fish: Effect on process-
ing variables on the nutritional and organo-
leptic qualities. Food Technol. 23: 85.

11. Bass, Janet L., and Caul, Jean F. 1972.
Laboratory evaluation of three protein
sources for use in chapati flours. J. Food.
Sci. 37: 100.

12. Gomez, F., Ramos-Galvan, R., Cravioto, J.
Frenk, S., and Labardini, I. 1958. Studies
on the use of deodorized fish flour in malnutrition. Bol. Med. Hosp. Infantil (Mexico)
15: 485.

13. Sidwell, V. D., Stillings, B. R., Knobl,
G. M., Jr. 1970. The fish Protein concentrate story. 10. U. S. Bureau of Commercial
Fisheries FPC's: Nutritional quality and use
in foods. Food Technol. 24: 40.

14. Nath, R. L., Dutt, Rama, Pain, S. K.
1960. Preparation of protein-rich biscuit
with fish flour. Bull. Calcutta Sch. Trop.
Med. 8: 161.

15. Nath, R. L., Ghosh, N. K., Dutt, Rama.
1961. Preparation of protein-rich biscuit
with fish flour from hammerhead shark
(Zygoena blochii). Bull. Calcutta Sch. Trop.
Med. 9: 12.

16. Thomson, F. A., and Merry, E. 1962.
Weight increase in toddler children in the

Federation of Malaya: A comparison of dietary
supplements of skim milk and fish biscuits.
Brit. J. Nutr. 16: 175.

17. Sidwell, V. D., Stillings, B. R., and
Hammerle, O. A. 1969. Use of fish protein
concentrate in foods: The physical character-
istics and sensory evaluation of pasta made
from wheat protein concentrate and semolina.
The 54th Annual Meeting of the American
Association of Cereal Chemists, Chicago,
Illinois, April 27-May 1.

18. Sidwell, V. D. 1967. FPC in foods.
Activities Report 19: 118.

19. Crisan, Eli V. 1970. The fish protein
concentrate story. 2. A demonstration program
in Brazil. Food Technol. 24: 90.

20. Baertl, J. M., Morales, E., Verastegui,
G., Cordano, A., Graham, G. G. 1966. Supplementation of a community with noodles enriched
with 10% fish protein concentrate. The VII
Intl. Cong. Nutr., Hamburg.

21. Baertl, Juan M., Morales, Enrique,
Verastegui, G., Graham, George G. 1970. Diet
supplementation for entire communities. Amer.
J. Clin. Nutr. 23: 707.

22. Woo, Choi Haynie, and Erdman, Anne Marie.
1971. Fish protein concentrate enrichment of
noodles. J. Home Econ. 63: 263.

23. Kapsiotis, G. D. 1968. The potential
utilization of FPC with special reference to
the Moroccan FPC. PAG Document R8/Add. 19.

24. Sidwell, V. D., and Stillings, B. R.
1972. Crackers, fortified with fish protein concentrate. Nutrition quality,

sensory and physical characteristics. J.
Amer. Diet. Assoc. 61: 276.

25. Rusoff, I. I., Goodman, A. H., Sommer,
J., and Cantor, S. M.   1964.   Protein fortification of doughnuts. Food Technol. 18:
131.

26. Rusoff, Irving I. Personal communication.

27. Contasso, Gustavo. 1965. Developments
of fish protein concentrate in Peru. Verando
process. WHO/FAO/UNICEF Meeting, Rome. PAG
Document 8/Add. 18.

XV
ENZYMATIC SOLUBILIZATION OF·FPC

M. C. Archer
S. R. Tannenbaum
and
D. I. C. Wang
Massachusetts Institute of Technology,
Cambridge, Massachusetts 02139

FPC prepared by solvent extraction of whole
fish is a highly denatured product which has
poor functional properties for incorporation
into food systems. It is not readily soluble
or dispersible, and it has poor wetting and
swelling properties. Although efforts have
been made to solubilize FPC,[1-6] a poor understanding of several process and kinetic factors has precluded the development of a continuous FPC solubilization process.

We have, therefore, examined in detail,
factors important for process design and have
described a process for the continuous production of kilogram quantities of soluble FPC per
day using enzyme digestion. (Part of the results presented here has been published elsewhere.)[7]

All experiments reported here utilized
"Monzyme", a mixture of neutral and alkaline
proteases obtained from <u>Bacillus</u> <u>subtilis</u>,
which was supplied by Monsanto Company, St.
Louis, Mo.; and red hake-FPC which was supplied by the National Marine Fisheries Service, College Park, Md.

Microbial Contamination during FPC
Solubilization

Few processes discussed in the literature deal
with the problem of microbial contamination.
FPC was solubilized in a continuous enzymatic
process in which sterilization of the input

streams was not possible. Microbial contamination of the feed streams and the reactor was
anticipated and indeed found. The problem was
tackled by attempting to define conditions
which would prevent growth of the organism(s)
    The contaminant tolerated temperatures up
to 60° C and pHs up to 8.0. At 70° C, however, there was no growth at any of the pHs
tested, and at pH 8.8 there was no growth at
any of the temperatures tested. The latter
finding is important because Monzyme possesses
proteolytic activities in the alkaline pH
region.[8]

Salt Accumulation during FPC Solubilization
Good enzyme activity and elimination of
microbial contamination were achieved by operating the enzyme reactor at pH 8.8. When
sodium hydroxide was used to maintain this pH
and to compensate for peptide bond cleavage,
however, undesirable salt formation resulted
when the product was neutralized. When
ammonia was used instead of sodium hydroxide,
the same degree of solubilization was obtained. Furthermore, dehydration of the final
product on a rotary evaporator completely removed the excess base, leaving a product with
a pH of 6.8 when resuspended in water.

Kinetics of FPC Solubilization
The Effect of pH and Temperature. A rather
flat profile for FPC solubilization over a pH
range of 6 to 10 was obtained as anticipated.[8,9] High activity was achieved at pH
8.8, a condition which also eliminates microbial growth.
    The temperature optimum for solubilization
of FPC for one hour at pH 8.8 was 50 to 60° C.

Enzyme Adsorption and Biphasic Kinetics. The
rate of reaction between a soluble enzyme and
an insoluble substrate has been shown to be

proportional to the amount of adsorbed
enzyme.[10] To test whether our system behaved
this way, 100 mg of Monzyme were allowed to
react with 10 g of FPC in a volume of 100 ml
at 40° C and pH 8.8. After five minutes of
reaction, the mixture was centrifuged; the
insoluble portion was washed with water, resuspended at pH 8.8 and 40° C, and allowed to
react for an additional 55 minutes. Figure 1
shows the amount of proteolysis measured by
base addition as a function of time. The
control (open circles) represents FPC acted on
by the full amount of enzyme for 60 minutes.
The degrees of solubilization corresponding to
points A, B, and C in Figure 1 are 30, 51, and
57 percent respectively. Thus, despite a
large difference in base addition, there is
little difference in the amount of protein
solubilized. This experiment was repeated using an initial reaction with varying amounts
of enzyme for two minutes followed by centrifugation, washing, resuspension, and reaction
for 58 minutes; these results appear in Table
1. Table 2 shows the effect of initial enzyme
concentration and equilibration time on the
distribution of Monzyme in the supernatant and
pellet.

Our findings indicate that the enzyme in-
teracts with FPC suspensions partly by rapid
adsorption onto FPC particles, leading to the
solubilization of insoluble protein, and partly by proteolysis of the protein fragments already in solution which have been cleaved by
the adsorbed enzyme. Once the enzyme equili-
brates with FPC, the remaining free enzyme can
be removed with little or no difference in the
yield of soluble protein.

Figure 2 shows typical solubilization
curves which were obtained during the digestion of FPC by Monzyme at pH 8.8 and 40° C.
The kinetics of these curves did not obey
simple integral order kinetics. The data

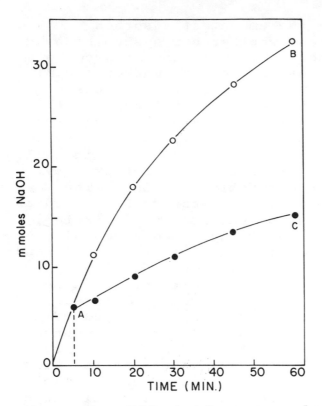

Figure 1. Effect of enzyme adsorption on base addition: (0) reaction with full amount of enzyme; (0) reaction with full amount of enzyme for 5 min followed by centrifugation and resuspension of pellet in water for 55 min. Reaction conditions: 100 mg/ml of FPC, 1 mg/ml of Monzyme, pH 8.8, 40° C. (Archer et al. 1972).

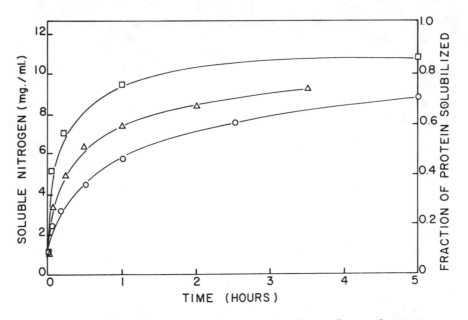

Figure 2.   Effects of enzyme levels of FPC
solubilization: (0) 0.4 mg/ml Monzyme; (Δ)
1.0 mg/ml Monzyme; ( ) 5.0 mg/ml Monzyme.
Reaction conditions: 100 mg/ml of FPC, pH
8.8, 40° C.   Archer et al. (0).

Table I. Effect of Enzyme Concentration on Adsorption

Enzyme Concentration, mg/ml	Solubilization[a,c]	Solubilization[b,c]
0.2	45	35
1.0	57	54
5.0	74	74

----

[a]Reaction with full amount of enzyme for 1 hr.
[b]Reaction with full amount of enzyme for 2 min, followed by centrifugation and resuspension of pellet in water for 58 min.
[c]Reaction conditions: 100 mg/ml of FPC; pH 8.8; 40° C.
(Archer et al. (7)).

Table II. Distribution of Monzyme in
Supernatant and Pellet

Enzyme Concentration, mg/ml	Fraction[a]	% Total Enzyme Activity (± 5%)[b]	
		2 min	10 min
0.05	sn	61	58
	p	39	42
0.10	sn	67	59
	p	33	41
0.20	sn	69	66
	p	31	34
1.0	sn	74	75
	p	26	25
5.0	sn	76	79
	p	24	21

----

[a]sn = supernatant, p = pellet.
[b]Reaction Conditions: 100 mg/ml of FPC, pH
8.8, 40° C. Each value is average of 3
determinations.
(Archer et al. (7)).

could be fitted, however, to a sequence of two first-order reactions. A combination of the first-order rate law and its integrated form yields:[11]

$$\ln dS/dt \; . \; \ln(-kS_0) - kt$$

where

S_0 = substrate concentration at time t = 0
S = substrate concentration at time t
t = time
k = first-order rate constant

An analysis of the solubilization rate by plotting the log of the rate versus time appears in Figure 3. The plot is distinctly biphasic with an initial fast reaction in the region designated as "a", followed by a slower reaction in the region designated as "b". Similar biphasic kinetics were obtained by Mihalyi and Harrington in their study of the tryptic digestion of myosin.[11]

The kinetics of FPC solubilization suggest a model in which the enzyme adsorbs to an insoluble protein particle and in a fast reaction, cleaves off polypeptide chains that are loosely bound to the surface. Solubilization of the more compacted core protein takes place more slowly.

The Continuous Production of Soluble FPC

An attempt was made to translate some of the process and kinetic considerations discussed above into a continuous operation for the production of soluble FPC.

A five-liter fermentation vessel was used as an enzyme reactor (Figure 4). Three four-bladed turbines with four stationary baffle plates were used to maintain a well-mixed FPC slurry of three liters with no vortex formation. One of the turbine blades was positioned just below the liquid surface in order to ensure that the solid was rapidly mixed as it fell into the reactor. A major problem with this system was that FPC settled in the

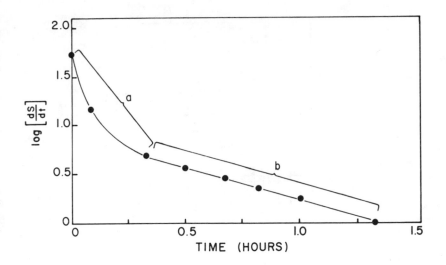

Figure 3. Log (rate) vs. time for
solubilization of FPC. Reaction conditions:
10 0 mg/ml of FPC, pH 8.8, 40° C, 5 mg/ml of
Monzyme. (Archer et al. (7)).

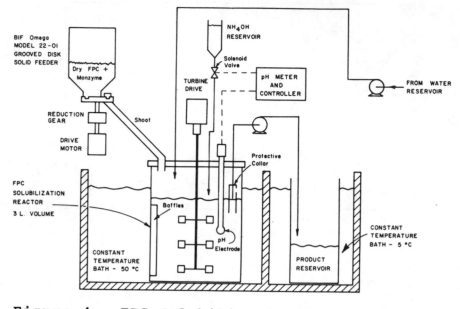

Figure 4. FPC Solubilization Reactor Layout.

holding tank and feed lines despite vigorous
stirring. This led to a variable solids content in the reactor. In addition, loss of
enzyme activity in the storage reservoir even
at 0° C was a problem.
     In order to eliminate the difficulty of
pumping an FPC slurry, we decided to feed FPC
into the reactor as a solid. A grooved disc
feeder gave a good reproducible metering of
FPC. The problem of enzyme activity loss in
the storage reservoir was solved by preblend-
ing the enzyme and FPC as solids in the
correct proportions prior to feeding them into
the reactor. This way the enzyme/FPC ratio
was automatically maintained at a constant
level throughout a run. No selective settling
of the enzyme or of the FPC occurred in the
hopper and the mixture remained well blended
throughout. Using batch kinetic data, an
enzyme/FPC ratio of 1 percent was chosen as a
compromise between high overall conversions
and the cost of enzymes, which are not recovered in this process.
     The product was removed from the reactor,
using a constant head tube connected to a
peristaltic pump operating at high speed. A
steel collar which dipped about four inches
under the liquid surface was fitted around the
constant head tube so that no unwetted, unre-
acted FPC was pumped off the surface. The
product was collected in a reservoir at 0 to
5° C.
     An example of results obtained from a
continuous run is shown in Figure 5. The
first hour of operation was a batch reaction
after which the run was continuous. Steady
state conditions were reached very quickly,
possibly after one hour residence time.

The Effect of FPC Concentration. Since a
major cost factor in the production of solubilized FPC is likely to be dehydration, we

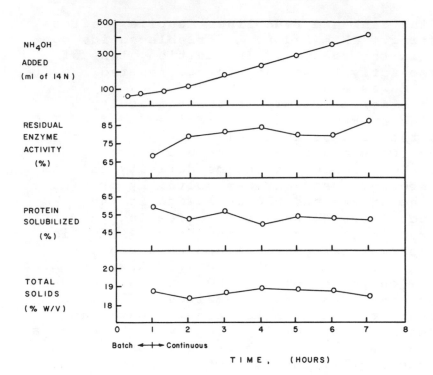

Figure 5. Continuous Solubilization of FPC
at 20% FPC Concentration, 1% Monzyme/FPC,
50° C, pH 8.8, 1 hour residence time.

investigated the use of high FPC concentrations in the reactor while maintaining the
enzyme/FPC ratio constant. The results are
shown in Figure 6. Thirty percent solids is
the upper limit for efficient operation of the
continuous reactor. We tried to obtain solids
of 35 to 40 percent by slowly and continuously
adding an increasing amount of FPC to the reactor containing partly digested 30 percent
FPC, but at over 30 percent the reaction mixture became pastelike in consistency and could
not be pumped to be stirred efficiently.
Maximum solid concentrations were about 10
percent higher in the continuous reactor than
in an equivalent batch reactor because the
viscosities of suspensions of partially digested material are lower than the limiting initial viscosity in a batch reactor.

The results show a marked drop in the overall conversion of FPC to a soluble product
going from 5 to 30 percent solids concentration. In the design of an FPC process, the
reduction in cost gained from a high solids
concentration in the reactor must be balanced
against the resulting increase in cost due to
lower conversion to a soluble product.

The Effect of Residence Time. The effect of
time on the yield of soluble FPC is shown in
Figure 7. After an initial fast rate of
digestion over a period of one to 20 hours,
the rate decreased rapidly with an increase of
about 10 percent in the soluble product over
the next two hours. The result was anticipated from our batch kinetic data. Two factors were responsible for this diminution in
rate: enzyme deactivation and biphasic nature
of the kinetics whereby an initial fast reaction is followed by a second slower reaction.
Forty to 50 percent of the initial enzyme
activity is lost during the first two hours of
reaction, but after that time activity is lost

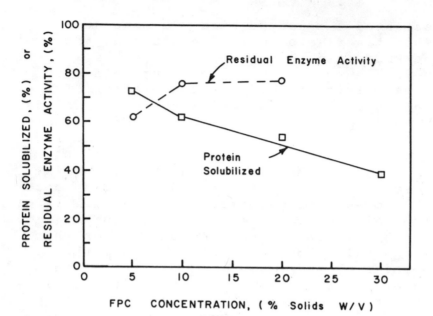

Figure 6. % FPC Solubilization and Remaining
Enzyme Activity at Various FPC Feed Concentrations.

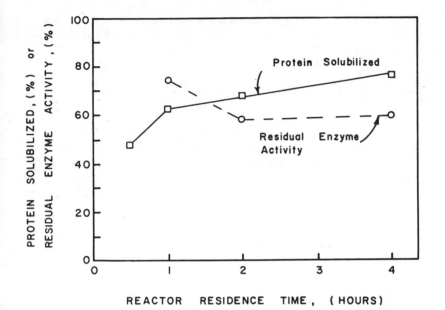

Figure 7. % FPC Solubilization or Remaining
Enzyme Activity at Various Residence Times.

slowly. This may be due to the stabilization
of enzyme activity by adsorption onto the protein particles.

Resuspension of Residue after Centrifugation.
Assuming that about 60 percent of the protein
in FPC (83.5 percent protein by weight) is
solubilized by one-stage enzymatic digestion,
a residue containing roughly 65 percent protein by weight is obtained after the removal
of the soluble material. This may be used as
a low-grade product possibly for animal feed.
However, since the enzyme is adsorbed to the
insoluble material during digestion, further
digestion can take place without the addition
of more enzyme.

Eighteen liters of digested FPC slurry containing 18.9 percent solids were passed directly into a Sharples Model M-47-11Y
Centrifuge with a bowl speed of 7500 rpm.
Twelve liters of centrifugate containing 11.2
percent solids were obtained. Sampling prior
to centrifugation indicated that 63 percent of
the protein was solubilized. The recovery of
soluble protein after centrifugation was
roughly 75 percent. The residue was recovered
from the centrifuge bowl and resuspended in
water. Three liters of this slurry containing
13 percent solids were then reacted for six
hours more at 50° C and pH 8.8. Figure 8
shows the time course for this reaction. At
time zero, 27 percent of the solids in the reactor was soluble and represented the soluble
material lost during centrifugation. A further 20 percent of the solids in the reactor
was solubilized in six hours. The residual
enzyme activity is a sum of activity due to
adsorbed enzyme and enzyme carried over with
the soluble solids. Expressed on a protein
basis and assuming no losses during centrifugation, the total yield of soluble product
after two hours residence time in the

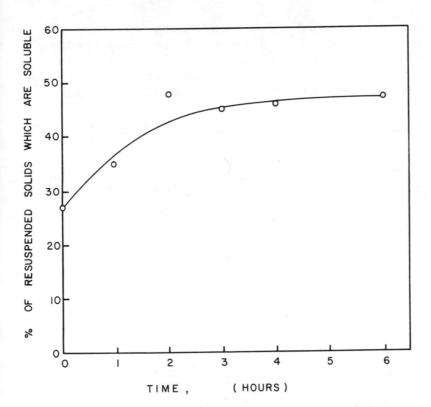

Figure 8.   Resolubilization of Residue
after Centrifugation of Digested FPC (13%
Solids, 50° C, pH 8.8).

continuous reactor plus six hours of resolubilization is 78 percent as compared to 63 percent before resuspension. The residue after resolubilization now contains roughly 50 percent protein by weight assuming no losses.

Enzyme Deactivation and Dehydration of the Product. Experiments indicated that spray drying of the product at drier outlet temperatures of 80 to 100° C did not destroy the proteolytic activity in FPC hydrolysates. A separate operation for the purpose of eliminating residual enzyme activity had to be designed.

The thermal denaturation curves for Monzyme in the presence of the substrate (hydrolyzed FPC) showed first-order kinetic behavior at temperatures above 60° C and gave an activation energy of 72 Kcal/mole for the deactivation process.

The FPC hydrolysate was pumped from the centrifuge directly through coils maintained at 90° C. After a two minute residence time at this temperature, zero protease and amylase activity was recorded.

The product was dehydrated in a spray dryer with a nozzle inlet. An inlet temperature of 220° C and an outlet temperature of 96 to 100° C were used. A dry, pale yellow product was obtained with no indication of browning. The product, which was freely soluble in water, had a moisture content of 3 to 4 percent and the pH of the material dissolved in water was 6.3. Further evaluation of the product has not been undertaken at this time.

References

1. Roels, O. A. 1969. Nutr. Rev. 27: 35.

2. Tannenbaum, S. R., Ahern, M., and

Bates, R. P.   1970.   Food. Technol. 24: 96.

3.   Tannenbaum, S. R., Bates, R. P., and
Brodfeld, L.   1970.   Food. Technol. 24: 99.

4.   Hale, M. B.   1972.   National Oceanic and
Atmospheric Administration, Technical Report,
NMFS SSRF-057.

5.   Rutman, M.   1971.   U. S. Patent No.
3,561,973.

6.   Cheftel, C., Ahern, M., Wang, D. I.C., and
Tannenbaum, S. R.   1971.   J. Agr. Food Chem.
19: 155.

7.   Archer, M. C., Ragnarsson, J. O.,
Tannenbaum, S. R., and Wang, D. I. C.   1973.
Biotech. Bioeng. 15: 181.

8.   Keay, L., and Wildi, B. S.   1970.
Biotech. Bioeng. 12: 179.

9.   Keay, L., Moser, P. W., and Wildi, B. S.
1970.   Biotech. Bioeng. 12: 213.

10.   McLaren, A. D.   1963.   Enzymologia 26:
237.

11.   Mihalyi, E., and Harrington, W. R.   1959.
Biochem. Biophys. Acta 36: 447.

XVI
ACCEPTABILITY OF FPC PRODUCTS

G. M. Dreosti
South African Fish Meal Producers Association
Limited, Cape Town, South Africa

The problem of making an extracted FPC with a
neutral odor and flavor, and of light tan
color, with a high protein content and quality
was solved in 1937 by the extraction with 92
percent ethanol of fish meal which was made
under hygienic conditions from fresh fish and
stored immediately after manufacture in an
inert gas until needed. However, the problem
of finding acceptable uses for FPC proved to
be much more difficult than its manufacture.
Little success was attained in trying to market a tasteless, odorless, shapeless product,
which was milled almost to dust and had no
functional properties, simply because it was
healthy. The food habits of underprivileged
people are firmly ingrained and, in any case,
they can hardly afford to buy fish meal, let
alone extracted FPC. For the time being, the
main purchasers of FPC would be large organizations such as governments and large mining
and manufacturing establishments for use in
food subsidization programs.

Uses in Africa
Our aim has been to produce the cheapest
possible FPC which would retain the protein
quality of the fish and remain undetected in
flavor and odor when added to products such as
brown bread at a level of 3 or 4 percent.
It has, therefore, always been made from fish
meal rather than by direct extraction of fresh
fish or press cake, since it is cheaper to use
a method which allows for extraction to proceed regularly throughout the year than one

which is geared to erratic fish landings.

Most of the FPC made in South Africa was incorporated into brown bread at up to 3 percent on a dry basis under subsidy from the government. The biological value of the wheat protein was considerably enhanced, and the volume, texture, elasticity, and toasting and keeping properties of the bread were improved. After using over 1200 tons of FPC in this way, however, the government subsidy on enriched brown bread was withdrawn as the FPC did not reach the target population. The underprivileged consumers preferred the more expensive white bread and the government was not prepared to subsidize its enrichment. In any case, FPC would have caused detectable darkening in white bread. The bread enrichment scheme was ill-conceived, as most of the underprivileged sections of the South African population consume little bread, the staple diet being a stiff maize porridge.

Smaller quantities of FPC (a few hundred tons per annum) were incorporated into Pro-Nutro, an inexpensive breakfast food also containing skim milk powders, defatted and heated soy beans, peanuts, food yeast, wheat germ, and added minerals and vitamins. Jacobsen claimed that none of the 1200 malnourished children to whom two ounces of ProNutro was fed daily over several years showed signs of kwashiorkor (a form of malnutrition), even though the children under test were all showing signs of malnutrition at the time of commencement of the test.

The NNRI (National Nutrition Research Institute) in Pretoria has developed a versatile enriching medium called PVM (for Proteine Verrykingsmedium) to be used on maize porridge or in soups or sauces at a level of about one ounce per small child per day. PVM contains cooked soy meal, skim milk powder, egg, minerals and vitamins, and 20 percent

extracted FPC. It also contains sodium
glutamate and curry powder, which impart a
slightly meaty flavor to the medium.

FPC has been used in a cancer hospital in
the form of a protein supplement for patients
who do not eat enough and consequently need
extra protein. There is also evidence to suggest (J. D. L. Hansen, private communication)
that it may be of value for patients who have
an intolerance to the lactose content of milk.
Experimental work at FIRI (Fishing Industry
Research Institute of South Africa) in Cape
Town has shown that FPC can be suitably incorporated into biscuits, provided that the sugar
content is kept low to avoid lysine damage
during baking due to Browning reactions. FPC
has also been successfully incorporated into
dried minced (crystalized) fruit, as well as
into soups, stews and sauces. Soup flavored
with curry, onion, sage, and to a lesser extent, with other herbs or spices could be made
even with imperfectly extracted FPC without
detection. The inclusion of inexpensive
digestive bran also masked the slight residual
odor and flavor in warm soup.

Human Preferences
The staple diet of malnouriched peoples usually consists of dishes made from cereals having
little flavor. In South Africa this is a
stiff porridge made from white maize. To a
taste panel consisting mostly of Africans
whose staple is porridge, even the most thoroughly multiple-extracted FPC was detectable
when added to the porridge. To a taste panel
consisting mostly of Europeans who seldom eat
porridge, the enriched porridge was indistin-
guished from the unenriched porridge. It was
found that the first-mentioned panel actually
preferred porridge containing 5, 10, or 20
percent fish meal, provided plenty of sugar
was added to the unenriched white maize

porridge. The second-mentioned panel found
this dish revolting.

We have found that, although extracted FPC
is useful for enriching foods having low
quality proteins without detection, we have
attained more success with fish meal whose
fats, phospholipids, and other odorous and
flavorous components have not been extracted.

Nonextracted FPC

Those who can only afford foods that consist
mainly of cereals generally try to find
flavorful additions to their bland diets. We
have, therefore, devoted our attention to the
production of nonextracted FPC, which is less
expensive, more nutritious, and more acceptable to those who need it.

Fish meal made from fresh fish has a fish
odor and flavor although it is not "fish
mealy" at the time of production. Therefore,
if it is stabilized immediately, it is possible to produce material that can be stored
for several years. We have done this by re-
placing the oil in fish meal with a more
stable lipid (a vegetable oil) and gas packing, and by means of an antioxidant (BHA) and
gas packing. Fish cakes made from material
stored several years were acceptable to both
taste panels at FIRI and were practically
indistinguishable from fish cakes made from
fresh fish. Such FPC made from fresh fish
after mechanical deboning should not be ground
very finely when it is intended for use in
fish cakes since the fiber and texture are of
considerable advantage in this product.

Ordinary unstabilized fish meal can be made
under hygienic conditions from fresh fish by
cooking, pressing, repressing, drying and
milling it. It should then be packaged
immediately in sealed containers and gas
packed to avoid oxidation. Such fish meal has
been tested in fish croquettes after prolonged

storage and found to be acceptable. Although
the product becomes rancid after the container
is opened, it is nevertheless acceptable to
those who are accustomed to far greater quantities of rancid oil in their diets. It could
be argued that the oxidation products may be
toxic; however, with an addition of about 3
percent FPC on a dry basis to the daily diet,
the amount of fish fat introduced to the diet
is about 0.3 percent, and the amount of oxidized fat is only about 0.1 percent on a dry
basis at maximum.

Nonextracted and Undried Products

The South African fishing industry has for
some years marketed canned, minced fish for
pets made from fresh pelagic fish. Much of
this has been eaten by human beings. The industry is, therefore, now also marketing
canned fish mince for human consumption as a
natural pack or spiced with chili. Although
this product would cost considerably more
than FPC on a unit of protein basis, it is,
nevertheless, relatively low in cost and useful as an alternative. The product is ready
for use and is acceptable to both well
nourished and malnourished communities. The
nutritional value considerably exceeds that of
extracted FPC and it is important that the
production of such a product needs no further
expensive research.

Some years ago, we prepared press cake from
fresh fish under hygienic conditions to which
we added sufficient salt to stabilize it. The
necessary salt content depended upon the moisture content, and products tested successfully
had salt contents varying from 14 to 18 percent and moisture contents from 43 to 49 percent. The press cake was kept in sealed
containers for many years after which it was
still in perfect condition. The test showed
that one could prepare press cake from fish

flesh, salt it immediately, add antioxidant if desired, and then prepackage it in plastic packages which could be packed in four or five gallon tins which are hermetically sealed. This product could be used for soups, stews and other dishes as an enriching medium. Bones could be ground finely and returned to the product if necessary.

In conclusion, more attention and more funds should be devoted to investigations concerning the preparation and use of other less expensive, stabilized or semistabilized fish products which would be readily accepted by those specific and differing groups who need such commodities most.

XVII
THE ENRICHMENT OF FOODS WITH FISH PROTEIN
CONCENTRATE

Enrique Yanez
Digna Ballester
and
Fernando Monckeberg
Laboratoria de Investigaciones Pediatricas,
Escuela de Medicina, Universidad de Chile,
Santiago, Chile

A great part of the world's population obtains
its daily protein requirements from sources
that are inadequate in both quantity and quality. Cereals, for example, constitute an important part of the diet of underdeveloped
countries in spite of their well-known deficiency in essential amino acids.

The nutritive value of the traditional
forms of cereal consumption would be significantly improved by the incorporation of animal
proteins, which contain a high concentration
of protein with an excellent amino acid
balance. It has been found that defatted fish
flour significantly improves the quality of
wheat, corn, and rice protein as evaluated by
the rate of growth and protein efficiency
ratio in rats.[1]

Based on our experience with the quality of
cereal protein,[2] it was decided to enrich some
foods widely consumed by the Chilean population with FPC made at Quintero, Chile.[3] The
most likely foods to be enriched with fish
flour were bread, pasta, cookies, high protein
mixtures for infants and preschool children,
and soups.

Bread
In a series of experiments, bread was enriched
with FPC at levels of 3, 6, 9 and 12 percent.

Table 1. Protein content and biological
quality of the protein of FPC-enriched bread

	Pro-tein	P %	NPUop[3]	NDp Cal %[4]
Bread	11.2	10.4	35	3.6
Bread + 3% FPC	13.0	12.5	-	-
Bread + 6% FPC	14.7	14.3	43	6.2
Bread + 9% FPC	16.5	15.6	-	-
Bread + 12% FPC	18.8	16.9	48	8.1
Bread + 12% dried skim milk	12.0	13.5	45	6.1

----

1. Percent by dry weight
2. Percentage of protein calories
3. Net protein utilization operative
4. Net dietary protein calories percent

It was observed that the loaf volume decreased
with increasing levels of FPC. The dough ab-
sorbed more water, altering the texture and
sponginess of the crumb, and crust coloration
increased, especially at the higher levels of
supplementation.

Although the protein value of the enriched
bread increased[4] (Table 1), the improvement
was less than expected, probably because of
protein damage during the baking process. The
addition of lysine to the 6 percent FPC-enriched bread improved its biological value up
to the expected levels, indicating that part
of the FPC lysine content was destroyed by
heat.

In acceptability tests, adults, including
university students, lactating women, and
workers, were asked to classify the enriched
bread as "acceptable", "as good as", or
"worse than" common bread.[5] Results showed
that at the 3 percent level there was no
significant difference between the nonenriched
and the enriched bread. At 6 percent, differ-
entiation became more apparent, and at 9 and
12 percent, the darker color caused considerable rejection. However, in a series of
assays done in a population of 300 school
children, bread enriched at 9 percent did not
show an increase in rejection, presumably because color was of less importance to children.

Pasta
Spaghetti, noodles, and macaroni are excellent vehicles for FPC. They remain unaltered
for long periods of time and are less likely
to suffer protein damage during production
than bread because the temperatures used are
lower than those used for bread baking.

The biological quality and acceptability of
spaghetti containing 10 percent FPC was
studied. Results showed that it was darker in

Table 2.   Protein Content and Biological
Quality of Spaghetti Enriched with FPC

	Protein[1]	P %[2]	NPUop[3]	NDp Cal %[4]
Spaghetti	11.5	11.9	38	4.5
Spaghetti + 10% FPC	18.0	19.1	47	9.0

----

1.   Percent by dry weight
2.   Percentage of protein calories
3.   Net protein utilization operative
4.   Net dietary protein calories percent

color--almost gray--and rougher in texture
than ordinary spaghetti, but the taste and
odor were the same. It was observed that
there was a significant increase in the percentage of calories, the biological quality
and the protein value as seen in Table 2.[6]
     Three acceptability tests were done: one
with adults and two with school children. In
the first test, 150 hospital personnel and 300
patients received one portion of enriched
spaghetti. In the second, 150 school children
received a portion of enriched spaghetti three
times a week for a three-month period. In the
third, 200 school children participating in a
school lunch program of the Office of National
Student Auxiliary and Scholarships received a
portion of enriched spaghetti twice a week for
a month and a half. In all three tests, the
spaghetti met with optimum acceptability as
measured by the quotient between the served
and the eaten.
     In summary, spaghetti enriched with 10 per-
cent FPC is adequate from both the point of
view of protein quality and technological
feasibility.

Cookies

Children eat large quantities of cookies in
spite of their low nutritional value. It
would therefore be of special benefit if a
high quality protein concentrate could be
successfully added to their composition.
     Following the traditional procedures of the
cookie industry in Chile, cookies were prepared with 4, 8, and 12 percent fish flour,
which was added in place of wheat flour. Results showed that the color, odor, and taste
of the enriched cookies were the same as the
control cookies, and those enriched at 8 and
12 percent levels were harder than the controls and those enriched at 4 percent.
     Several acceptability tests were done with

groups of school children at different ages
enrolled in primary and high schools, as well
as with college students and adults. In every
test the acceptability was excellent.

Table 3 shows values of protein content and
protein efficiency ratio of regular cookies
and cookies enriched with FPC at different
percentages. The protein efficiency ratio of
regular cookies was in the range of 0 to 0.72,
while those with 10 percent FPC had PER values
ranging from 2.50 to 3.30.[7]

High Protein Mixtures for Infants and Preschool Children

In Chile, infant foods consumed by the majority of the low income population are of low
nutritive quality. They are basically composed of cereal flours, and therefore, their
protein content is low and the quality poor.
The protein value of these foods would be improved by the incorporation of a protein such
as FPC. Various mixtures were prepared to be
fully comparable to animal proteins as seen in
Tables 4 and 5.[6,8,9]

Mixtures given to infants for three months
and preschool children for ten months (mixtures 18 and 23) had excellent acceptability
with tolerance similar to cow's milk.[9] The
acceptability of Leche Alim was assayed for
twelve months in 1100 children from two to
five years old, who lived in both urban and
rural areas. Children under two continued receiving their powdered milk from the National
Health service as usual. All subjects were
weighed and measured once a month. At three
and twelve months, acceptability was found to
be satisfactory; it was lower than that of
powdered milk containing 12 percent fat and
similar to that of dry skim milk.

Soups

A variety of soups generally prepared with

Table 3. Protein content of regular cookies
and cookies enriched with FPC

	Crude Protein	PER
Cookies	5.7 - 8.2	0 - 0.72
Enriched cookies	10.3 - 10.4	2.50 - 3.30

Table 4. Proximate chemical composition (%)
and biological quality of ingredients of
protein-rich mixtures

	H_2O	Ether ex- tract	Ash	Crude fiber	Pro- tein	Avail- able lysine	NPU
Fish flour	7.3	0.2	15.9	-	75.8	8.6	67
Sunflower meal	6.8	1.7	8.7	10.8	42.8	2.8	51
Toasted wheat flour	4.2	1.9	2.2	0.9	13.4	-	34
Milk powder	7.2	12.0	6.8	-	32.0	7.5	76

Table 5. Protein quality of protein-rich
mixtures containing FPC

	P %	NDpCals %	PER
Mixture 18	35	12.3	-
Mixture 23	40	12.8	-
Leche Alim	29	14.7	2.56

vegetables, noodles, bones, or meat is a
major part of the Chilean diet. It was therefore decided to prepare powdered soups based
on legumes with the addition of 10 percent
fish flour. In comparison to other powdered
soups, the color of this product was slightly
darker; the texture varied slightly. No fish
odor was noticed, and the cooking process
caused no changes in color or odor. It was
assayed for three months with 20,000 children
registered in a school lunch program. The
acceptability was normal for that type of
product.

In summary, we think that our results indicate that it is possible to incorporate
FPC in a variety of foods based on cereals and
legumes significantly increasing the protein
quality without substantially modifying their
characteristics. This could contribute to the
solution of the shortage of good quality proteins that now affects millions of people in
every continent, especially young children in
developing countries.

References

1. Sure, B. 1957. The addition of small
amounts of defatted fish flour to milled
wheat flour, corn meal and rice. Influence on
growth and protein efficiency. J. Nutrition
61: 547.

2. Ballester, D., Tagle, M. A., Donoso, G.
1962. Utilization proteica neta de trigo,
maiz y algunos derivados de consumo popular.
Nutr. Bromatol Toxicol. 1: 235.

3. Yanez, E., Barja, I., Monckeberg, F.,
Maccioni, A. and Donoso, G. 1967. Quintero
fish protein concentrate: protein quality and
use in foods. Food Technol. 21: 1604.

4.   Donoso, G., and Yanez, E.   1963.   Valor
proteico del pan enriquecido con harina de
pescado.   Bol. Ofic. Sanit. Panamer. 55: 520.

5.   Donoso, G., Munoz, M., Barja, I.,
Durán, E., Urrea, M., and Santa Maria, J. V.
1963.   Enriquecimiento de pan con harina de
pescado de consumo humano.   1. Estudio de
panificacion y pruebas de aceptacion aguda.
Nutr. Bromatol. Toxicol. 2: 72.

6.   Yanez, E., Ballester, D., Maccioni, A.
Spada, R., Barja, I., Pak, N., Chichester,
C. O., Donoso, G., and Monckeberg, F.   1969.
Fish protein concentrate and sunflower press-
cake meal as protein sources for human con-
sumption.   Am. J. Clin. Nutr. 22: 878.

7.   Monckeberg, F., Ballester, D., and Yanez,
E.   1972.   El pescado y la reduccion de las
deficiencias nutricionales en paises en
desarrollo.   En: Seminario Internacional de
desarrollo pesquero-industrial.   Proceedings
of the meeting, Lima, Peru.

8.   Ballester, D., Barja, I., Yanez, E., and
Donoso, G.   1968.   Protein rich mixtures for
human consumption based on fish flour, sunflower presscake meal, dried skim milk and
wheat flour.   Br. J. Nutr. 22: 255.

9.   Vega, L., Gattas, V., Barja, I., and
Donoso, G.   1968.   Introduccion de mezclas
proteicas semi-convencionales en la alimenta-
cion habitual del pre-escolar.   Nutr. Bromatol. Toxicol. 7: 5.

XVIII
EFFECTS OF PROCESSING PARAMETERS ON THE
CHEMICAL AND FUNCTIONAL CHARACTERISTICS OF FPC

David L. Dubrow
College Park Fishery Products Technology
Laboratory, National Marine Fisheries Service,
National Oceanic & Atmospheric Administration,
U. S. Dept. of Commerce, College Park,
Maryland 20740

One of the problems of solvent extraction of
fish is the effect of the solvent temperature
and of the alcohol itself on the characteristics of the proteins.[1-4] In most cases, the
extraction temperature is at or near the boiling point of the solvent used. Extractions
using IPA (isopropyl alcohol) are made at
close to 80° C; however, most proteins undergo
changes in solubility characteristics at about
40 to 60° C.

Experiments were conducted at the Fishery
Products Technology Laboratory to determine
the lipid and protein characteristics of FPC
when it was extracted at 20, 40, and 50° C.[5]
Similar experiments were conducted to determine the effects of drying temperature and of
steam desolventization on the chemical and
functional characteristics of FPC.[6]

Extraction Temperature
A five-stage counter-current process was used
to determine the effect of the extraction temperature on lipid extractability from red hake
(Urophycis chuss).[7] The solvent to raw fish
ratio was 2:1 w/w or 10:1, based on a lipid-
free, moisture-free solid. Before bringing
the miscella up to extraction temperature, it
was chilled to 3° C to remove lipids from the
solvent system prior to contact with the raw
fish. Final wet solids were vacuum dried at

40 to 50° C, milled, and analyzed.

The 20° C (room temperature) extraction failed to remove enough lipids to meet the FDA specification of less than 0.5 percent. (Figure 1). Although the first cross-current run produced FPC with less than 0.5 percent, in subsequent counter-current runs, the residual lipids increased to a steady state condition of about 1 percent.

Other experimental evidence indicates that a first-stage cross-current dehydration followed by four counter-current stages will reduce the lipid level to about 0.35 percent, but this procedure requires more solvent. It may be possible to meet the 0.5 percent residual lipid level at or about room temperature by adding extra stages; by partially vacuum-evaporating the moisture prior to extraction; or by using better separation techniques than those used in these experiments.

The 40 or 50° C extraction can reduce the lipid content to below 0.5 percent in four stages and possibly in three, given better separation techniques. Therefore, it should be possible to lower the solvent losses which occur through high temperature volatilization.

Salt soluble protein from FPC extracted at 80° C ran at about 5 percent. Extraction at 20° C yielded nondesolventized FPC containing about 27 percent soluble protein; the contents decreased to 19 percent at 40° C; and 8.5 percent at 50° C. There was also a subsequent increase in the pH of the FPC as the temperature increased. Thus, the amount of soluble protein showed a negative correlation with the pH, $r = -0.8466$.

The emulsion stability was affected in the same manner as the soluble protein. FPC extracted at 20° C retained a heat stable emulsion, whereas FPC extracted at 40 and 50° C did not. Of course, laboratory tests are one thing, and actual food preparations may show

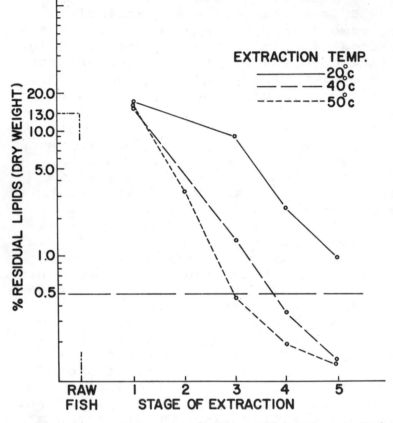

Figure 1.   Effect of Temperature on Extraction of Lipids from Whole Red Hake with
Isopropyl Alcohol (5 Stage Counter-Current).

different results. Dr. Anglemier's group at
Oregon State University prepared a weiner
product with various fish proteins, either
modified or as FPC. It was of interest that
the satisfactory product was made with standard IPA-extracted FPC where the normal temperature for extraction is 80° C.

Drying Time and Temperatures

The stage following extraction is the removal
of excess alcohol by drying. In order to
determine the effect of drying on the chemical
and functional constituents of FPC, several
drying times and temperatures were tested.
The protein solubility was shown to decrease
step-wise with temperature increase when last-
stage wet solids were dried for either 30 or
120 minutes at the temperatures indicated in
Table 1. The emulsion stability of FPC with
oil and water was considered good in all but
the treatment at the highest temperature.
Those emulsions showed a complete breakdown.
As indicated in Table 2, neither the drying
temperatures nor the amount of exposure to
temperature had any real effect on reducing
the residual IPA level to less than the 1 to 3
percent obtained from low temperature drying.

Desolventization

Steam desolventization of FPC solids can reduce the residual IPA to levels meeting
specifications of 250 ppm. However, when the
solids are subjected to steam desolventization, different results are obtained for dry
and wet solids. Whole Atlantic menhaden were
extracted by a five-stage cross-current process at room temperature. In the last stage,
the wet solids were divided into two portions:
one portion was desolventized while wet, and
the other portion was first low-temperature
aid dried. Desolventizing was performed by
steam stripping in an autoclave at 2 to 3 psi.

Table 1. Effect of Drying Temperature and Time on the Salt Soluble Protein and Emulsifying Capacity of FPC

Temperature °C	Time Hr.	Kjeldahl soluble nitrogen Mg N/ml	Soluble protein (N x 6.25) % dry wt	$\bar{x}$	Emulsifying capacity % water separated
Wet solids	-	1.17 ± .08[1]	36.56	36.56	0.0
Ambient	16	2.10 ± .04	36.43	36.43	0.0
40-50	0.5	1.80 ± .08	31.33		0.0
	2.0	1.76 ± .08	29.99	30.66	0.0
60-70	0.5	1.44 ± .03	24.06		0.0
	2.0	1.81 ± .11	31.46	27.76	0.0
90-100	0.5	1.76 ± .09	28.92		0.0
	2.0	1.62 ± .10	26.88	27.90	0.0
110-120	0.5	1.31 ± .04	21.64		0.0
	2.0	1.29 ± .03	21.42	21.53	-
140-150	0.5	0.84 ± .01	13.55		100
	1.0	0.77 ± .01	12.19		100
	2.0	0.73 ± .02	11.70	12.48	100

[1]standard deviation.

Table 2. Effect of Drying Temperature and Time on the Total Volatile and Residual Isopropyl Alcohol Contents of FPC

Temperature °C	Time Min.	Total volatiles %	Residual isopropyl alcohol %	x̄
Wet solids		50.00		
Ambient	16	9.94	2.00 ± .09	
40–50	30	10.25	2.47 ± .09	
	120	8.30	3.05 ± .17	2.76
60–70	30	6.50	2.85 ± .13	
	120	10.10	2.40 ± .14	2.62
90–100	30	4.90	2.75 ± .19	
	120	5.85	2.32 ± .13	2.53
110–120	30	5.40	2.55 ± .06	
	120	5.90	2.30 ± .14	2.42
140–150	30	3.20	1.50 ± .14	
	120	2.45	1.40 ± .18	1.45

Table 3. Effect of Steam Desolventizing FPC Wet Solids and FPC Dry Solids on the Salt Soluble Protein, Emulsifying Capacity, Color and Volatile Content

Sample	Time Min.	Salt soluble protein % of dry wt	Emulsifying capacity % water separated	Color L	a	b	Residual IPA ppm	Total volatiles %
Wet solids								
Non-desolventized	-	32.29	-	-	-	-	-	-
	0	9.49	20.01	62.02	+.30	+11.72	30,000	7.76
	5	8.57	24.31	52.94	+.35	+11.76	200	5.29
	10	10.52	20.71	50.83	+.71	+11.22	75.5	4.91
Dry solids								
Non-desolventized	-	28.23	0.0	-	-	-	55,000	11.44
	0	26.70	0.0	65.65	-.60	+10.75	24,500	6.38
	5	12.71	5.01	62.12	-.07	+12.15	1,000	5.35
	10	10.68	15.01	61.71	-.08	+12.50	367	4.91

1Separation into three phases: water, solids, emulsion.

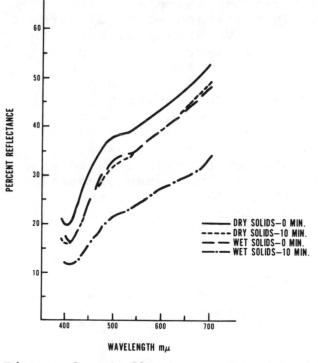

Figure 2.   Reflectance Scan Results.

The results of these tests are shown in Table
3. The wet solids contained about 32 percent
soluble protein prior to steaming, but within
the short period of come-up time, they lost a
major portion of this fraction. The dry
solids decreased in soluble protein as well,
but at a slower rate. The emulsion stability
of FPC samples also decreased with steam
desolventization, and the emulsions showed
complete separation into three phases.

The residual IPA was further reduced when
wet solids were steamed than when dry solids
were steamed. After five minutes, the residual alcohol in wet solids was reduced to 200
ppm, while in dry solids it was only reduced
to 1000 ppm.

In the area of color, wet solids darkened
considerably more than dry solids, as indicated by the L and a (redness) values in Table
3. This is also seen in Figure 2, where a
reflectance scan from 700 to 400 mu of FPC
desolventized for up to ten minutes. The dry
solids for each time period were lighter than
corresponding wet solids.

References

1. Herskovits, T. T., Gadegbeky, B., and
Jaillet, G. 1970. On the structural stabili-
ty and solvent denaturation of proteins. J.
Biol. Chem. 245: 2586.

2. Herskovits, T. T., and Jaillet, H. 1969.
Structural stability and solvent denaturation
of myoglobin. Science 163: 282.

3. Gerlsma, S. Y. 1968. Reversible denaturation of ribonuclease in aqueous solutions as
influenced by polyhydric alcohols and some
other additives. J. Biol. Chem. 243: 957.

4. Joly, M. A physico-chemical approach to the denaturation of proteins. New York: Academic Press.

5. Dubrow, D. L., and Kramer, A. Effect of temperature on lipid extraction and functional properties of fish protein concentrate (FPC). To be submitted to Food Science 38: 1012.

6. Dubrow, D. L. 1973. Effect of drying and desolventizing on the functional properties of fish protein concentrate (FPC). Submitted to Fishery Bulletin 71: 99.

7. Brown, N. L., and Miller, Harry Jr. 1969. Experimental production of fish protein concentrate (FPC) from Mediterranean sardines. Com. Fish. Rev. 31: 30.

XIX
UTILIZATION OF FISH PROTEIN CONCENTRATE OR
MARINE PROTEIN CONCENTRATE

Amara Bhumiratana
Institute of Food Research and Product
Development, Kasetsart University, Bangkok

Most Thais do not have a large enough income
to supply themselves with an adequate daily
diet, particularly in the form of proteins.
The situation has been exacerbated over the
years due to the rising cost of foods containing proteins, and especially animal proteins.
Research has been done to develop protein from
cereals; however, this source of protein must
be supplemented. For example, Kaset Protein,
Formula 18 contains 9 percent FPC and Kaset
Noodle contains up to 10 percent FPC.
     The problem of protein deficiency in Thai-
land begins in infancy. Babies have been fed
sweetened condensed milk, which has been declared to be unfit by the Ministry of Public
Health. Pounded rice, containing 5 percent
incomplete protein, has been used as a weaning
food. A weaning food using 100 parts pounded
rice, 25 parts full fat soy flour and five
parts FPC has been developed and is presently
being used in trial studies at the infant care
center in Amphoe Mae Rime, Chiengmai, Sirirai
Hospital, and at Ramathibodi Hospital.
     Attention is also being given to the
development of Marine Protein Concentrate from
cuttle fish and sea mussels, which are available in great quantity at very low cost. It
is difficult to use marine sources for direct
consumption due to transportation costs and
spoilage; and salting, fermenting, or pickling
limits the general applicability of the protein. Therefore, the development of a new
form of concentrate from local marine

resources will be an important aid to the
problem of protein deficiency in Thailand.

XX
STUDIES ON THE CHEMICAL MODIFICATION OF FISH PROTEIN CONCENTRATE

(Technical Paper #3352, Oregon Agriculture Experimental Station)

A. F. Anglemier
and
H. J. Petropakis
Department of Food Science and Technology,
Oregon State University, Corvallis, Oregon
97331

This report summarizes the work performed at Oregon State University during 1969-71 on the chemical modification of fish protein concentrate (FPC). The major objective of the research was to alter FPC to improve its functional properties.

Experimental

Materials. FPC samples were supplied by the National Center for Fish Protein Concentrate, NMFS, College Park, Maryland. Two types of FPC material were studied rather extensively. One type was the standard isopropyl alcohol (IPA) extracted material from ground, whole hake. This FPC had a proximate analysis of protein 87.7 percent, ash 11.9 percent, volatiles 2.1 percent, and lipid 0.1 percent. The other sample (B103/11) was prepared by less harsh extraction procedures; the second through fourth extractions were completed at room temperature rather than at 170°F, and the step of steam stripping to reduce the residual IPA at the end of process was omitted. Proximate analysis of this material was protein 84.9 percent, ash 13.8 percent, volatiles 3.2 percent, lipid 0.3 percent, and IPA 1.9 percent.

Two other types of FPC which were examined briefly will be described later.

Methods. A modification of the hot alkali procedure of Tannenbaum et al.[1] was used to hydrolyze FPC. Although varying amounts of FPC were mixed with different concentrations of aqueous sodium hydroxide, only the optimum conditions are given below.

Either 5 percent of standard-FPC or 5 percent of B109/11-FPC in 0.1N or 0.2N NaOH were hydrolyzed at 95-100°C for 10 to 15 minutes in a closed system with continuous agitation. After heating, the hydrolysis mixture was cooled to ambient temperature and centrifuged at 1,000xG for 20 minutes. The pH of the clear supernatant was adjusted from 12.5 to 4.5 by the addition of 6N HCl or 7 percent sulfurous acid with continuous agitation. At pH 4.5, isoelectric precipitation occurred and either centrifugation (15,000xG, 20 minutes) or careful decanting was used to recover the protein. The latter was then washed 3-4 times with water or water adjusted to pH 4.5 with sulfurous acid, which helped to bleach the final product. After washing, the protein was dispersed in water by continuous agitation and the addition of 1N NH_4OH until a pH range of 6.8-7.2 was achieved. The resulting solution was spray dried to yield a fluffy material hereafter referred to as M-FPC.

The supernatant retained from the isoelectric precipitation of the hydrolyzed FPC contained soluble protein which was collected by precipitation with sodium hexametaphosphate.[2] The latter material was added to these solutions to obtain final concentrations of 0.0005 M, 0.005 M or 0.01 M of the phosphate compound. The resulting solutions were adjusted to the desired pH by the addition of either 6N HCl or 2N NaOH. The

precipitated protein was collected by
centrifugation (15,000xG, 20 minutes) and
dried in vacuo. The dry material was dispersed in water and subsequently dissolved
when the pH was adjusted to 7.0 by the addition of NH_4OH. This solution was spray dried
and hereafter designated as HMPh-FPC.

Varying amounts of different edible vegetable colloids were used to improve the
dispersibility of M-FPC.

Selective gas chromatographic analysis[3]
was used to determine the dimethylamine (DMA)
and trimethylamine contents of standard-, M-
and HMPh-FPC's.

Results and Discussion
Greater yields of modified material were obtained when hydrolysis was carried out with
0.2N than with 0.1N NaOH. Optimum times of
hydrolysis for the two types of FPC varied
according to the original extraction procedures. A hydrolysis time of 15 minutes at 95
to 98°C was found to be optimal for 5 percent
standard-FPC in 0.2N NaOH as contrasted to 10
minutes for the B103/11-FPC.

Characteristics of the FPC hydrolyzed and
treated as above described are summarized
below.

Color and Odor. When 6N HCl was used for the
isoelectric precipitation, a light yellowish
material was obtained having a slight odor of
ocean water. Use of H_2SO_3 to adjust pH to
4.5 produced an almost white and practically
odor-free powder. The latter material was
slightly superior in color and odor to that
precipitated by HCl. Sulfurous acid was more
effective in bleaching and deodorizing the
final product. However, relatively large
volumes of H_2SO_3 were required to achieve an
equivalent amount of protein precipitated by
HCl; therefore, the former procedure would be

more costly and laborious to use. Further
work was completed in which both acids were
combined into one treatment to retain their
respective benefits. It was found that the
isoelectric precipitation could be completed
with 6N HCl, followed by washing the precipitated protein 3 to 4 times with water adjusted
to pH 4.5 with sulfurous acid, thereby obtaining the desired degree of bleaching.

Yield. About 65 to 70 percent of the original
FPC-protein can be recovered from the modification process. An additional 7 to 10 percent soluble protein can be recovered from the
sodium hexametaphosphate isoelectric precipitation of the supernatant of the original
hydrolyzate. A concentration of 0.01 M hexametaphosphate and a final pH of 3.5 are optimal for this recovery step.

Solubility. Hydrolyzed FPC precipitated
isoelectrically by either HCl or H_2SO_3 showed
very similar solubility properties. Both
types were fairly soluble in water at pH below 3.5 and above pH 5.5. A zone of insolu-
bility occurred in a pH range of 3.5 to 5.5.
The modified FPC could be dissolved in water
by gentle agitation up to levels of 4.5 to 5
percent in 8 to 10 minutes to form clear solutions. At levels of 6 percent or higher,
particulate matter began to form which gradually precipitated. The modified FPC was alkali labile. At pH 11.5 or higher, considerable
deamination occurred which caused the protein
to precipitate and become insoluble at pH
values on the acid side of the isoelectric
zone (pH 5.5 and below).

Protein and Ash Content. The protein content
(N x 6.25) of the modified FPC exceeded 94.5
percent. Mineral content of the M-FPC was
approximately 1 percent, indicating a

significant reduction from the initial level
of 12 percent.

Taste. The bitter or salty taste usually
associated with hydrolysis products was
noticeably absent in the M-FPC. The lack of
salty taste may have been due to the use of
NH_4OH during re-solubilization of the isoelectric precipitate and the subsequent spray drying.

Other Properties. In using a model system for
evaluating emulsifying capacity, a 3 percent
salt extract of the M-FPC had approximately
50 to 70 percent greater emulsifying capacity
than a 3 percent salt extract of lean beef
muscle. The over-run and foam stability of a
5 percent M-FPC in water solution, pH 7.0,
were equivalent to that of a 5 percent egg
albumin-water solution.

Protein precipitated with hexametaphosphate
was similar in color, taste and appearance to
the M-FPC.

The addition of V-7-E hydrophilic colloid
(Burtonite Co.), at a level of 1 percent of
the M-FPC dispersed in water (pH 6.8 to 7.2)
just prior to spray drying, improved the subsequent solubility properties. When this
dried material was added to water to make a 4
percent solution, complete solubilization
occurred in 3.5 minutes with gentle agitation,
as compared to the 8 to 10 minutes required to
solubilize M-FPC spray dried without V-7-E.
Final pH of the latter was 5.4, as compared to
an ultimate pH of 6.4 for the former solution.
This difference in pH may have contributed to
the higher solubility.

Brief studies were also conducted on the
modification of FPC extracted by the standard
IPA procedures from deboned hake, and that
prepared from deboned fish but extracted at
room temperature with omission of the

desolventizing and fluid energy bed grinding
procedures. The latter, sample B109/1, was
the least denatured of all material examined.
The deboned-FPC reacted similarly to the
standard-FPC extracted from whole fish during
alkali hydrolysis. However, difficulties
were encountered in hydrolyzing the less
harshly processed material (sample B109/1).
At concentrations exceeding 4 percent in 0.2N
NaOH, excessive swelling, increased viscosity,
and subsequent gelatinization occurred before
completion of a 10 minute hydrolysis period.
   Other work completed in our laboratories
indicated that standard IPA-extracted FPC
could be added to meat emulsions at levels of
1 to 3 percent in place of soy protein isolate without detracting from the quality of
the finished product. However, under mildly
acidic conditions, nitrites can react with
secondary amines to yield a class of
carcinogenic compounds, the nitrosamines.[4]
Thus, certain samples of FPC were analyzed
for their secondary amine contents. These results were:

	Dimethylamine	Trimethylamine
Standard FPC	150 ppm	5 ppm
Modified FPC	25 ppm	5 ppm
HMPh-FPC	30 ppm	5 ppm

Although chemical modification of FPC appre-
ciably reduced the secondary amine contents,
the amount remaining may still pose a potential hazard when allowed to come into contact
with nitrites.

References

1.   Tannenbaum, S. R., Ahern, M., and Bates,
R. P.   1970.   Solubilization of fish protein
concentrate.   I. An alkaline process.   Food
Technol. 24: 96.

2.   Spinelli, J., and Koury, B.   1970.
Phosphate complexes of soluble fish proteins:
Their formation and possible uses.   J. Agr.
Food Chem. 18: 284.

3.   Miller III, A., Scanlan, R. A., Lee,
J. S., and Libbey, L. M.   1972.   Quantitative
and selective gas chromatographic analysis of
dimethyl- and trimethylamine in fish.   J. Agr.
Food Chem. May/June.

4.   Magee, P. N., and Barnes, J. N.   1967.
Carcinogenic nitroso compounds.   Adv. Cancer
Res. 10: 163.

XXI
FISH PROTEIN CONCENTRATE IN THE TREATMENT OF MALNOURISHED CHILDREN AND IN THE FIELD, TECHNOLOGY OF UTILIZATION, PREPARATION, AND ACCEPTABILITY

Juan Manuel Baertl
Department of International Health, School of
Hygiene and Public Health, The Johns Hopkins
University, Baltimore, Maryland 21205, and
Instituto de Investigacion Nutricional, Lima,
Peru

We have evaluated Fish Protein Concentrate
(FPC) under four different conditions: 1) in
the diet therapy of severely malnourished
children at the Matabolic Unit of the Instituto de Investigacion Nutricional, formerly of
the British American Hospital; 2) in a five-
year food supplementation program of several
entire village populations of the northern
coast of Peru; 3) as a significant source of
protein in a preschool children's supplementation program carried on during four years in
one of these villages; and 4) in miscellaneous
trials in methods of food preparation and
acceptability.

In this presentation we are mainly concerned in discussing our experience in the
forms of preparation and the regimens by
which we utilized FPC to feed the hospitalized
malnourished children and the preschoolers on
the food supplementation program, the ways in
which it was recommended to be used by the
people in the field supplementation study, and
the acceptability of the different groups.

In the management of malnourished children
in the metabolic unit, FPC was used either as
the sole source of protein or in a 10 percent
FPC-90 percent wheat flour mixture. It was
administered in sufficient amounts to provide

a diet isonitrogenous with the control diets.
A modified milk preparation* was used as our
reference diet. The proportions of nonprotein
calories (Fat 53 percent and CHO 47 percent)
of the modified milk preparation were always
maintained by adding the necessary amounts of
sucrose (cane sugar) and cottonseed oil when
increasing the caloric content of the diet.
When FPC was the only source of protein, two
grams of cornstarch/kg/day were given as part
of the carbohydrate allowance which permitted
better mixing of ingredients providing a
smoother consistency in the final product.
Suitable mineral and vitamin mixtures[1] were
given to insure minimum requirements.

The preparation of the constant diets was
as follows: the required amount of ingredients as determined by daily calculations was
cooked in water for ten to fifteen minutes and
then blended; water was added to complete the
prescribed constant total volume; finally it
was distributed in as many bottles as feeding
times had been indicated for each child. The
bottles were stored at 4°C, and warmed just
before each serving time.

Our evaluation[3] of FPC in the treatment of
malnourished children has consisted mainly of:
"Comparative" metabolic studies, done on daily
recalculated isocaloric, isonitrogenous diets
of milk, fish protein concentrate and FPC-
wheat mixture; "Initial "metabolic studies, on
FPC alone or in the 10 percent combination
with wheat, by giving either one, as the only
protein source to newly admitted malnourished
children following the same dietary program as
with the control diets[3]; and "Long-Term"
studies, by the continuous administration of
FPC alone or in combination with wheat as the

----

*Similar with Iron, supplied by Ross
Laboratories, Columbus, Ohio.

only source of protein for several months.

As an illustration of our metabolic data obtained during the treatment of malnourished children 7 to 54 months of age, we are presenting in Table 1 the results of the "Comparative" metabolic studies of 6 malnourished children given isocaloric and isonitrogenously diets based on milk or 10 percent FPC-90 percent wheat flour combination. The first two females illustrate similar apparent nitrogen retention as with milk; less weight gain; greater decrease of serum albumin by 10F and less by 4F. The next three males depict almost the same apparent nitrogen absorption as with milk; apparent nitrogen retention and weight gain were slightly better than with milk in two of the children (12M-16M) and significantly less in the other (17M); serum albumin decreased in 12M, slightly increased in 16M and 17M and, in all three, its increments were larger on milk. The last patient (6M) was studied at lower levels of protein intake (1.5 g protein and 130 Kcal/kg/d . 4.6% Kcal from proteins). He demonstrates equal apparent nitrogen absorption and similar apparent N retention as with milk; one-half body weight increments; and greater decrease of serum albumin.

Table 2 illustrates the metabolic data of two newly admitted malnourished children to whom the 10 percent FPC-90 percent wheat flour mixture was given from the start, as the only source of protein, to provide 2 gm of protein/kg/d. Calorie content of the diet was progressively increased from 75 to 150 Kcal/kg/day. The apparent nitrogen absorption was as good or better than with milk. The apparent nitrogen retention progressively increased in time with the caloric increments of the diet as have been previously reported by us on control diets.[4] One of my patients (14M) remained in apparent negative nitrogen balance during the

Table 1. Apparent nitrogen balances (N Balances) absorption (Abs.) and retention (Ret.) as % of intake (% of Int.); gains in body weight (B. wt.) and changes in serum albumin (Ser. Albumin), compared with those while receiving a modified cow's milk preparation (M) at comparable levels of % Kcalories from protein. Data within parenthesis indicates children's weight age in months.

Daily Diet Protein Source	% Kcal	No. Days	N Balances No. Days	mg/kg/d Intake	% of Int. Abs.	Ret.	B. Wt. g/kg/d	Ser. Albumin g/100 ml	Final
#4F:	Hosp. day 90;		10 months,	4.59 Kg	(1.2 mo.)				
M	5.3	27	3	331		48	8.0	-0.65	3.78
WF	5.3	24	6	320		42	7.0	-0.26	3.52
#10F:	Hosp. day 72;		10 months,	5.59 Kg	(2.6 mo.)				
M	5.3	27	9	320		49	8.9	-0.26	3.26
WF	5.3	29	9	288		48	3.0	-0.38	2.93
#12M:	Hosp. day 19;		7 months,	4.61 Kg	(1.2 mo.)				
M	5.3	38	18	321	76	33	5.8	0.57	3.43
WF	5.3	29	9	300	82	37	5.2	-0.47	2.96
#16M:	Hosp. day 38;		31 months,	6.14 Kg	(3.8 mo.)				
M	5.3	22	15	320	88	43	6.2	0.27	4.10
WF	5.3	30	12	320	86	45	6.4	0.16	4.26
#17M:	Hosp. day 50;		15 months,	4.66 Kg	(1.4 mo.)				
WF	5.3	31	12	320	74	27	2.9	0.11	3.18
M	5.3	55	18	318	79	45	5.2	1.47	4.65
#6M:	Hosp. day 48;		13 months,	6.47 Kg	(4.5 mo.)				
M	4.6	32	12	246	83	37	6.2	-0.13	3.80
WF	4.6	27	6	245	83	34	3.9	-0.40	3.40

Metabolic Evaluation of 10% FPC-90% Wheat Flour (WF) Mixture in Recovering Malnourished Children

Table 2. Apparent nitrogen balances (N Balances), absorption (Abs.) and retention (Ret.); as % of intake (% of Int.); changes in body weight (B. Wt. Δ) and in serum albumin (Ser. Albumin Δ) during consecutive dietary periods on this protein source at a constant protein intake of 2 gm/kg/day and progressive calorie increments, therefore, the % Kilocalories from proteins (K calories % Prot.) progressively diminished. And a final dietary period on a modified cow's milk preparation (M) was followed iso-caloric and iso-nitrogenously. Data within parenthesis indicates the corresponding weight age (in months) of each child.

Daily Diet				N Balances				B. Wt. Δ	Ser. Albumin g/100 ml	
Protein Source	Kcalories /kg	%Prot.	No. Days	No. Days	mg/kg/d Intake	% of Int. Abs.	% of Int. Ret.	g/kg/d	Δ	Final
#14M:	13 months,	5.30 Kg		(2.2 mo.)						
WF	75	10.7	10	3	320	75	Neg.	-3.5	-0.35	3.10
WF	100	8.0	9	3	321	64	Neg.	-2.2	-0.29	2.81
WF	130	6.1	30	12	320	78	23	1.9	0.21	3.02
WF	150	5.3	27	9	312	73	19	4.7	-0.40	2.62
M	150	5.3	24	12	320	78	47	8.1	1.07	3.69
#19M:	54 months,	5.18 Kg		(2.0 mo.)						
WF	75	10.7	10	10	319	92	37	1.2	0.30	3.43
WF	100	8.0	35	27	320	85	34	0.4	0.77	4.20
WF	130	6.1	16	6	320	89	50	3.1	-0.25	3.95
WF	150	5.3	33	11	320	83	48	5.5	-0.22	3.73
M	150	5.3	55	24	320	84	52	6.3	0.74	4.47

Metabolic Evaluation of 10% FPC-90% Wheat Flour (WF) Mixture in Newly admitted Malnourished Children

initial 19 days and until the caloric content
of the diet was increased to 130 Kcal/kg/d.
He demonstrated more than 100 percent increase
in apparent nitrogen retention when given an
isocaloric and isonitrogenous milk diet. On
the other hand 19M showed only 15 percent increase when given milk. Gain of body weight
paralleled caloric increments of the diet, as
have been reported by us on control diets.[3]
There was a considerably larger increment of
body weight in both children when given the
milk diet. Serum albumin significantly increased after the milk period in both bases,
as had been previously reported.[5]

Table 3 summarizes the metabolic data of a
10 month-old female with 0.8 months weight
age, who was given FPC as the only source of
protein from the start of her hospitalization
and continued on it or in combination with
wheat for 10 consecutive months. Only one 16-
day period of a milk diet was administered
starting on hospital day 60. She was started
on a diet that provided 2 gm of protein and
75 Kcal/kg/d. The protein was increased to
2.5 gm/kg/d on day 4. Progressive caloric
increments were given. Isocaloric and
isonitrogenous balance periods were carried
on FPC alone or in combination with wheat, and
also on milk. Her metabolic data illustrates
that she had adequate apparent nitrogen retention, but a substantially better one on
milk. Rate of weight gain was also markedly
greater on the milk diet. Serum albumin had
marked fluctuations while on the FPC based
diets, and it was substantially increased during the two weeks on milk.

It should be pointed out that the amount of
protein intake, and especially the level of
the % kilocalories from proteins under which
our studies have been carried out, are quite
low; they are lower than those used by most
other authors. This is probably the most

Table 3. Apparent nitrogen (N Balances), retention as % of intake (% of Int.); changes in body weight (B. Wt. Δ) and in serum albumin (Ser. Albumin Δ), during consecutive dietary periods on this protein source alone or in combination with wheat (WF), and one on modified cow's milk preparation (M). During one of the dietary periods of 10% FPC-90% wheat mixture (WF*), 20 mg/kg/d of methionine were added to the diet. Data within parenthesis indicates patient's weight age (0.8 months) at start of study.

| Daily Diet | | | No. | N Balances | | | B.Wt. Δ | Ser. Albumin g/100 ml | |
Protein Source	Kcalories /kg	%Prot.	Days	No. Days	mg/kg/d Intake	% of Int. Retention	g/kg/d	Δ	Final
F	75	10.7	1	0	320		−40.0		3.13
F	100	8.0	2	2	321	19	8.5	−0.12	3.01
F	100	10.0	6	6	400	24	4.3	0.60	3.61
F	125	8.0	9	3	401	23	− 0.2	−0.15	3.46
F	150	6.7	41	27	401	15	2.5	−0.51	2.97
M	150	6.7	16	3	401	50	10.1	0.80	3.77
WF	150	6.7	9	9	400	25	5.0	0.55	4.32
F	150	6.7	15	15	401	Neg.	2.5	−0.59	3.73
WF	150	6.7	27	18	400	28	5.7	−0.44	3.29
WF*	150	6.7	48	15	400	33	3.8	0.34	3.63
F	150	6.7	16	9	395	33	4.2	0.19	3.82
F	75		9	6	16	Neg.	− 5.5	0.12	3.94
F	100	8.0	45	6	320	20	− −	0.55	4.49
F	125	6.4	34	0	320		4.0	0.63	5.12
F	125	6.4	30	0	320		2.1	−0.52	4.60
F	100	8.0	63	0	320		0.1	−0.90	3.70

Metabolic Evaluation of Fish Protein Concentrate in a Newly Malnourished Child
#73F: 10 months, 4.25 Kg (0.8 mo.)

likely explanation why our results favor milk.
But it is also worth emphasizing that at the
same time we have shown a very fair performance of FPC along at these levels and a
better one when combined with wheat.

In the field food supplementation studies,
the whole population of one village was given
1/2 kg of 10 percent FPC-enriched noodles per
person per week. There was no fish flavor in
final products, and villagers were not informed that the supplementing protein was
fish. We utilized 10 percent FPC-enriched
noodles of two types; spaghetti and "angel
hair", a fine noodle given to young children
throughout Peru, usually prepared in soup.
Village dwellers were given a short instruc-
tion course in several ways of noodle preparation. People stated they were "accustomed"
to eating noodles with meat, probably really
meaning that this was the way, they thought,
for adults to eat noodles. We stressed that
these noodles were good enough by themselves,
that they did not require meat to go with
them. We advised them just to season the
noodles with the different locally available
and commonly used spices and vegetables,
such as aji, which is a Peruvian chili,
culantro, known as fresh coriander, garlic,
onion, tomatoes, etc. and to add some fat
after cooking, (oil, margarine, butter,
etc.). Instructions were also given to prepare puddings and gruels for children:
noodles could be crushed into powder and
cooked with cane sugar and cooking oil for
about thirty minutes with sufficient water,
or they could be cooked in water first and
then blended; this latter process could not
be done by many since blenders are rare.
Some of the few people that had ice-boxes
froze these gruels and puddings and made FPC-
enriched "ices" which were fun for many and a
source of money for a few.

Since results of this supplementation study
have been published, I will only summarize by
stating that it was difficult to demonstrate
that the supplementation had a clear effect on
the heights and weights of the population, but
a lowering of mortality rates for infants and
preschoolers was seen.[6] A dental survey was
undertaken on all children 4 to 14 years of
age in the supplemented villages and in one of
the control villages after 4 1/2 years of the
10 percent FPC-enriched noodle food supplementation program. It disclosed no evidence of
fluorosis in any of the 3 populations
studies.[7]

The preschool supplementation program was
designed for all children 6 to 30 months old
in one of the villages. They were to receive
a daily dietary supplementation to provide
them with 2.5 gm of protein and 80 Kcal/kg.
This was to be accomplished by offering the
youngsters two meals a day under our direct
observation and by using adequate food preparations commonly used by those people to
feed children of this age group. Two food
preparations were selected (Table 4) and made
with FPC: a soup (based on the 10 percent
enriched-angel hair noodles) that provided
per serving an almost similar amount of protein and 50 percent more Kcal than a glass
of cow's milk; and enriched wheat flour
cookies, each of which provided approximately the per g daily requirements of protein
and 80 percent of the Kcalories for children
of this age group. Part of the program included also a gruel based on cottonseed flour
which provided per serving (150 ml) a slightly greater amount of protein than a glass of
cow's milk and twice the calories. These
food preparations were designed to provide a
similar proportion of kilo-calories from
carbohydrate, fat and protein as does human
milk.

Table 4

Food Preparations	Vol ml	Prot gm	Kcal
Cookie	one	1.6*	69
Soup	240	6.5*	240
Gruel	150	9.0	320

----

*50% from FPC

The soup was prepared following typical
local customs of soup preparations: first
frying onions, tomatoes and other seasoning
items in some of the calculated amount of
oil; then pouring in the measured amount of
hot water; and upon boiling, the calculated
amount of noodles and the rest of the oil was
added to provide enough soup for the number of
expected children with the prescribed composition.

Children were to be brought to the feeding
station twice daily by their mothers to be fed
by them. Shortly after the start it became
evident that the mothers were too busy to
bring their children and therefore sent them
with their older siblings who also fed and
took care of them. The soup was very well
accepted from the start by children and
mothers; the gruel was well accepted by most
children but poorly by mothers due to the dark
grayish color. The cookies did not seem to
appeal to children as much as had been expected; they played a lot with them losing
large portions as they crumbled.

The average child attendance for the group
was 46.1 percent. There was no correlation
of age with attendance of the children to the
feeding station (Table 5). Of those who
attended, consumption seemed to increase with
age as illustrated in Table 6. Mean consumption for the group was 73 percent. The
correlation coefficient of consumption and
attendance was 0.30 suggesting some relationship between consumption and attendance.
Several children ate more than their prescribed allowance, pointing out the great
acceptability by mothers and children of food
items enriched with FPC.

A nutritionist working on her thesis[8] in
our research unit also evaluated acceptibili-
ty, satiety, hypersensitivity, and toxicity
in children by feeding them several food

Table 5.   Children group attendance during one
of the months of the study is presented broken
down in 4 (6 months) age groups, illustrating
no relation of age and attendance.   There is a
normal frequency distribution curve.

Attendance

Age group months	Average %	Frequency Distribution %	No.
6-12	38.6	0	6
13-18	45.4	21-40	11
19-24	56.3	41-60	12
25-30	44.3	61-80	14
6-30	46.1	81-100	-7
		0-100	57

r.   Attendance & Age = 0.13

Table 6. Food consumption of children (during one of the months of the study) increased
in the 2 older age groups, giving a correlation with age of 0.36. Food consumption and
attendance have a correlation coefficient of
0.30.

FOOD CONSUMPTION

Age group months	Average %	Frequency Distribution %	No.
6-12	67	0	6
13-18	52	1-20	0
19-24	80	21-40	1
25-30	87	41-60	9
6-30	73	61-80	14
		81-100	19
		101- +	8
		0-100+	57

r.   Consumption & Age = 0.36

r.   Consumption & Attendance = 0.30

Table 7. Food Preparations Containing FPC

SOUPS   PASTAS   BREADS   CEREAL DISHES

PUREES:

        POTATOE   CASAVA   PUMPKIN

        SPINACH   SWISS CHARD   OLLUCO

DESSERTS:

    ARROZ CON LECHE   (RICE PUDDING)

    MAZAMORRA CON MANZANA   (APPLE PUDDING)

    MAZAMORRA DE CHANCACA   (MOLLASES PUDDING)

    BUDIN DE PAN   (BREAD PUDDING)

    TORTA   (CAKE)

    ARROZ ZAMBITO   (RICE AND MOLASSES
                               PUDDING)

    MAZAMORRA DE GELATINA   (GELATIN PUDDING)

    BIZCOCHUELO   (SPONGE CAKE)

    HELADOS DE FRUTA   (FRUIT-FLAVOR ICE-
                               CREAM)

    GELATINA DE LECHE   (MILK JELLO)

    MAZAMORRA DE SEMOLA   (SEMOLINA PUDDING)

    MAZAMORRA DE LECHE   (MILK PUDDING)

preparations containing FPC. A summary of her
findings and of our related experience is
shown in Table 7. Soups, pastas, cereal
dishes, purees, and desserts were made as typical Peruvian dishes. She found that acceptability was great; that satiety was more
complete when cereals (wheat noodles) were
enriched with FPC; and that no allergic or
toxic effects were observed.

Conclusions

In our studies, FPC has been shown: a) to be
a good source of protein for human consumption alone or in combination with wheat or
other protein foods; b) to continue and maintain recovery in malnourished children started
on milk diets; c) to be easily included in
practically all Peruvian traditional (folklore) dishes with great acceptability; and d)
to cause no evidence of toxicity, fluorosis
or allergic reactions.

Acknowledgment

This study was supported by Grants AM-04635,
AM-05935 and AM-09137 from the National
Institutes of Health, USPHS.

References

1. Snyderman, S. E., et al. 1959. The
essential amino acid requirements of infants:
Lysine. Amer. J. Dis. Child. 97: 175.

2. Graham, G. G., Baertl, J. M., and
Cordano, A. 1965. Dietary protein quality in
infants and children. I. Evaluation in rapidly growing infants and children of fish protein concentrate alone and in combination with
wheat. Amer. J. Dis. Child. 110: 248.

3.   Graham, G. G., Cordano, A., and Baertl,
J. M.   1963.   Studies in infantile malnutrition.   II. Effect of protein and calorie intake on weight gain.   J. of Nutr. 81: 249.

4.   Graham, G. G., Cordano, A., and Baertl,
J. M.   1964.   Studies in infantile malnutrition.   III. Effect of protein and calorie intake on nitrogen retention.   J. of Nutr. 84:
71.

5.   Graham, G. G., Cordano, A., and Baertl,
J. M.   1966.   Studies in infantile malnutrition.   IV. The effect of protein and calorie
intake on serum proteins.   Am. J. Clin. Nutr.
18: 11.

6.   Baertl, J. M., Morales, E., Verastegui,
G., and Graham, G. G.   1970.   Diet supplementation for entire communities: Growth and
mortality of infants and children.   Amer. J.
Clin. Nutr. 23: 707.

7.   Baertl, J. M., Pomareda, J., Beltran, P.,
Verastegui, G., and Graham, G. G.   Dental
Survey of Rural Peruvian Children 4 to 14
years old after 4 1/2 Years of Daily Consumption of FPC Enriched Foods.   To be published.

8.   Ysela Wimpon Salinas.   1966.   Aplicacion
de la harina de pescado en la recuperacion de
ninos desnutridos.   Thesis for graduation as
Dietitian.   Escuela de Dististas del Hospital
de la Caja del Seguro Social Obrero.   Lima,
Peru.

Part V

ECONOMICS

XXII
THE ECONOMICS OF FISH PROTEIN CONCENTRATE

James A. Crutchfield and Robert Deacon
Department of Economics, University of
Washington, Seattle, Washington

Research conducted on fish protein concentrate
(FPC) in the past has been concerned primarily
with processing technology and nutritional
evaluation. Efforts to evaluate the economic
role of FPC in world markets have been few by
comparison. Although such research has been
of generally high quality, it has often been
limited in scope. Some analyses have focused
upon single locations for production and consumption and have examined FPC in light of a
single specific use; others have looked at
potential markets with little or no analysis
of economic aspects of production; most reports have evaluated FPC on the basis of present technology and have not tried to assess
potential gains from further research.
    A more global approach to the problem,
considering production, marketing and the
allocation of research effort is needed.
Since private markets allocate too few resources to research and are heavily oriented
to specific, mission-oriented work with short
term, identifiable payoffs, the more global
approach would probably be conducted by
government research. When the government con-
ducts successful research and distributes the
knowledge generated to industry, the social
benefit of the research will be reflected in
lower prices for final products. Thus, in
order to survey the proper directions for
government research on FPC, one must address
the following questions. What is the nature
of foreign and domestic markets for protein at
present, and what are present indications of
future developments? What are the critical

physical and economic qualities needed to compete in these markets? Given present technology, what conclusions can be drawn about
the costs and qualities of FPC, and what are
the potential markets for such a product?
Given the above considerations, what are the
implications for further FPC research--i.e.,
what crucial problems need solving, and which
directions for research appear most promising?

Our purpose is to investigate briefly each
of the areas outlined above and to present the
preliminary implications of this comprehensive
view of FPC. Some areas of concern are given
less attention than others because our knowledge in these areas is relatively limited.
For example, the analysis of potential markets for FPC will be rather general and less
detailed than the investigation of the economic aspects of production.

The Product Group

A necessary part of an economic study of any
product is an investigation of the environment
in which that product must compete. In the
case of FPC this calls for an evaluation of
the present market for protein ingredients and
an examination of the characteristics of the
products currently being used. The nutritive
and functional properties of these products
and the prices which they command are of prime
importance to the successful development of
FPC. Furthermore, indications of future
trends in the demand for protein and the long
run supply prospects for alternative sources
are essential for even tentative conclusions
concerning the future potential of FPC.

A survey of world markets for protein
supplements reveals that present usage of protein ingredients is largely restricted to
"developed countries", despite the fact that
most of the world's population lives in
"developing countries" where problems of

inadequate protein consumption are most acute.
This dichotomy is partially depicted by two
considerations: 1. two-thirds of the world
population living in developing countries
command about one half of the world's protein
(most of which is cereal protein); and 2. the
one billion people in "developed countries"
use practically as much cereal to feed animals
as the two billion people in developing countries use directly as food.[1]

Oilseeds. The most important protein additives in developed countries are derived from
oilseed and dairy products. These products
are used for consumption both directly and indirectly via use in animal feeding. The oilseeds yield oil for industrial purposes and
meal which may be processed into a variety of
protein-rich products. A large portion of the
meal extracted is used in the feeding of livestock and poultry, a market in which fish meal
is a major competitor. It is significant that
these markets are closely related; oilseed and
fish meal are easily interchangeable in their
most important use, the feeding of livestock
and poultry.[2] In the U. S. oilseed and fish
oils are largely used as drying agents in the
manufacture of paints, caulking compounds,
etc., but the degree of interchangeability is
less evident for drying agents than for meals.
    These factors indicate that the price
ratios between oilseed and fish meal should
remain fairly stable over time since the major
users of these products will alternate between
them until price ratios are such that livestock and poultry growers are indifferent to
alternate sources of protein.
    In terms of direct human consumption the
soybean is easily the most important oilseed.
In developed countries, protein products extracted from soybeans include soy flour and
grits, soy concentrates and isolates, and

textured items including extracted and spun
soy protein products.

The U. S. is a major producer of soybeans
and soy products. Price quotations from one
of the larger domestic producers[3] were 6 to 9¢
per pound for soy flour which is guaranteed 50
percent protein and suitable for human consumption. The higher values are for fatted or
lecithinated products, while lower prices in
the 6 to 7¢ range are for a defatted product.
These prices have remained fairly stable over
the last fifteen years. Rapid growth in demand has produced corresponding increases in
farm production and processing capacity.
Virtually all case exports of this commodity
are made to developed countries (primarily EEC
nations), although substantial sales are also
made to the U. S. government for use in AID
(Agency for International Development) programs to developing countries such as India,
Pakistan, and African nations. In addition to
soy flour, price quotations were obtained for
the following items[3]: soy concentrates (70
percent protein--dry basis)--20 to 26¢ per
pound; soy isolates (88 percent to 90 percent
protein)--42 to 50¢ per pound.

Foreign production of soy products for human consumption is small by comparison. The
Japanese manufacture some soy flour, concentrates, and isolates; and a plant in Spain
currently manufactures soy flour.

Soy protein ingredients are used in the Far
East where the bitter, "beany" taste of soy is
appreciated. Sauces and pastes made from soy
beans have long been used in Oriental countries and a variety of beverages fortified
with soy protein are currently being marketed
in Hong Kong and elsewhere.[4]

In the United States, soy protein ingredients are used in a variety of products including, among others, baby foods, baked
goods, breakfast cereals, processed meats,

and pet food. The volume of soy ingredients
used in the U. S. in 1969 was about 192 million pounds.[5] The USDA projects rapid growth
in the use of soy protein as extenders and
analogs for meat products and estimates that
by 1980, 1.7 to 3.7 billion pounds of red meat
products will be replaced by soy protein
products. In addition, 27 to 55 million
pounds of soy protein products are expected to
find use as replacements for poultry
products.[6]

These estimates were derived from projections of total consumption of meat products
with varying assumptions about the percentage
of total meat replaced by soy products (estimates of meat replaced ranged from 10 to 21
percent for processed meats and from 3 to 6
percent for major pountry products.) Figures
for pounds of meat replaced can be roughly
converted to pounds of soy protein used by
dividing by four, since soy protein is combined with water and fat in a ratio of about
3:1 (water:soy).

The figures above correlate fairly closely
with information provided in the report by
Call and Hammonds.[5] This report projects
rapid growth for the use of extenders and analogs in canned and processed meat and estimates a potential market of about 500 million
pounds of protein by 1980.

As indicated above, prices of soy flour,
meal and grits have been remarkably stable
over the past fifteen years.[3] In 1971, 43
million acres of soybeans were harvested in
the U. S. and the USDA projects that an addition of only 330 to 990 thousand acres would
be required to meet projected use by 1980, so
that little or no effect on the price of soybeans is expected despite the rapid growth in
demand. In general, their projections to 1980
indicate that the price of soybeans will remain near recent levels. Anticipated

economies in processing are expected to offset
or at least moderate any upward movement in
the cost of producing soy proteins.[6]

Use of other oilseed proteins is small compared to soy, although the manufacture of
cottonseed protein products has aroused interest in the U. S. At present, one company
is producing cottonseed flour marketed under
the name of "Proflo." This product is 55 percent protein and sells for 11¢ per pound
(f.o.b. Texas) in carlots.[7] Major users of
this product are bakeries (for use in bread,
doughnuts, cookies, etc.), and noodle and
macaroni producers. It is believed that this
is the only commercial operation in the world
producing high-grade cottonseed flour.

This product was initially used as the
major protein ingredient in Incaparina, but
was later replaced by a cheaper, low-grade
cottonseed meal produced in Central America.
More recently, the cottonseed in Incaparina
has been replaced by soy flour grown locally
in Central American countries. Acceptability
problems and high cost were cited as reasons
for discontinuing the use of cottonseed
flour.[8]

Under the sponsorship of AID, a pilot plant
using the "liquid cyclone" process for making
70 percent protein concentrate from cottonseed was placed in operation at Hubli, India.
A Texas corporation has recently invested $1.5
million in a 25 ton per day plant using the
same process to remove gossypol from cottonseed and to produce a high-grade protein
product.[9]

Because this is a relatively new product,
speculation about future prices and utilization is difficult. Work has been done on
developing strains of cotton which are free of
gossypol. Some of this product has been grown
in Texas, but low yields appear to more than
offset any reduction in processing costs. The

U. S. appears to be the only country producing
human-grade cottonseed flour in significant
quantities. Taking the domestic f.o.b. price
of 11¢ per pound and adding 1¢ per pound for
transport yields 12¢ per pound as an estimate
of the current price of human-grade cottonseed
flour.

   It is possible that lower prices may be
attainable in foreign countries where cotton
is grown. However, the fact that INCAP abandoned cottonseed in favor of soy flour in
Incaparina indicates that the foreign cost of
producing acceptable cottonseed flour is above
the current price of soy flour.

   Speculation about the future course of
cottonseed prices must rest on the nature of
the product. Cottonseed flour is a by-product
(and a relatively minor one) obtained in con-
junction with cotton fiber and cottonseed oil.
In the past ten years, cotton has been subjected to severe competition from synthetics
with the result that U. S. production of fine
all-cotton broadwoven fabrics decreased from
1.5 billion linear yards in 1960 to less than
0.5 billion linear yards in 1970.[5] USDA ex-
pects cotton to continue to lose potential
markets to synthetics in the future. Thus it
seems reasonable to expect the relative price
of cotton fabric to decline which, in the absence of major technological progress, will
result in a relative increase in the price of
cottonseed flour.

Dairy Products. The recent turnaround in
world dairy markets has had a drastic effect
upon two major protein supplements, NFDM (nonfat dry milk) and casein. The increase in
world prices for NFDM was so dramatic that
several European countries dropped export subsidies and imposed export taxes on NFDM to
prevent sharp increases in domestic price.
World NFDM prices have increased from about

7.5¢ per pound in 1969 to 27¢ per pound in
1971.[10]

A variety of factors, including droughts in
1970 and 1971 in two major dairy producing
countries (Australia and New Zealand) and gra-
dual depletion of surplus stocks of dairy
products in many areas of the world contributed to the price increases. This trend is expected to continue. U. S. exports of NFDM in
1971 were down 15 percent from their 1970
levels to 358 million pounds. Although cash
exports increased, NFDM donations declined
enough to more than offset these sales.[11]

Current high prices for NFDM may cause dis-
continuation of its use for calf feeding in
Europe, and in other uses for which substitutes exist. Thus, prices will probably fall
below the current price of 28¢ per pound.

The same pressures that have raised prices
for NFDM have caused prices for casein to increase rapidly in the last two years. New
Zealand and Australia provide most of the
world supply of casein; little is produced in
the U. S. U. S. imports of casein in 1970
totaled 135.3 million pounds--almost 50 percent of total world production. In response
to higher prices in 1971, domestic imports
declined to 105.9 million pounds. The use of
casein in food products, where it is valued
for its functional properties, has risen
rapidly in the last two decades. These markets now account for about half of U. S. consumption of casein and caseinates.[10]
Industrial uses (in adhesives, plastics, and
synthetic fibers) and animal feeding make up
the balance of domestic consumption. The
areas of most rapid growth have been in human
grade food products and in milk replacers for
calf feeding.

Although the very high current prices for
dairy proteins probably will not persist, a
return to the low levels of the late 1960s

seems highly unlikely. The price of NFDM is
expected to settle somewhere below the current
price of 29¢ per pound and for the purposes of
this paper a price of 20¢ per pound will be
used. The price of casein has risen from its
1970 level of 26.6¢ per pound to the current
figure of 64.8¢ per pound,[10] and in the next
few years the price will probably fall somewhere between these extremes.

Synthetic Amino Acids. Most of the research
now being done on development of synthetic
amino acids is being financed by private companies. For this reason information on these
products and their development is exceedingly
scarce.

One domestic producer, Merck and Co., Inc.,
is producing synthetic lysine and marketing it
for $1.95 per pound, but information on volume
of production and usage are not available.[12]
Dupont invested substantial sums in research
on synthetic amino acids but has abandoned the
project.[13] The Japanese appear to have a
comparative advantage in the production of
synthetic amino acids (primarily lysine and
methionine). One firm (Kyowa Fermentation
Industry and Co., Ltd., Japan) is manufacturing lysine and methionine by fermentation of
glucose and yeast.[14]

Estimates of current prices for amino acids
per pound of material are as follows: L-
lysine, $1.00; L-threonine, $7.50; and DL-
tryptophan, $5.90.

Various writers have suggested that these
prices, especially for threonine and tryptophan, will decline. Estimates of the eventual
equilibrium price of threonine go as low as
$3.00 per pound.[1] The trend in prices has
been downward; the price of human grade lysine
has fallen from $1.14 per pound in 1969 to its
current level of $1.00.[15] Although no quota-
tion for human grade methionine could be

obtained, an estimate of $1.00 per pound
seems reasonable in light of the fact that
both lysine and methionine were selling for
$1.14 per pound in 1969. Information con-
tained in this section is summarized in Table
1.

Protein Supplementation in Developing Countries

The preceding section identified major protein
supplements now in use and presented data on
current prices and usage, and indications of
future trends. We now turn to the markets for
protein supplements. The properties which a
protein source must offer to be competitive in
these markets are identified and preliminary
conclusions are drawn as to the potential role
of FPC vis-a-vis other additives. This section of the analysis is preliminary and somewhat conjectural and the conclusions herein
should be viewed as topics for more intensive
study. The investigation has been divided into sections on potential markets in "developing" and "developed" countries. Since the FPC
program was initially designed to provide a
highly nutritious, low cost product to combat
protein malnutrition in developing countries,
this market is discussed first.

The general dimensions of the world protein-calorie malnutrition problem have been
described in the MIT study[15] and elsewhere.
Interest was initially centered on protein
deficiencies alone, but recent evidence suggests that calorie deficiencies are equally
important. In the future, however, the major
increases in food production are expected to
come from greater production of cereals which
are typically deficient in certain essential
amino acids. Thus the long term "protein
problem" is still very real.

Recent History of Protein Supplementation. A

Table 1. Summary of Protein Supplement Prices

Supplement	Current U. S. Price f.o.b. ¢/lb.	Current World Price ¢/lb.	Expected Future Price
DAIRY PRODUCTS:			
NFDM	28	28.8	11-29--should decrease from present levels
Casein	64.8	64.8	26.6-64.8--should decrease from present levels
SOY PRODUCTS:			
Soy Flour	6-7.5[1]	7-8.5[5]	stable
Soy Concentrate	20-26[2]	21-27[5]	possible slight decrease
Soy Isolate	42-50[3]	43-51[5]	possible slight decrease
COTTONSEED PRODUCTS:			
Cottonseed Flour	11[4]	12[5]	possible slight increase
SYNTHETICS:			
Lysine	195	100	probable decreases from present levels
Methionine	?	100	probable decreases from present levels
Threonine	?	750	probable decreases from present levels
Tryptophan	?	590	$3.00 probable decrease from present levels

[1] Quote from ajor U. S. producer--defatted 50% protein.
[2] Quote from major U. S. producer--70% protein.
[3] Quote from major U. S. producer--88.5-90% protein.
[4] Quote from major U. S. producer--55% protein.
[5] U. S. f.o.b. price plus 1¢/lb. shipping charge.

brief review of the history of food
supplementation programs and the involvement
of government and private industry provides
some insight into the nature of the problem.

Official concern in the U. S. over world
malnutrition became evident in the early 1960s
and spread to industry. By late 1966, most of
the major international food companies had
initiated laboratory research on low cost protein foods. In 1968, a dozen such food items
(e.g., baby foods, imitation milks, candies,
snacks, soups and noodles) were being marketed. The more recent history of these
attempts indicates the range of problems encountered; as Berg[16] points out, the wide-
spread belief that industry and technology
could solve the world malnutrition problem was
founded upon assumptions that often proved
erroneous. The fact that processing and refining invariably raise the price of the final
product above that of the staple ingredients
was neglected. For example, the widely her-
alded Incaparina, marketed in Colombia and
Guatemala, costs 20¢ per pound--about four
times as much as the corn meal it replaces.
By 1966 it had attained an annual distribution
of 4.7 million pounds[17] which is the recommended daily dosage for about 0.3 percent of
the combined population of these two countries. At present prices it seems unlikely
that this product is reaching the low income
people who need it most. Even in cases where
these high protein foods have reached the
needy, the effect has not been uniformly beneficial. In Pakistan, for example, a variety
of high protein baby foods was marketed so
successfully that low income people substituted it for the cheaper local cow's milk.[16]

Few of the food companies involved in these
programs have found them profitable. In addition to predictable problems such as lack of
"effective demand" and difficulty in applying

tested marketing skills to new and diverse
cultures, these companies have faced unex-
pected problems such as competition from
institutional feeding programs (U. S. subsidized CSM (corn-soy-milk) vs. privately marketed Incaparina, for example) and a tendency
for foreign governments to protect local food
industries.

From this experience, Berg[16] draws the conclusion that government aid is needed if food
supplementation programs are to achieve their
desired goals. There is real promise in programs funded by government but operated under
contract by private companies (the "Bal Ahar"
program in India and CSM in the U. S. are
examples).

It has been noted by Devanney et al.[15] and
elsewhere that the basic protein-calorie
problem is largely one of distribution, not
total supply. Thus, selective supplementation
to low-income persons has been proposed as a
less costly way of upgrading the nutritional
intake of malnourished persons. The apparently simple and obvious truth of this generali-
zation proves illusory under closer
examination, however. A basic assumption
underlying government food supplementation
programs must be that government agencies know
what is best for low-income populations--pre-
sumably because the agencies have better
information than the consumers. Total reli-
ance upon individual tastes and preferences
would call for an income supplementation program, leaving undernourished people to solve
their individual nutritional problems in the
market place. While we accept the assumption
underlying government distribution, we believe
it has serious implications for programs aim-
ing at target populations either free or at
heavily subsidized prices. Many recipients,
viewing this as an increase in income, could
be expected to trade or resell it to members

of higher income groups. The extent of this
phenomenon under present programs is unknown,
but it is certainly worthy of investigation.
Furthermore, such target programs always run
the risk of having their products identified
as "poor people's food"; the history of marketing "Incumbe" in South Africa and its subsequent rejection on these grounds is a case
in point.[18]
     It is widely accepted that protein-calorie
malnutrition has its most severe and irreversible effects upon children from birth to
five years. Although it is difficult to find
controls other variables such as socioeconomic backgrounds, availability of close
social contacts at early ages, deficiencies of
other nutrients such as vitamins and minerals,
etc., and genetic traits, there is evidence
that protein-calorie malnutrition and its
attendant ills leads to the "...production of
underweight babies, many of whom will die before reaching two years of age, whilst among
the survivors, there will be some who never
reach their full physical or mental potential."[19] The contention that severe protein-
calorie malnutrition has its most drastic effects during the period when growth is most
rapid (six to thirty months) has been documented by Cravioto.[20] Thus, specific supplementation through school lunch feeding is
likely to come too late to avoid permanent
physical and mental impairment in a high
proportion of the most important target group.
     Proposals to supplement the diets of in-
fants through high protein baby foods developed in research laboratories to meet
nutritional standards often run afoul of rigid
dietary customs in target countries. As
Foster points out, food shortages frequently
cause competition for food within families.[21]
Weanling infants are often fed small portions
of the adult diet;[22] thus any protein

supplement aimed at infants in these areas
must also meet the approval of adult populations, especially mothers. Peasants often
fail to see the proper line of causation
between eating habits and health.[21] A healthy
child is fed because he has a good appetite;
a child who loses his appetite often has his
ration cut. Hence, it is important that
acceptance is gained by children as well.

This is all compounded by superstitions
such as humoral pathology, which explains ill-
ness in terms of some alleged effect which
various foods have upon body temperature.
Some combinations of acceptable foods will not
be eaten regardless of taste or nutrition.
The result is to magnify the acceptance problem.

These problems suggest two tentative conclusions about food supplementation programs
in general. First, in a large number of situations, universal supplementation of staple
items in the local diet is likely to be the
only way to reach those persons most needing
better nutrition.

Second, the diversity and rigidity of
dietary habits in developing countries indicates that no single supplementation formula
will work in all areas of the world. Feeding
programs must be geared to the customs of
individual target populations.

Relative Efficiencies of Alternative Proteins
in Universal Supplementation. These considerations indicate that the feasibility of
introducing FPC into staple items of various
diets in a scheme of universal supplementation should be investigated. Information provided by the MIT study was taken as a starting point for the analysis.[15]

In the MIT report, a computer program was
utilized to construct universal fortification
schemes which would provide a target

individual (a 10 month old child) with
adequate calorie intake as well as sufficient
protein to meet, alternatively, 100, 150 and
200 percent reference protein requirements as
determined by FAO. Basal diets of wheat,
rice and corn; Chilean mixed diets based upon
wheat and other local foodstuffs; and a mixed
diet of cassava, corn, beans, and honey were
examined.

The MIT investigators found that basal
diets of rice and wheat, when fortified with
synthetic lysine, required less of the country's resources than any other supplement
considered. These results held up even when
prices of lysine were modified to reflect
transport costs and the scarcity value of
foreign exchange required for importing. In
both bases, soy flour was the second cheapest protein source; FPC and dry skim milk were
found to the most expensive alternatives.[15]
This case illustrates the advantage of fortification with synthetics when a single amino
acid is limiting in a diet composed entirely
of a basal food. However, as the authors
later point out, no one eats a diet of 100
percent corn, wheat, or rice. Even in cases
where nonbasal foodstuffs make up relatively
small shares of one total diet, the above results may not hold.

The whole problem of mixed diets is interesting. Suppose we know that a population
is not eating a purely basal diet and that two
specific diets are fairly representative of
eating habits in general. To ensure adequate
nutrition through universal supplementation,
protein must be added to a staple item in a
manner that ensures adequate nutrition for
users of both diets. Suppose we wish to
supplement Chilean nutrition to 150 to 200
percent of the FAO/WHO protein requirements.
The MIT study has provided supplementation and
cost information on two typical Chilean

diets.[15] With each diet, information is provided on the amount of various supplements
needed to reach the nutritional target. Since
we do not know who is eating which diet, it is
necessary to use the maximum amount of each
supplement needed for either of the two diets
to guarantee adequate nutrition for all.

The diets both contain large amounts of
wheat (bread), vegetables, sugar, fruit and
other foods. One diet contains 28.7 percent
milk, and in the other, potatoes and farinas
have been substituted for most of the milk.
Using the price information in Table 1 and
assuming that the price of ingredients in the
diet is, on average, one-fourth of the price
of FPC, it is possible to construct break-even
costs for FPC vs. other supplements.

Figures in Table 2 are interpreted as
follows: Items in column two show the cost of
FPC at which FPC and the alternative supplement require equal amounts of the nation's resources for supplementation--the lower the
break-even cost, the lower the cost FPC must
be if it is to be a competitive source of protein. Fortification with synthetics is now
the most expensive alternative (at 200 percent
FAO levels) and soy flour and peanut flour are
the least expensive. The decline in the position of synthetics in this case is the result
of two factors: 1. with one of the mixed
diets, two amino acids, lysine and methionine,
are limiting, and 2. since we cannot identify
precisely which persons are eating which
diets, it is necessary to "over-fortify" some
diets to ensure adequate nutrition for the
population.

The concentration ratios shown in the third
column of Table 2 are included to give some
idea of the relative acceptability problems
that various supplements may present. Note
that these are the percentages of supplements
in the total diet. However, the relevant

Table 2.   Break-even Cost of FPC Universal
Supplementation of Two Chilean Diets[14]

200% FAO/WHO Requirements

Supplements	Supplement Cost* $/lb	Break-even Cost of FPC	Concentration of Supp. in Diet**
Dry Skim Milk	.21	$.29	7.8%
Peanut Flour	.06	$.09	23.9%
Cottonseed Flour	.12	$.21	9.4%
Soy Flour	.08	$.14	10.2%
Lysine & Methionine	1.01	$.53	0.6%

150% FAO/WHO Requirements

Supplements	Supplement Cost* $/lb	Break-even Cost of FPC	Concentration of Supp. in Diet***
Dry Skim Milk	.21	$.36	2.5%
Peanut Flour	.06	$.11	6.6%
Cottonseed Flour	.12	$.22	3.0%
Soy Flour	.08	$.17	3.3%
Lysine & Methionine	1.01	$.21	0.2%

----

*All prices include 1¢/lb. transport charge.
**FPC supplements requires 2.5% concentra-
tion.
***FCP supplements requires 0.8% concentra-
tion.

figures are the concentration ratios in staple
items of the diet (see Table 3).

Assuming that supplements are incorporated
into flour and thus used in bread, spaghetti
and flour in Diet I, and in bread only in Diet
II, the concentrations of various supplements
in the staple items can be calculated.

The figures in Table 3 point out a distinct
advantage of FPC and synthetics over alternate
protein sources--their high degree of concentration. Peanut flour requires concentrations
about 8 to 10 times and soy flour about four
times as high as FPC to achieve the nutritional goal. Peanut flour may look attractive in
terms of the dollar cost of supplementation,
but the prospects for inducing a population to
eat flour containing 60 to 70 percent peanut
flour (for 200 percent of FAO/WHO standards)
or even 17 to 20 percent peanut flour, when
peanuts do not already form a staple part of
the diet, appear doubtful. Even soy flour, a
strong competitor in terms of price may face
acceptability problems if introduced into a
staple item at 10 to 30 percent concentrations. The familiar problem of flavor reversion when soy is used in concentrations
greater than 3 to 5 percent has been noted by
Call and Hammonds[5] and elsewhere. Present
technology can produce a purely flavorless soy
protein product, but not for 6 to 7.5¢ per
pound; these flavorless items are the sophisticated spun and extruded proteins used as
meat analogs and are much more expensive.

In summary, the evidence that diets are
typically composed of a variety of foods, even
in the poorest countries, together with the
fact that diets vary among individuals within
countries (probably within local towns and
villages), raises serious doubts about the
general effectiveness and fortification with
synthetic amino acids. This is not to say
that synthetic fortification should be ruled

Table 3.   Concentration in Staple Foods[1]

Supplement	Diet I 150% FAO	200% FAO	Diet II 150% FAC	200% FAO
Dry Skim Milk	7.5%	23%	6.5%	20%
Peanut Flour	20%	71%	17%	62%
Cottonseed Flour	9%	28%	7.8%	24%
Soy Flour	10%	30%	8.6%	25%
Lysine & Methionine	0.6%	11.8%	0.52%	1.5%
FPC	2.5%	7.5%	2.1%	6.2%

----

[1]From Devanney et al.[15]

out. On the contrary, there are in all
probability substantial populations for
which supplementation with synthetics is the
"best" program. But, by the same reasoning,
FPC supplementation should not be rejected
on the ground that it is not "cost effective"
on a diet which virtually no one eats. The
importance of the fact that fish protein,
oilseed proteins, and dairy proteins are
nutritionally more complete than synthetics
is worthy of emphasis. When one fortifies a
stable item with 100 units of FPC, he is
supplying 8 units of lysine to those persons
deficient in lysine, 1 unit of tryptophan to
segments of the population deficient in
tryptophan, 4 units of threonine to individuals deficient in threonine, etc. To some
extent this is true of all oilseed and dairy
proteins. In general, however, the balance
of essential amino acids in animal proteins
(and in FPC in particular) more closely
approximate human requirements than do oilseed and other vegetable proteins.

There is still the possibility of educating the undernourished populations of the
world to eat unfamiliar but nutritions foods.
However, the cost of educating particular
populations must be weighed against the cost
of supplementation with the cheapest, readily
acceptable protein source.

When the MIT study compared supplementation costs for a purely basal diet, fortification with synthetics was found to be "cost
effective" where basal diets were composed
of 100 percent wheat or rice and thus were
limiting in one amino acid only.[15] However,
when the basal diet is corn, two amino acids
(tryptophan and lysine) are limiting and the
high cost of tryptophan ($41.00 per pound at
the time of the study) ruled out supplementation with two synthetic amino acids. In this
case, soy flour was determined to be the least

costly supplement, even with prices adjusted
to reflect shipping charges and foreign exchange losses from importing. In general, the
basal diet of corn appeared most favorable to
supplementation with FPC.

Efficiency under Varying Assumptions. MIT investigators assumed the following in deriving
their results: 1. levels of world prices for
FPC and other protein additives; 2. equal
availability of protein from all alternative
sources; 3. levels of world prices for basal
items (wheat, corn, rice); 4. equal acceptability of all supplements at concentrations
in which they are actually used. It is in-
structive to examine each of these assumptions
in light of currently available information to
assess their validity and their importance to
the conclusions reached.

Recent trends in prices of alternative
supplements could not have been foreseen at
the time of the study; and price changes that
have occurred do not alter significantly the
conclusions reached. The 300 to 400 percent
increase in prices of NFDM served only to increase the already high cost of this protein
source. The price of synthetic lysine has
fallen from $1.14 per pound to about $1.00 per
pound and prices of soy products have remained
nearly constant. We have been unable to obtain price quotations for foreign cottonseed
flour, primarily because the U. S. appears to
be the only major producer of this product.
The price of cottonseed flour used in the MIT
report was obtained from a Central American
firm supplying flour for use in Incaparina,
and we have been unable to determine whether
or not this firm is still operating. For this
reason, the domestic price of 11¢ per pound
plus 1¢ per pound for transport was used as
the world price of human grade cottonseed
flour. We have also been unable to obtain

information on the production or price of
human grade peanut flour, and for this reason
have used the MIT estimate of 5¢ per pound
plus 1¢ per pound for shipping. Using these
data and other price estimates in Table 4 the
break-even costs of supplementation for various basal diets were recomputed.

The relative cost advantages of lysine,
soy flour and peanut flours are evident, although the analysis of varied diets should be
taken into account when considering the
desirability of lysine. As noted in the last
place of column 3 in Table 4, supplementation
with lysine alone cannot achieve the nutritional goal in corn diets. This is because
corn is limiting in tryptophan as well as
lysine. On considerations of current costs
alone, the price of FPC must fall to 16 to 17¢
per pound before it would be competitive with
soy and peanut flours.

The second assumption of equal availability
may be invalid if there are differential
losses in processing or cooking foods with
alternative protein supplements. Studies comparing such protein losses are scarce. In one
study, FPC prepared at the Quintero plant in
Chile was introduced at 6 percent into
"marraqueta" (a small loaf bread consumed by
Chileans) and compared to marraqueta enriched
with 12 percent skim milk powder.[23] After
baking, it was noted that net dietary protein
calories and protein scores were similar for
both samples. Protein scores of both samples
were much lower than before baking on indication that the "Maillard reaction" may have
rendered some of the protein unavailable.
Similar tests conducted with pasta and roasted
whole wheat meal resulted in only slight protein losses for both samples.

Stillings et al. conducted studies to
determine the relative supplemental value of
FPC and lysine when added to wheat flour, both

Table 4. Break-even Cost of FPC Universal
Supplementation of Purely Basal Diets to 150%
FAO/WHO Requirement for 10 Month Old Child*,**

Prices in ¢/lb.

	Wheat	Rice	Corn
Dry Skim Milk 21¢/lb	43	36	65
Peanut Flour 6¢/lb.	16	13	21
Cottonseed Flour 12¢/lb.	32	28	40
Soy Flour	17	13	16
Lysine $1.01/lb.	9	9	x***

----

*Adapted from [14, top pg. 86a] and current
world prices--see preceding section.
**All prices reflect 1¢/lb shipping charge--
no scarcity price on foreign exchange.
***Requirements cannot be met through lysine
supplementation.

before and after processing into bread.[24]   In
rat feeding studies, mixtures containing
alternatively FPC and lysine were added at a
1.6 percent nitrogen level to diets that were
iso-caloric. A diet containing 1.6 percent
nitrogen from casein was used as a control.
Their results show that 6 to 16 percent of the
L-lysine HCl theoretically available could not
be accounted for in the bread and was apparently lost during processing. On the other
hand, lysine in bread fortified with FPC was
within 3 percent of the amount theoretically
available. However, PERs of bread fortified
with FPC were lower than unprocessed mixtures,
indicating that other amino acids were partially lost or rendered unavailable in processing.

Recently Sidwell has undertaken studies to
determine the effect of cooking upon various
staple foods enriched with FPC, dry skim milk,
soy flour, and lysine.[25] All supplements
were added in ratios such that the percentage
of protein added by each was equal. Pasta
enriched with FPC and soy flour showed slight
increases in PERs after cooking although these
were not statistically significant. Slight
decreases in PERs of samples fortified with
dry skim milk, and large significant decreases
were noted with lysine supplementation, indicating that lysine may be prone to leaching.

Thus, it appears that synthetic lysine may
be subject to processing losses on the order
of 10 to 20 percent when used in pasta and
bread. However, these studies have not compared processing losses from all supplements
when used in the relative concentrations required for a particular diet. The concentrations required will probably vary with
different diets, and the percentage of protein
lost in cooking may not be constant with varying concentrations. For these reasons, more
analysis is needed on processing losses for

all protein supplements, when used at varying
concentrations in dietary staples. Besides
losses due to processing and cooking, protein
may be lost because food is not eaten. The
magnitude of these losses will be directly
related to acceptability, which is discussed
below.

Assumptions about the price of the dietary
bases (wheat, rice and corn) are important
because the general nutrition problem is one
of both protein and calories. A protein
supplement that provides calories as well will
permit a decrease in the amount of the base
needed in the total diet. The importance of
this phenomenon will depend upon the value of
the base and the amount of calories which the
protein supplement provides. The more expensive the base, the greater the value of
calories provided by a supplement. The MIT
study rather arbitrarily assumed that the
price of the base was one fifth the cost of
FPC, which translates into about 5¢ per
pound.[15] Data provided by FAO indicate that
the price of wheat flour in international markets
has averaged about 3.8¢ per pound in recent years, and the price of maize has been in
the 2.7 to 2.8¢ per pound range; prices for
both commodities have been markedly stable.[26]

To examine the sensitivity of break-even
costs in Table 4, these figures were recomputed using various assumptions about the
price of basal foods and world prices of
supplements. Because corn appeared most
favorable to FPC fortification, the figures
were recomputed for a corn-based diet only.
Data on the amounts of corn and various
supplements needed to attain 150 percent of
the FAO/WHO standard were taken from the MIT
report.[15] Figures in Table 5 show break-even
costs of FPC under two assumptions about the
cost of supplements (where the shadow price of
foreign exchange is 1.0 and 1.3 respectively)

Table 5. Break-Even Costs of FPC: Universal Supplementation to
150% FAO/WHO Requirement for 10 Month Old Child--Varying Assumptions
about Base Prices and Costs of Supplements (all figures in ¢/lb.)

Supplement	CORN DIET World Prices Supp - A[1]	Break-even Costs AI[2]	Break-even Costs AII[3]	World Prices Supp B[4]	Break-even Costs BI[5]	Break-even Costs BII[6]
Cottonseed Flour	12	47.0	50.0	15.6	61.2	65.0
Soy Flour	8	16.7	17.0	10.4	21.6	22.1
Peanut Flour	6	27.1	30.1	7.8	35.3	39.2

[1]Adapted from [15, top pg. 86a] and current world prices (see preceding
section) -- prices include 1¢/lb. transport cost.
[2]Assuming price of maize = 3¢/lb.
[3]Assuming price of maize = 2.5¢/lb.
[4]Same as 1 but multiplied by 1.3 to reflect foreign exchange loss from
importing.
[5]Same as 2.
[6]Same as 3.

and two assumptions about the price of corn
meal. The break-even cost associated with soy
flour is relatively insensitive to the price
of the base, because soy flour provides only
small amounts of calories. The effect for
peanut flour and cottonseed flour is more
dramatic since both of these supplements supply calories to the total diet in significant
amounts. Under what we consider to be more
realistic prices for basal items, the advantage of supplements supplying calories is
substantially reduced.

The fourth assumption concerning equal
acceptability of all supplements in concentrations in which they occur is the most
difficult to assess. Some indication of the
relative problems that acceptability may present can be gleaned from the break-even cost
figures in Table 6. The concentration ratios
shown apply only to a diet consisting of pure
basal food items (100 percent corn, wheat, or
rice). The relevant concentrations are the
concentrations of supplement in the staple
dietary item. If for example the total diet
consisted of 50 percent staple food and 50
percent nonstaple food, and if the nonstaple
food supplied calories only (no protein) then
the concentration ratios in Table 6 would be
doubled to yield the concentration of supplement in staple foods. In general, concentrations about twice as large as those shown
in Table 6 would seem to be more relevant to
the actual situation; hence the problem of
acceptability becomes even more important.

As in the case with protein availability,
studies comparing acceptability of staple
foods fortified with alternative protein
sources are rare. In 1967, Kwee et al.
evaluated the quality and nutritive value of
various pastas fortified with FPC and soya.[27]
Although no specific analysis was made to
compare acceptance of FPC vs. soya, the

Table 6. Break-even Costs* of FPC and
Concentration Ratios of Supplements for 150%
FAO/WHO Requirement for 10 Month Old Child--
Prices as Indicated

Supplement	Wheat Cost ¢/lb	Wheat Conc. %	Rice Cost ¢/lb	Rice Conc. %	Corn Cost ¢/lb	Corn Conc. %
Dry Skim Milk 21¢/lb	43	5.5	36	4.9	86	12.4
Peanut flour 6¢/lb	16	9.5	13	8.5	30	16.7
Cottonseed flour 12¢/lb	32	7.0	28	6.3	50	9.4
Soy flour 8¢/lb	17	4.8	13	4.4	16	3.5
Lysine $1.01/lb	9	0.18	9	0.6	X	X
FPC	X	2.1	X	1.8	X	1.7

---

*Using world prices and assuming cost of base
is one fifth the per pound cost of FPC.

results of sensory evaluation are interesting.
American panel members were critical of both
texture and tannish appearance when FPC was
added at 20 percent. Indonesian panel members, however, seemed much less critical of
the texture of the 20 percent FPC samples
and in general seemed unaffected by tannish
samples as compared to pale samples. This
underlines the fact that there is no substitute for field testing of various protein
supplements.

In 1969, Bass and Caul conducted sensory
evaluations of chapati, a coarse unleavened
bread prepared from wheat flour, which is
widely eaten in West Pakistan and India.[28]
Alternative supplements used were FPC,
CPC (cottonseed protein concentrate), and
SPC (soy protein concentrate) containing 79.8
percent, 60.1 percent and 66.9 percent
(N x 6.25) respectively. The samples were
evidently not controlled to be iso-caloric or
to have equal amounts of protein available in
the final product. Sensory evaluation was
reported for various concentrations of alternative supplements. As a rough approximation
to iso-nutritious mixtures the results of
fortification with 5 percent FPC, 15 percent
CPC, and 10 percent SPC can be compared. In
the MIT study it was shown that about 3.5
times as much cottonseed flour (50 percent
protein) and 2.3 times as much soy flour (50
percent protein) as FPC were needed to meet
150 percent FAO/WHO nutritional requirements.
Although comparison is difficult, it appears
that both FPC and SPC surpass CPC in both
performance and flavor when all are supplemented in an iso-nutritional fashion. Evaluations of FPC and SPC reveal no marked
differences in the two. This study suffers
from failure to identify in detail the specific FPC, SPC and CPC used. It is known that
the FPC was obtained from a commercial

supplier and held for 18 months before use so
that these results should not be extrapolated
to other types of FPC currently being investigated.

Sidwell recently examined sensory characteristics of wheat-based staple items fortified with FPC, soy flour and dry skim milk.[25]
In general, she found that introduction of
soy flour into bread decreases loaf volumes
about 13 percent when added in 6 percent concentration, whereas fortification with 3 percent FPC caused only about a 1 percent
decrease in volume. She also found that
introduction of both supplements into pasta
(on an equal protein basis) caused cooking
times for both samples to increase; moreover,
the increase for the soy products was about
twice that for the pasta fortified with FPC.
While these studies are not substitutes for
actual acceptability tests in the field, they
do show that significant differences exist
which should be investigated. The extent to
which these results would carry over to similar staple items made from corn is unknown.

Present information does not permit objective evaluation of differentials in acceptability among various supplements. However,
this area is likely to be surprisingly important when supplementation programs are
initiated. The high concentration of protein
in FPC prepared by IPA (isopropyl alcohol)
extraction could provide a substantial advantage.

In mixed diets that vary among individuals
in a given population, the effect of the high
concentration of protein may be magnified by
the good balance of essential amino acids in
FPC. As Table 6 shows, the concentrations of
soy flour required are about twice as high as
those of FPC when a purely basal diet is considered. As noted earlier, however, in mixed
diets (e.g. Chilean diets I and II)

concentrations of soy flour required are four
times as great as those of FPC. The extent to
which these results would apply to other mixed
diets is unknown, but will obviously be of
sufficient importance in actual application to
warrant careful investigation.

Before examining potential markets in
developed countries, it should be noted that
the present IPA-FPC is a highly refined,
harshly extracted material that has been
developed with the USFDA (Food and Drug Administration) standards as a constraint. In effect, the product has been made to conform to
domestic tastes and preferences as interpreted
by the FDA. Preferences in most parts of the
world are likely to be very different, as the
following example indicates.

In the early 1960s, Thomson and Merry conducted nutrition and acceptability tests on
toddler children in Malaysia with alternative
sources of protein: dry skim milk; deodorized
undiluted fish meal; and biscuits containing
12 to 14 percent fish meal, millet, ground nut
flours and sugar.[29] Malays relish the taste
of fish and a small dried salted fish is a
common part of the diet of children and
adults. For this reason, acceptability was no
problem when straight deodorized fish meal and
the fish biscuits were fed to the local children. Nutritional analysis of two groups fed
equivalent amounts of protein in dry skim milk
and fish biscuits respectively showed significantly greater weight gains for the latter
group.

These findings reinforce the recognized
importance of developing a variety of FPCs.
Dietary patterns and tastes vary widely in
different parts of the globe, and it makes
little sense to expect a single supplement,
let alone a single variety of FPC, to be
"best" for all people. Although the extent of
such taste patterns is unknown, it is true

that the practice of feeding dried salted fish
to children is not limited to Malaysia. As
Swaminathan has pointed out, this practice is
widespread in Central Africa, Bangladesh, the
Philippines, Thailand, and South Vietnam.[22]

Delivery Systems in Developing Countries.
There are two general categories of marketing
structure that helps define the delivery problem. The first, perhaps best illustrated by
the Latin American economies, involves a large
mass of urban and rural poor, who are woefully
deficient in proteins and often in calories,
in nations whose middle and upper income citizens support a modern commercial marketing
system for foodstuffs. Although there are
exceptions, the majority of the diet-deficient
target group sell their services or commodities for money and purchase at least some portion of their food requirements through retail
stores or open markets. A substantial proportion of even the very poor purchase some processed foods. Both the form in which food is
consumed and the ways in which it is delivered
to the buyer provide "bottlenecks" at which
protein supplementation is technically possible in a sufficiently large scale for commercial operation. Given the factors that make
universal supplementation a necessity in some
regions, such bottlenecks are absolutely
essential if large blocs of people are to be
reached at minimum cost.
     Unfortunately, a large part of the world's
poor and needy do not live in this kind of
economy. For example, more than 100 million
people in Black Africa south of the Sahara
live in a purely subsistence economy, or produce cash crops only for minimal purchases of
manufactured goods. Even when they are incorporated into a rudimentary market economy in
the larger cities, a remarkably high proportion of these people still walk, cycle, or

ride buses to homes outside the urban area
where they can grow their own food. Trade
flourishes, of course, even in subsistence
societies, but it consists largely of barter
or very simple money exchanges in periodic
open markets. A similar living pattern is
common in many parts of Asia.

There is simply no best--or even any very
good--solution to protein malnutrition in
these communities. There is seldom a focal
point where additives can be incorporated in
bulk; most food is eaten unprocessed or is
processed as required in the household or
village. Purchased foods are likely to be
luxury items, acquired intermittently. Under
these conditions, sophisticated comparisons of
protein products in terms of cost-effective-
ness are simply pointless. Even where the
typical dietary pattern might suggest that
synthetics or soy flour would be most desirable, for example, there is literally no way
in which either product could be utilized on a
broad scale. NFDM and FPC have physical properties that make them much easier to distri-
bute to the urban poor in these areas, but the
delivery of protein supplements to the rural
needy--usually a much larger segment of the
population--remains intractable.

The only logical points of attack appear to
be the small but growing clusters of institutional concentration: schools, hospitals,
mobile clinics, and prisons. Introduction of
protein additives to the diets of these "captive consumers" and perhaps some educational
effort to extend their use warrant careful
investigation, case by case. But the extent
to which such programs might reach back to the
real target--the weanling child--is not encouraging.

Protein Supplements in Developed Countries
Although the FPC program was initially

intended to provide low cost protein to low
income countries, it had been recognized that
a number of possible uses in the domestic
force industry might provide an important
market. The potential of fish protein for use
in high income developed countries may be
judged less important, from the standpoint of
social welfare, than its potential for feeding
starving populations, but the benefits from
providing high income countries with lower
cost protein additives are still very real.
More than forty major U. S. food processing
firms have requested samples of FPC for use in
product testing and development. These firms
included major soft drink manufacturers, producers of baby foods, canned fruits and vegetables, breakfast cereals, baked goods, and
processed meats, as well as major distributors
of soy proteins and casein. As one might expect, given recent developments in prices of
dairy products, a major U. S. distributor of
casein for animal feed and human consumption,
expressed the greatest interest in acquiring
FPC for testing.

To date, the technical feasibility of producing "functional" fish protein concentrate
from whole fish has not been demonstrated. In
the absence of even rough estimates of processing costs, we can only speculate about the
potential role of functional FPC in the food
industries of developed countries. Because of
this lack of information the following section
will be confined to a review of literature on
domestic markets for protein and on research
aimed at the development of functional FPC.
Wherever possible, the results of research on
functionality will be related to potential
uses in the U. S. food industry.

The Potential Market. Hammonds and Call conducted a thorough investigation of present and
potential utilization of protein ingredients

in the U. S. food industry.[5] We summarize
below the more salient findings in that report
and relate their conclusions to some of the
on-going research on the utilization of FPC in
domestic foods.

Perhaps the most impressive finding reported in this study is the variety of functional properties which various protein
ingredients impart to final products and the
importance of these properties in the demand
for such proteins. In addition to acceptable
taste and nutritional value, the ability to
absorb fat and water, stabilize an emulsion,
bind other ingredients, carry flavors and
colors, and improve texture are highly valued
in the food industry. Hammonds and Call[5]
estimated wholesale trade by product class in
the U. S. food industry and then examined
specific product ingredients to find the percentage of functional protein in various
products (functional protein is defined in
this context to include protein added to improve physical properties of the end product
as well as the portion of total nutritional
protein content added in ingredient form).
These percentages were then applied to the
trade volume data to estimate a potential
volume of functional protein (i.e., protein
in foods which could be replaced by alternative protein ingredients) of 3.1 billion
pounds annually. From this figure they subtracted their estimate of the volume of functional protein currently used (0.9 to 1.1
billion pounds) to arrive at a figure of 2.0
to 2.2 billion pounds as the maximum potential untapped market for functional protein.
Of the 3.1 billion pound gross potential,
approximately 600 million pounds could be
relatively unsophisticated items, while the
remaining 2.5 billion pounds would require
higher degrees of functionality.

The most important protein products in

current use are milk protein products (NFDM,
dry whole milk, casein and sodium caseinate);
soy protein products (meal and grits, flour,
concentrates and isolates); egg proteins; and
hydrolized vegetable proteins. Of these
ingredients, nonfat dry milk is easily the
most important, in terms of both physical and
dollar volume, but its position is expected
to decline significantly.

A bland or unobjectionable taste is a very
important factor in the ingredients market in
the U. S. The characteristic flavor of soy,
evident when used in concentrations greater
than 4 to 5 percent, has apparently hindered
its use in foods now using milk protein, even
though soy products possess many desirable
functional characteristics and cost much less
per pound of protein than NFDM and casein.

An FPC with good nutritional quality and
very bland taste may be able to compete with
NFDM in the market for baby food, breakfast
food, candy, and diet drinks with a combined
potential to absorb 22.6 million pounds of
protein (as of 1969). A concentrated fish
protein with the ability to absorb fat might
be able to compete with NFDM and soy concentrates and isolates in the large market for
canned and processed meats where slightly
objectionable tastes can be masked by the
addition of spices.

The concept of using comminuted fish
products for human consumption is not new.
Many products made from fish processed in this
way have already been marketed successfully.
In Japan, for instance, the production of fish
sausages and "hams" grew from 81,269 metric
tons in 1959 to 170,660 metric tons in 1964.
In India, fish sausage has gained acceptance
and "fish fingers" developed in the United
Kingdom have apparently been successful.[30]
However, most of these products are prepared
from large fish which have been skinned,

eviscerated and deboned. Utilization of
small, "trash fish" appears unfeasible unless
efficient flesh separating devices are developed for use on small fish of mixed sizes
and species.

Most of the work done on developing a
functional fish protein concentrate from
trash fish has attempted to modify the standard IPA-FPC to produce a soluble product.
FPC solubilization can be achieved by several
processes. The use of direct biological conversion by microorganisms has been reviewed
by Roels,[31] and the direct use of enzymes has
been investigated by Hale.[32] Cheftel et al.
have worked on enzymatic solubilization of FPC
in a process of continuous operation that re-
covers the enzymes for re-use.[33] In two
articles, Tannenbaum et al. described the use
of sodium hydroxide and high temperatures to
achieve a high yield of FPC solids.[34] Research undertaken at Texas A & M University
has produced a process of preparing a functional FPC using ethanol and hexane to extract
lipids from comminuted fish (golden
croaker).[30] Other significant research has
been undertaken at the NMFS laboratory in
Seattle to develop an extraction process that
would produce a functional FPC.[35]

Anglemier has investigated opportunities
for incorporating unmodified IPA-FPC into
snack crackers, candy and processed meats.[36]
Encouraging results were obtained with all
three products. IPA-FPC was added at 1 percent to wieners and Polish sausage (prepared
in the laboratory) and compared to samples
containing 1 percent soy protein concentrate.
Taste panels were generally unable to detect
significant differences in the two products,
although the FPC sausage and wieners were
rated slightly better than those containing
soy protein. Similar experiments were conducted using 3 percent FPC or soy protein

concentrate with ice to replace 12.5 percent
of the meat in weiners. FPC products were
judged significantly better than wieners containing soy protein concentrate. When FPC
and soy protein concentrate were used at 4
percent with ice to replace 25 percent of the
meat in Polish sausage the results of sensory
evaluation were mixed. It is significant that
no flavor problems were encountered when 25
percent of the meat in sausages was replaced
by FPC, although the characteristic red color
of the original product was dulled somewhat.
It was also noted that FPC did not undergo
flavor reversion with prolonged storage as soy
often does.

These results with processed meat must be
qualified, since the meat ingredients used
were of rather high quality and possessed
better natural binding properties than the
lower grade meats used by commercial processors. Even so, it is encouraging that the
functional characteristics of unmodified FPC
were as good as or better than soy when used
in concentrations close to those actually
employed by industry (1.6 to 3.3 percent
functional protein). This market consumed
over 66 million pounds of protein in 1969,
which was principally from soy protein concentrates and isolates (at 27 to 42¢ per pound
protein) and nonfat dry milk (at 40 to 50¢ per
pound protein).[5] The FDA is currently working
on standards of identity for meat extenders
and analogs, and present indications are that
these products will be required to duplicate
meat in all nutritional aspects.[6] Such
standards should further enhance the position
of FPC vis-à-vis soy protein in this important
market.

Production Costs of FPC
The preceding analysis has been largely independent of economic considerations involved in

processing FPC. The species to utilize, location of the processing activity, and other
factors bearing on FPC costs are considered in
this section. Because detailed cost figures
from actual commercial scale operation are
unavailable, it is necessary to rely on various engineering estimates for much of the
analysis.

Operating Experience. Technological methods
for producing FPC from whole raw fish may be
categorized into chemical, physical, and biological. These processes have been described
in detail elsewhere.[37-40] Recently NMFS researchers have been working on a process of
aqueous phosphate processing that shows promise especially for processing fatty fish.[41]
To date three specific processes have been
developed to the point of commercialization:
the VioBin process developed by Levin in
which lipids are extracted from comminuted
fish with ethylene dichloride; the Astra process which uses a press cake made from deboned eviscerated fish and removes lipids by
alcohol extraction; and the IPA process which
utilizes successive extractions with IPA moving in a direction counter current to the raw
material.[39-44]
    In 1968, the BCF (Bureau of Commercial
Fisheries) awarded a contract to Ocean Harvesters (a joint enterprise of SWECO and Star-
kist Foods, Inc.) to construct and operate
an experiment and demonstration plant using
the IPA process developed by the BCF. The
objectives of the contract were to: gain
engineering knowledge through design, construction and operation of the pilot plant;
provide FPC for experimental use; and provide
a vehicle for conducting research on the
methodology of manufacturing FPC.[43] Raw
material to be used in the plant was ocean
hake caught off the coast of Washington.

During the summer of 1971, the technical
feasibility of producing FPC from hake using
the BCF process was clearly demonstrated.
By late 1971 some 90,000 pounds of final
product had been certified as meeting FDA
specifications on protein content (no less
than 75 percent), residual IPA (less than 250
ppm), fluoride content (less than 100 ppm),
lipids (less than 0.5 percent) as well as
standards for ash and moisture content,
bacteriological count and nutritive value.[43]

Although this measure of success was
achieved, the plant was plagued with raw
material shortages and frequent mechanical
breakdowns. Equipment problems are to be expected in a pilot operation, especially when
capital costs are subject to a binding constraint on funds; but the recent decline in
the availability of Washington hake was not
foreseeable. As a result, the rate of production rarely approached capacity (50 tons
per day input) and was never sustained long
enough for the system to reach an operating
equilibrium. Furthermore, it was initially
planned to utilize an adjacent fish meal plant
to process soluble proteins, fish oil and the
bone fraction removed from hake by deboning.
Unfortunately, the fish meal plant terminated
operation before the feasibility of processing
by-products could be examined.

The EDP (Experimental and Demonstration
Plant) showed that deboning was necessary with
hake if FDA standards for fluoride were to be
met. This was a prime cause for the relatively low yields of 7.5 to 8.1 percent realized
(weight of FPC as percentage of weight of
whole fish). Deboning removed about 15 percent of the protein in raw fish, and of the
protein remaining, 71 percent was recovered in
the form of high quality FPC (over 95 percent
protein) and well within FDA standards for
fluoride. Protein losses are also believed to

be related to the length of time fish are
stored. The protein content of fish entering
the plant (most of which had been stored in
chilled brine 1 to 7 days) averaged about 12.6
percent, considerably lower than the 14 to 15
percent normally found in freshly caught hake.
This represents about a 15 percent loss in
protein before the fish are even deboned. It
is obvious that improved storage techniques or
elimination of extensive storage by operating
near a day fishery are of prime importance.
Where deboning is required, the 15 percent
losses in protein to the bone fraction should
be at least partially recoverable, since the
bone fraction contains about 50 percent high
quality protein and could probably be processed into animal feed.

Thus, the fish actually entering the EDPs
extraction process contained about 73 percent
of the protein in whole fresh fish. Of this
amount, about 71 percent was recovered. Protein lost in processing included 15 percent in
the bottom of the distillation column, 9 percent in sludge from the centrifuge used to
clarify spent miscella and 5 percent in fine
protein.[43] The use of decanters to replace
the screens and presses now employed to
separate liquids from solids has been considered as one method of cutting the amount
of fine protein going into the miscella and
eventually being discarded in the form of
sludge at the clarifying centrifuge.[45]
Furthermore, the length of time spent in brine
storage seems to have an effect on the way
protein behaves in processing; decreasing
storage time may reduce the fraction of protein that becomes soluble in processing. The
material collected in the bottom of the distillation column contains fish oil and soluble
fish proteins. Recovery of these by-products
will be important to the economic feasibility
of the process.

Problems with solvent recovery were also
encountered during operation. These losses
averaged about 0.1 pound IPA lost per pound
of FPC produced (which represents about 6¢ per
pound FPC in solvent costs). These losses
were believed to be primarily the result of
mechanical breakdown--i.e., losses resulting
when pumps and lines are unclogged, etc. It
is believed that losses of 0.025 pound IPA per
pound FPC (or about 1 1/2¢ per pound FPC in
solvent cost) could be attained in a commercial scale plant.[45]

The operation at Aberdeen was by no means
the first attempt at commercial scale processing of FPC. In 1970 Astra Nutrition, a
Swedish firm, began processing a high grade
FPC (over 90 percent protein) from press cake
produced aboard a factory ship.[46] Cardinal
Proteins of Canada constructed a 200 ton per
day (input) plant in Nova Scotia to process
FPC using alcohol extraction. Its designers
planned to satisfy a large part of their input
requirements with sanitary fish trimmings
from an adjacent food fish processing plant.[47]
The Peruvian firm of Carlos Verrando reportedly made a low grade FPC from Peruvian hake,
using hexane vapors to extract lipids from
comminuted and heat dehydrated fish.[48] In the
late 1960s Alpine Marine Protein Industries,
Inc. of New Bedford, Massachusetts, was en-
gaged in processing FPC using the VioBin process, but it has since discontinued
production. Other attempts at commercial
scale manufacture of FPC have been described
by Knobl.[37]

Engineering Cost Estimates: The General
Oceanology and MIT Data. Unfortunately, information on processing costs from commercial
manufacturers is not available; and useful
estimates of cost cannot be constructed as yet
from data generated by the pilot plant at

Aberdeen. Thus, it is necessary to rely on
engineering estimates. The most widely used
estimates are those provided by SWECO for an
IPA extraction plant with capacity to process
180 metric tons of raw fish per day. These
estimates were adopted by General Oceanology,
Inc. (GO) in their studies of the "Commercial
Feasibility of Fish Protein Concentrate in
Developing Countries".[49] In studying the
feasibility of FPC in Chile, GO estimated that
raw material (local hake) could be purchased
for $22.00 per metric ton and would be suffi-
ciently available to permit the plant to
operate 200 days per year. Although $22.00
per metric ton is the purchase price of hake,
the true cost of using Chilean hake in FPC is
somewhat higher; utilizing hake for FPC would
necessitate diverting it from the fish meal
industry which produces primarily for export.
Exporting fish meal earns foreign exchange for
the economy and since foreign exchange is
scarce in Chile (as it is in most developing
economies) its value to the economy is greater
than the par value of the currency. This
scarcity premium was estimated at 30 percent
in the Chilean situation, hence the cost of
hake to the economy was placed at $28.60 per
metric ton. According to GO estimates, the
cost of raw material represented 28 percent of
production costs minus the scarcity premium on
foreign exchange, and 33 percent when the premium is included. Thus, ignoring foreign exchange losses, a small change of x% in the
price of raw material will bring forth a .28x%
change in the cost of the final product. All
these estimates are based on costs of production before taxes and profits.

Other items of cost included in the GO figures are "fixed costs" (primarily payments for
labor, supervision and maintenance, depreciation, and annual outlays for interest and loan
amortization). The labor components of "fixed

Table 7. Costs of Producing FPC in Chile -- Re-estimates of General
Oceanology[49] Figures

Cost Parameters - Value of plant, $3,628,000; Value of depreciable assets,
$3,200,000; life of assets, 5 years; interest rate, 10%; cost of raw
material, $22.00/MT; solvent loss, 5%; oil content of fish (as % of whole
weight), 3%.

I. Nonvariable Costs:
    A. Interest - $362,800/year, P.V. interest @ 10%
        for 5 years $ 1,375,012
    B. Depreciation - P.V. of $3,200,000 @ 10% after
        5 years $ 1,987,200
    C. P.V. of Nonvariable costs $ 3,362,212

II. Variable Costs:
    A. Raw material -- $146.70/MT, FPC - $792,800/yr.,
        P.V. raw material @ 10% for 5 years $ 3,004,712
    B. Other materials (except solvent) $81.60/MT FPC
        or $440,640/year
    C. Solvent loss (5%) $325,000/year
    D. Fixed cost (labor, etc.) $362,400/year
    E. B + C + D. $1,129,840/year, P.V. @ 10% for 5
        years $ 4,282,113

III. P.V. all costs @ 10% for 5 years $10,649,037
IV. P.V. of total rev.: 27MT FPC/day for 200 days/year
     = 5400 MT/year = 11,880,000 lbs/year
     P.V. of total rev. = P.V. at (11,880,000) x (Price/
     lb) = 45,025,000 x (Price/lb)
     set P.V. (total rev.) = P.V. (total cost) and
     solve for price =   23.65¢/lb.
     subtract credit for by-products =   1.89
                                                                 21.76¢/lb.*

*This is about 1% lower than the GO estimate.

cost" as termed above are normally variable
(varying with the rate of output, number of
days of operation, etc.) but the custom in
Chile is to pay workers an annual wage regardless of the amount of time worked. In other
situations it is probably more realistic to
consider these costs as variable. Interest
and amortization costs are independent of the
rate of output; to the extent that depreciation is due to obsolescence, these costs will
also be invariant to the rate of output.

The distinction between "variable" and "
"nonvariable" costs was drawn so that the importance of certain variables assumed to be
critical to the cost of the final product
could be examined. To derive an estimate of
"nonvariable" costs of production, the following assumptions were made on the basis of the
GO figures: 1. The total capital cost of the
plant is $3.628 million; 2. The estimated
total write-off in five years on depreciable
assets is $3.2 million; 3. The interest rate
is 10%. We are not necessarily defending the
validity of these assumptions; rather we are
using them to examine the structure of costs
within the General Oceanology framework.

Since the amount of interest and amortization payable in any given year will depend
upon specific loan arrangements, we assume
that the entire $3.628 million is borrowed
initially at 10 percent compounded annually
and is payable at the end of the fifth year of
production. This assumption has the conven-
ient feature of incorporating both interest
payments and depreciation costs in the same
context. The total cost of interest payments
is the present value of interest payments in
each year (at 10 percent) on $3.628 million
for five years. At the end of year five, all
nondepreciable assets are sold for $428,000
and the balance of the loan ($3.2 million) is
paid. Thus, total depreciation cost under

this arrangement is the present value of $3.2
million (at 10 percent) five years hence. The
figures in Table 7 display the importance of
"nonvariable" costs in the total cost of the
final product. The life of productive assets
chosen by GO was rather short, apparently because it was felt that advances in technology
would make the process and some of the extraction equipment obsolete within that time
period. Thus depreciation is not due to wear
and tear and will not be directly related to
the rate of operation. The same is true of
the opportunity cost of invested capital (or
interest payments if loan financing is used).
Thus a y% increase in the number of days the
plant can operate will result in a 0.32y% decrease in the cost of producing the final
product. Once again, these figures do not include tax payments or profit for the entrepreneur. To the extent that tax payments are
fixed, annual charges and profits are a return
to invested capital, inclusion of these components would only magnify the importance of
"nonvariable" costs.
     Cost estimates provided in the MIT study[15]
were adopted from the same SWECO production
plan and are of the same general order of magnitude. Significant differences between GO
and MIT assumptions are: 1. MIT estimates are
based upon 150 operating days per year;
2. Opportunity costs of capital and depreciation costs were adjusted to reflect foreign
exchange losses since they estimate that about
two-thirds of plant capital will be imported;
3. A ten year life of productive capital was
used; 4. An interest rate of 12 percent was
assumed. Evidently, revenue from the sale of
by-products (fish oil and soluble protein) was
not credited against production costs when
estimating the final cost of FPC.
     In the MIT report, all costs were reported
as costs to the economy (with foreign exchange

valued at 130 percent of par value). Raw
material accounted for about 33 percent of
total cost, and "nonvariable" capital and depreciation costs contributed about 26 percent
to the cost of the final product. Again, the
importance of raw material costs and the number of operating days per year are evident.

Modification of Cost Data: Other Supply
Sources. In light of these facts, it seems
odd that the MIT study did not analyze the
problem in terms of alternative, low cost,
regularly available supplies of fish. FPC, as
produced by present technology, is a highly
concentrated product from which as much as 85
percent of the bulk and weight of the raw
material is removed by processing. The final
product is a high value, low bulk and weight
commodity that is storable and easily transported. Efficient production of such commodities generally calls for location of the processing facility close to the best possible
source of raw material and shipment of the
final product to markets for consumption.
The possibility of locating an FPC plant at
the most globally efficient location(s),
regardless of local nutritional problems, and
producing for export to those countries which
can best benefit from FPC remains to be explored. The tendency to view FPC as a means
of developing new employment opportunities for
depressed or nonexistent industrial fishing
industries has also obscured the economic
evaluation of FPC.
     There are several possible reasons why the
approach outlined above has not been utilized.
First, at the time the MIT study was undertaken, hake was the only species of fish that
had been approved by the U. S. Food and Drug
Administration. Since then, menhaden and
herring have been approved and it is anticipated that anchovy will soon be added to the

list. Thus, if one were bound by FDA
regulations to use hake, Chile might be a good
locational choice. However, these standards
seem irrelevent when considering supplementation for undernourished populations. A second
possible reason has to do with the general
scarcity of foreign exchange in developing
countries. Importing FPC from a foreign producer would involve spending valuable foreign
exchange, thus (apparently) magnifying the
cost of FPC supplementation to the economy.
However, the decision to produce FPC domestically also involves foreign exchange losses.
As both the GO and MIT studies point out, fish
used in the manufacture of FPC will generally
have to be transferred from the production of
fish meal that is produced for export.
Furthermore, as the MIT study noted, a substantial portion of the plant capital would
probably be imported from industrial countries. Both of these factors involve foreign
exchange losses.

An estimate of the net loss in foreign exchange involved in importing FPC vs. producing
it domestically can be derived from the MIT
cost figures. Consider two hypothetical
countries for which the opportunity costs of
fish, labor, capital, etc. are identical
(Tables 8 and 9). In country A, foreign exchange commands a 30 percent scarcity premium,
while in country B, foreign exchange is valued
at par. Applying the MIT cost figures to both
cases, the cost of FPC to the economy of
country A is 25.4¢ per pound--identical to the
MIT estimate. In country B, the cost of FPC
to the economy is about 22.1¢ per pound. If
country A imports FPC from country B at 23.1¢
per pound (which includes a 1¢ per pound shipping charge), the cost of imported FPC to
economy A is 30.0¢ per pound, the value of
foreign exchange lost; this is 18 percent
higher than the cost of producing at home. In

the example given above, country A should
import if it can find a producer who will sell
FPC at a price which is at least 18 percent
lower than production cost in country A.
Thus, the net foreign exchange losses involved
in importing FPC are not as great as they
might appear at first glance.

   With these considerations in mind, various
potential locations were surveyed. In an unpublished report Crutchfield et al. summarized
present and potential fisheries for reduction.[50] From among several likely possibilities, two fisheries, the Peruvian anchoveta
fishery and the lightly exploited Northern
anchovy fishery located off the coast of
Southern California, were chosen for more
intensive investigation. It was deemed
desirable to investigate production costs in
one domestic (U. S.) site as well as at an
efficient foreign location. The two fisheries
were chosen for several reasons: fish are
presently landed at both locations at relatively low cost; climatic conditions in both
areas permit fishing virtually year round; and
behavioral patterns of both species (schooling
and migration habits) permit landing both
species throughout the year. It is true that
neither species has been given FDA approval
for human consumption, although it is believed
that this approval will soon be forthcoming
for Northern anchovies. In any event, FDA
standards may well be of little consequence to
foreign nations.

   The future course of any clupeoid fishery
is inherently uncertain; as Crutchfield et al.
point out, the collapse of the California sardine, Atlanto-Scandian herring, and other
fisheries of the same type is a sobering consideration.[50] However, Paulik has described
the anchovy as a possible "fish of the
future," noting that the stocks are most productive when fishing intensity is high.[50] He

Table 8. Costs of Producing FPC in Chile--Re-estimates of MIT[15] Figures Costs to Chilean Economy (30% scarcity value on foreign exchange)

Cost Parameters—Value of plant $3,955,000 (with premium on foreign exchange); value of depreciable assets $3,955,000; life of assets, 10 years; interest rate 12%; cost of raw material $28.60/MT.

I.   Nonvariable Costs
     A. Interest and depreciation—Present Value $ 3,955,000
II. Variable Costs:
     A. Raw material - $191.00/MT or $895,500/year
        P.V. @ 12% for 10 years $ 5,059,575
     B. Other variable costs (except solvent) $81.60/MT
                                       or $376,200/yr
     C. Solvent cost (5% solvent loss) $325,000/yr
     D. Fixed cost (labor, etc.) $362,400/yr
     E. B + C + D $1,063,600/yr
        P.V. for 10 years @ 12 % $ 6,009,340
III. P.V. all costs @ 12% for 10 years $15,023,915
IV. P.V. of total cost: 30MT/day for 150 days/year =
     9,900,000 lbs. per year
     A. P.V. of total rev = P.V. of (9,900,000) x (Cost/lb)
        = 55,935,000 (Cost/lb)
     B. Equate A to P.V. of all costs (III) and solve
        for cost/lb.   26.86¢/lb.*
     C. Credit Sale of by-products (at scarcity value of
        foreign exchange) 2.46¢/lb FDC   24.40/lb.**

*This is about 6% above MIT estimate
**This is about 4% below MIT estimate

Table 9.   Costs of Producing FPC in Chile--
Re-estimate of MIT[15] Figures Production Costs
(no scarcity premium on foreign exchange)

I.   Nonvariable Costs $ 3,274,000
        A. P.V. interest and
            depreciation $ 3,274,000
II.   Variable Costs
        A. P.V. raw material $ 3,891,820
        B. P.V. other variable
            costs $ 6,009,340
III.   P.V. all costs $13,175,160
IV.   Production cost of FPC   23.65¢/lb
        Credit for sale of by-
        products (1.89¢/lb)   21.76¢/lb

Note: Figures in Tables 7 and 8 were used as
a framework for analyzing MIT costs. For
example, to estimate production costs in MIT
figures, take the difference between the
figure 26.86¢/lb (Table 7) and 23.65¢/lb
(Table 8) as the foreign exchange cost. This
figure is subtracted from the MIT figure of
25.4¢/lb to derive an estimate of production
costs in the MIT context. This is 22.1¢/lb.

draws this conclusion from the facts that
growth of the species is most rapid at early
ages, and there seems to be no strong
relationship between the number of spawning
adults and subsequent recruitment. This is
not to imply that the stocks are not capable
of being fished to a degree that poses a real
threat; given the right set of climatic and
economic conditions, the fisheries could be
rapidly depleted. However this seems likely
with anchovies than with most other species.

Cost Analysis for FPC from Peruvian Anchoveta. Catch and price statistics for the
Peruvian anchoveta fishery were obtained from
the Instituto del Mar del Peru.[52] During
the period from 1966-1969, the reported
average annual price varied from $9.31 to
$11.92 per metric ton. Landings in 1966
were 8.5 million metric tons and reached a
peak of 10.3 million metric tons in 1968
(this represents 18 to 20 percent of the
estimated total world catch of all species
for that year). The price statistics have
been challenged by various experts in the
field who point out that most Peruvian purse
seiners are owned by fish meal companies and
reported payments for landed fish are merely
crew shares. The true cost of landing anchoveta in 1969 has been estimated at $11.00 to
$15.00 when capital costs are included.[53]
     Since the price of fish is crucially im-
portant to the feasibility of FPC, the problem of obtaining a reliable estimate of price
was investigated further. Roemer provides an
excellent study of Peruvian fishing and fish
meal industries.[54] He has estimated cost
functions for producing fish meal as well as
average yields (pounds of fish meal per pound
of fish) for processors. Using these data,
one can work backward from the price of fish
meal to derive an estimate of the cost of fish

in any particular year. Applying this
technique to the 1969 price of fish meal
(f.o.b. Peru), produces an estimate of $11.20
as the cost per metric ton of landing anchoveta. It is known that in periods when fish
cannot be found close to port, the seiners
may stay out two or three days between landings. This may cause deterioration of fish
stored on board so that shipboard refrigeration may be necessary in some instances. The
frequency of this phenomenon is unknown, but
it is not believed to be too important. Estimates of the cost increases one could expect
from installing refrigeration equipment
aboard a modern seiner are in the 10 to 15
percent range. Thus, a price of $12.50 per
metric ton will be used as the cost of landing Peruvian anchoveta in subsequent analysis.

Data obtained from the Instituto del Mar
del Peru,[52] showed that the fish supply was
sufficient to provide daily input capacity for
a 200 ton per day plant eleven months in 1969.
Examination of catch data showed that this was
also the case in 1968. The closed season ex-
tends from June through August, but it does
not apply to fishermen in southern ports who
are allowed to land fish throughout the year.
In the months of February and March, fishing
is restricted to weekdays only, but this
should be no problem for a plant with three
day storage capacity.

Aside from low costs and regularly available supplies of fish, other factors considered important to the efficient production
of FPC are an operating fish meal industry
and a labor pool possessing the technical
skills needed to operate an FPC plant. Locating adjacent to an existing fish meal plant is
considered important because such a facility
could absorb temporary excess fish supplies at
the FPC plant[49] and could also process bone
and skin fractions obtained when FPC is

manufactured from deboned fish, as well as
other by-products such as fish oil and fish
solubles. This is no problem in either Peru
or Southern California.

   With regard to skills available in the
labor pool, Ocean Harvesters, Inc., the firm
operating the NMFS (formerly the Bureau of
Commercial Fisheries) pilot plant in Aberdeen,
indicates that crucial personnel requirements
are: supervision and administration requiring
engineering and administrative skills; quality
control requiring laboratory technicians;
production personnel requiring a few boiler-
making or related activities; and laborers who
could be trained on the job. Labor pool
requirements are obviously no problem in
Southern California; as for Peru, Roemer[54]
cites encouraging evidence that supervisors in
the fish meal industry generally hold engineering degrees and almost all are Peruvian
citizens. Skilled mechanics, electricians,
etc. are also required in the sugar and chemical refining industries. Quality control
personnel should be no problem given the
existence of a vigorous sugar refining industry.

   FPC has been produced at the NMFS laboratories from a variety of species, including
the Northern anchovy. The process used was
the usual four-stage, counter-current IPA extraction and did not differ from that used on
hake.[38] We are not aware of any commercial
scale production of anchovy-FPC using the IPA
process, although the pilot plant in Aberdeen
did operate on anchovies for one month in
1972. The fish, which had been frozen and
shipped from California, were thawed three to
four days in brine before use. This caused
some problems since conditions of storage
directly affect the behavior of the protein
during processing. Even so, the normal four
stages of extraction used on hake were

sufficient to extract FPC from anchovies.[45]
The ratio of solvent to fish requires some
adjustment when going from lean to fatty fish,
but this caused no serious problems. Yields
were slightly less than those experienced
with hake, but this was probably because the
fish had to be frozen and subsequently thawed.
The end product was slightly darker than that
produced from hake and had a reddish-brown
color. However, limited laboratory work has
shown that the final product can be lightened
by the use of hydrogen peroxide in one of the
extraction phases. The nutritive value and
acceptability of anchovy-FPC have been investigated, but discussion of these aspects is
reserved for later.

    With this information in hand, the MIT cost
figures were adopted to the Peruvian situation
in the following manner. We start by assuming
that the wage rates paid to labor and supervision are equal in Chile and Peru. Furthermore, we assume that the costs of productive
capital, production materials (solvent, elec-
trical power, water, fuel oil, etc.) and taxes
are equal in both countries. Thus, the major
differences between the Peruvian and Chilean
situations is the cost of raw material and the
number of days the plant can operate. Payments for labor, supervision, maintenance, and
taxes are assumed to vary directly with the
rate of output. Since we are considering producing FPC in Peru for export to other countries, the operation will earn foreign
exchange for the Peruvian economy. Thus we
have not placed a scarcity premium upon fish
diverted from the fish meal industry or upon
the cost of imported capital. As noted earlier, production costs in Chile were estimated
at 22.1¢ per pound using MIT figures and were
based upon $22.00 per metric ton as the cost
of raw material and 150 days of operation.
Taking this figure as a starting point,

production costs in the Peruvian situation
were estimated as shown in Table 10.

The figures in Table 10 show production
costs in a variety of Peruvian situations,
assuming that all factors except the number of
operating days, value of foreign exchange, and
cost of fish are identical to the situation in
Chile. The figure of 250 operating days per
year will be used as a bench mark in further
sensitivity testing since it appears to be a
conservative estimate of the number of days
that fish of suitable quality could be available in Peru. Thus, within the context of MIT
cost estimates, a figure of 16¢ per pound
seems a reasonable estimate of production
costs in Peru. We are less certain about the
absolute level of production costs than we are
about the effect which variation in certain
parameters has upon cost. Thus, the most important figure in Table 10 is the 5.4¢ per
pound decrease in production cost that is realized by moving the operation from Chile to
Peru.

Taking the figure of 16¢ per pound as the
most likely Peruvian production cost (within
the MIT framework) we tested the sensitivity
of this figure to the rate of interest and the
life and cost of productive capital. A 12
percent rate of interest, a ten year life for
productive assets and a cost of $3.274 million
for plant capital was used in the MIT study.
Table 11 shows the effect upon production
costs of allowing the interest rate to vary
from 6 percent to 14 percent (given a ten year
life of assets), and the effect of varying the
cost and useful life of assets given a 12 percent rate of interest.

Production costs are rather insensitive to
assumptions about interest rates and the cost
and life of capital assets over plausible
ranges; using a 6 percent rate of interest instead of 12 percent reduces costs by less than

Table 10.   Production Costs, FPC from
Peruvian Anchoveta and Chilean Hake (MIT
Data)[15]

Operating days per year	Cost of Fish $/MT	Prod. Cost of FPC (¢/lb)	Prod. Cost + 1¢/lb Shipping	Location
150	22.00	22.1*	23.1*	Chile
150	12.50	19.1	20.1	Peru
200	12.50	17.6	18.6	Peru
250	12.50	16.7**	17.7**	Peru
300	12.50	16.2	17.2	Peru

----

*MIT estimate of "production cost" in Chile
(no scarcity premium on foreign exchange).
**250 operating days per year seems most like-
ly for Peru.

Table 11. Sensitivity of Production Costs of FPC from Peruvian Anchoveta (From MIT data)[15]

Effect of interest rate		Effect of life of assets		Effect of non-variable costs	
Interest rate %	Production cost including 1 cent/lb shipping* cents/lb	Life of assets yrs	Production cost including 1 cent/lb shipping** cents/lb	Non-variable costs million $	Production cost including 1 cent/lb shipping*** cents/lb
6	16.9	6	19.1	3.274	17.7
8	17.2	8	18.2	3.500	17.9
10	17.5	10	17.7	3.750	18.2
12	17.7	12	17.4	4.000	18.5
14	17.8	14	17.2	4.250	18.7

*Based on 250 days/year; 10-year life of assets; $12.50/MT anchoveta; present value of nonvariable cost $3,274,000.
**Based on 250 days/year; 12% interest; $12.50/MT anchoveta; present value of nonvariable cost $3,274,000.
***Based on 250 days/year; 12% interest; 10-year life of assets; $12.50/MT anchoveta.

1¢ per pound. This is due primarily to the
assumption of a rather short life for durable
capital, and the fact that the process is not
very capital-intensive. As one might expect,
the cost of fish and the number of days the
plant can operate are the crucial variables.

To provide a partial check on the validity
of these results, similar analysis was performed on the cost estimates provided in the
General Oceanology study. The method used
for deriving estimates within the cost structure of the GO report was outlined above.
When these costs were modified to reflect
lower raw materials costs and expanded days of
operation, the results in Table 12 emerged.
These figures assume a 10 percent interest
rate and a five year life on productive assets
and a value of $3.628 million for plant capi-
tal.

Analysis of other effects on production
costs showed the effect of interest rates to
be small. Production costs are quite sensitive to depreciation periods in ranges near
the five year figure chosen by GO; in the
range of 8 to 12 years however, the effect is
minimal. As with the MIT figures, the cost
of raw material and the length of the annual
operating season are of prime importance.

One interesting feature of the GO study is
the estimate of by-product revenues from fish
oil and fish solubles. Since that study
assumed the use of hake as raw material, the
choice of 3 percent oil yield (weight as percent of weight in whole fish) was appropriate.
However, the oil content of anchoveta and
other fatty fish is considerably greater.
Oil content will vary from season to season
and average content for Peruvian anchoveta
has been estimated at 6 percent. For other
species, such as the Northern anchovy, this
figure may range closer to 9 percent depending
on the season chosen for fishing operations.

Table 12. Sensitivity of Production Costs of
FPC from Anchoveta (GO data)[49]

No of operating days	Cost of fish	Production cost of FPC + 1 cent/ lb shipping	Location
	$/MT	¢/lb	
200	22.00	23.10	Chile
200	12.50	20.22	Peru
250	12.50	18.23*	Peru
300	12.50	16.73	Peru

----

*250 days operation seems likely in Peru.

Table 13. Value of Byproducts from FPC
Processing

Oil content	Value of oil*	Value of fish solubles**	Value of byproducts
%	¢/lb FPC	¢/lb FPC	¢/lb
3	1.15	.85	2.00
6	2.30	.85	3.15
9	3.45	.85	4.30
12	4.60	.85	5.45

----

*At 1971 price of 5.75¢/lb.
**At 1971 price of 2.35¢/lb.

Table 13 assumes a 100 percent recovery of
fish oil and solubles and shows the gross
value of by-products per pound of FPC.
    The recovery of marketable fish oil from
commercial operation of the IPA process remains to be demonstrated. Thus, the figures
in Table 13 are included merely to provide an
indication of the importance of by-product
recovery.

Production Costs Using Northern Anchovy. The
Northern anchovy is an attractive domestic
fish stock since it can easily be exploited as
a day fishery by purse seiners operating out
of the San Pedro area in a climate that is
conducive to year round operation. However,
the fishery is regulated by the California
Department of Fish and Game, which allows
fishing from mid-September through mid-May
with an annual quota of 110,000 tons. These
restrictions have been promoted by an active
lobby of sport fishermen, primarily in the belief that summer anchovy fishing would inter-
fere with the sport fishery by depleting and
scattering game fish forage. Maximum sustainable yield has been estimated at 1.0 to 2.0
million metric tons.
    With the exception of a closed summer
season, anchovies are available throughout the
year. Monthly fluctuations in landings occur,
but these are probably caused more by variances in fishing effort directed at anchovies
than by fluctuations in their availability.
The present catch is used for reduction into
fish meal (although a small portion is canned
or used for bait). The hypothesis that total
catch and availability are not directly related is supported by data shown in Table 14.
Relatively small landings in the months of
October-December and April are associated with
high catch per unit effort.
    The closed summer season is a definite

problem. Tillman and Paulik[55] point out that
school sizes are larger and the fish school
closer to shore in the summer than at other
times of the year; thus anchovies are at least
as accessible to fishing effort during the
closed season as at other times of the year.
Furthermore, the oil content of anchovies
reaches a peak in the summer months. The
economic feasibility of FPC processing in
California will depend heavily upon development of a rational regulatory scheme such as
individual annual quotas for vessels to replace the present closed season.

Since there is no fleet fishing solely for
anchovies, the cost of supplying raw material
on a year round basis is difficult to estimate. The boats moving out of tuna and
mackerel fishing when these species are unavailable were not specifically designed to
fish for anchovies; hence reported prices may
not reflect at all accurately the cost of capture for efficient vessels specifically designed for anchovy fishing. The problem of
estimating attainable fish cost was approached
by examining estimates of cost for vessels in
the San Pedro wetfish fleet. This information
was gathered by Perrin and Noetzel[56] and has
been further analyzed by Paulaha.[57]

Paulaha estimated the marginal cost of
landing anchovies, assuming an optimally designed and regulated fleet operating 200 days
per year, at $14.50 to $18.50 per ton. The
range of estimates is due to two factors:
uncertainty about how the stock would react
under intense pressure; and whether or not the
season could be altered to include the summer
months. To this range of figures must be
added the $2.00 per ton state landing tax,
yielding a range of $16.50 to $20.50 per ton.
Extension of the season into the summer months
when the oil content in anchovies is high may
cause fish meal plants to bid up the price of

Table 14.   Catch and Catch Per Unit (C.P.U.)
Effort in the Northern Anchovy Fishery

	1965/1966 Season		1966/1967 Season	
	Catch	C.P.U. Effort	Catch	C.P.U. Effort
	tons		tons	
October	N.A.	N.A.	2,911	7.2
November	43	8.7	2,560	13.0
December	47	7.4	6,151	14.9
January	2,183	5.5	11,250	8.6
February	2,170	6.1	6,771	5.3
March	6,173	6.6	5,868	3.8
April	6,031	9.0	3,084	6.0

Source: 58

anchovies in order to obtain the valuable oil.
Paulaha estimates that this could cause the
price of anchovies to go as high as $22.50 per
ton. However, since meal factories currently
demand anchovies only when offal obtained as a
by-product from other species is unavailable
(in the winter and early spring) estimation of
what these factories would be willing to pay
at other times is uncertain. For these reasons, a range of raw material prices of $18.50
to $22.50 is considered with $20.50 assumed
most likely.

   Based on the amount of anchovies supplied
to fish meal plants in recent year, it should
be feasible to supply 200 tons per day to an
FPC plant for eight months of the year. Landings were considerably smaller in 1969 and
1971, but this is certainly due to lack of demand rather than of available fish. An operating season of 200 days per year will be used
as a conservative estimate of the number of
days an FPC plant could operate in California.

   The cost of producing FPC in California was
estimated by adapting cost information provided in the GO report on the potential role
for FPC in Korea.[49] The primary factors considered in adapting these figures to the situation in California were labor costs, solvent
loss costs, and the cost of raw material. The
cost of plant capital was adjusted to reflect
lower shipping costs. Solvent costs were
adjusted in accord with current estimates of
attainable solvent losses[45] and solvent
prices. A summary of cost information is included in Table 15.

   The methods used to estimate cost per
pound of FPC are the same as those employed in
analysis of Peruvian operation. Manufacturing
costs shown (primarily labor) assume 200
operating days per year. When considering
longer operating seasons, these costs are
allowed to vary.

Table 15. Production Cost Elements -
California Anchovies

I.   Plant Construction and
      Start-Up*   (x$1,000)
         Processing Equipment   1,500
         Support Equipment   575
         Freight   100
         Site and Site Development   100
         Buildings/Enclosures   200
         Special Structures and
         Foundations   100
         Services/Utilities   50
         Erection   150
         Engineering and Consulting   100
         Start-Up Expense   400
         Contingency   300
         Working Capital   350
         TOTAL (rounded) $ 3,900

II.   Manufacturing Costs (Annual costs
      assuming 200 operating days per year)
      Personnel   (x$1,000)
      Supervision   66   3 persons
      Office   54   6 persons
      Control Lab   28   2 persons
      Maintenance   44   4 persons
      Others   48   4 persons
      Production   140   14 persons
      Subtotal-Personnel $380   33 persons
      Maintenance
      supplies   55
      General Expenses   25
      Insurance   50
      TOTAL $510**

----
*Input capacity - 200 tons raw fish per day
vs. 180 tons per day for the plant described
by GO in the Chilean study.
**Excludes taxes.

III.   Direct Costs   ($/ton FPC)
        Raw Material   136
        Solvent loss   35
        Electricity and fuel
        oil   75
        Production contin-
        gencies and losses   50
        Other   10
        TOTAL   305

In deriving a reference point for further
sensitivity testing, the following values were
assumed: 200 operating days per year; 10 percent interest rate; an eight year write off on
depreciable assets of $3.9 million; $20.50 per
ton as the cost of raw material. Under these
assumptions a cost of 25.6¢ per pound was derived.

Table 16 shows the sensitivity of production cost to raw material cost, alternative
operating seasons, life of capital assets,
cost of plant capital, and interest rates.
All figures are production costs before taxes
or profit.

Under the most favorable conditions considered, (250 operating days, $18.50 per ton
for raw fish, 10 percent interest and 10 year
life of assets) production costs could be as
low as 23¢ per pound. In general, unit costs
in the 24.5¢ per pound to 26.5¢ per pound
range seem more likely. As expected, the
sensitivity of cost to variations in parameters (interest rate, depreciation period and
operating season) over plausible ranges corre-
lates closely to that observed in the Peruvian
case. Costs which vary directly with the
length of the operating season (primarily payments for labor and raw materials) are more
important in the California situation so that
the sensitivity of unit cost to the length of
the operating season is diminished.

It seems likely that extension of the anchovy season could affect production costs in
a manner not analyzed above. By allowing
anchovy vessels to operate over an extended
season, the capital invested in boats and
fishing gear could be used more intensively,
thus decreasing fishing costs per ton of
anchovies. The magnitude of this effect, however, has not been explored.

The figures shown in Table 16 have not been
adjusted to reflect the value of by-products

Table 16.   Sensitivity of Production Costs of
FPC from California Anchovies

Variable tested	FPC Production cost* Cents/lb
Raw material cost ($/ton)	
18.56	25.0
20.50	25.6
22.50	26.3
Operating Season (days of year)	
175	26.5
200	25.6
225	25.0
250	24.4
275	24.0
Interest rate (%)	
6	24.8
8	25.2
10	25.6
12	26.1
14	26.8
Depreciation period (years)	
6	27.0
7	26.2
8	25.6
9	25.2
10	24.8
Non-variable costs (present value)	
$3,500,000	25.0
3,750,000	25.4
3,900,000	25.6
4,250,000	26.1
4,500,000	26.5

----

*Does not include taxes or profit.

which may be recoverable from the process.
Although the feasibility of by-product recovery has not been demonstrated in a commercial
plant, data in Table 13 indicate the potential
importance of this factor.

These figures assume 100 percent recovery
and no additional costs of processing by-
products. The cost data in Table 15 allegedly
include the cost of recovering by-products
which would make the above figures the net
value of by-products to be credited against
FPC production costs. However, since recovery
of by-products from a commercial scale IPA
plant has not been demonstrated, these figures
can be taken as upper limits on the value of
by-products.

The oil content of Northern anchovies
varies by season. Dr. Rubin Lasker at the
NMFS laboratory in La Jolla, California, indicates that oil content is low (about 3 percent) in late winter and reaches a peak of up
to 13 percent in late summer. For an annual
average, a value in the 6 to 9 percent range
would be appropriate.

Nutritive Value and Acceptability of Anchovy-FPC

If the SWECO engineering estimates are reasonably accurate, production costs in the 16¢ per
pound range appear quite attainable in Peru.
Under plausible assumptions, production costs
of 24.5¢ per pound to 26.5¢ per pound seem
likely for an operation located in Southern
California. However, these figures pertain to
anchovy-FPC, while the analysis of FPC vis-a-
vis other protein supplements in earlier sections invariably referred to the product
manufactured from hake. As noted, there
appears to be no problem in adapting the IPA
process for fatty fish, anchovy in particular,
but before drawing conclusions about the
potential for FPC in the family of protein

additives, the nutritive value and acceptability of anchovy-FPC must be considered.

The composition of FPC prepared from various species using the IPA process has been compared by Knobl et al.[38] They have shown that anchovy-FPC compares very favorably with red hake-FPC. Sidwell et al.[58] have examined the pattern of essential amino acids occurring in FPC manufactured from red hake, Northern anchovies and other species. The results obtained showed that the patterns of essential amino acids were quite similar, although there were some significant differences.

It seems possible that the amount of FPC required to supplement a given diet could vary among different FPCs depending upon which amino acid is limiting. However, we are not aware of any studies that have investigated this phenomenon.

Sidwell et al. have also investigated the acceptability of various FPCs when incorporated into a variety of foods.[58] In pasta fortified at the 10 percent level, they found that anchovy- and herring-FPC produced a grayish product. The meaning one should attach to results of 10 percent supplementation are questionable since our earlier analysis found that 5 to 7 percent was normally adequate, even with mixed diets. Aside from the color of the product, no differences among different FPCs were noted. FPC was also added to sugar cookies at 5 and 10 percent concentrations. At 5 percent, no significant differences from control samples which contained no FPC, were noted in any of the FPCs. At 10 percent, cookies containing anchovy-FPC were significantly darker in color compared to those containing hake-FPC.

In general, the color of anchovy-FPC appears to be the only factor which could affect its acceptability vis-a-vis other FPCs. The anchovy-FPC prepared at the pilot plant in

Aberdeen did not have a fishy taste, although
a slight taste of "bouillon" was evident, but
it did retain a characteristic reddish-brown
color.

In summary, the problems of acceptability
do not appear insurmountable, and are clearly
swamped by the dominant effect on cost of using low priced, abundant, regularly available
raw materials. The importance of developing
an acceptable FPC from anchovies and other
fatty fish is likely to increase in the future
as the trend toward utilizing lean fish for
direct human consumption continues.

Conclusions

With regard to supplementation programs in
developing countries, we feel that government
subsidies will be needed to deliver adequate
nutrition to target populations. Supplementation almost always raises the cost of staple
items in the diet and consumers do not seem to
demand "nutrition" as such; custom and inertia
are more important in shaping eating habits.

Competition for food within families and
the widespread practice of feeding weaning infants small portions of the adult diet indicate that universal supplementation to all age
groups will, in most cases, be the only way to
ensure adequate nutrition for the critical
target group (weaning infants.) School feeding programs, though useful, will probably
reach children after much of the irreparable
damage of protein-calorie malnutrition has
been done.

Although low cost supplementation schemes
can be devised to utilize cheap sources of
protein that provide calories as well, these
plans often require a change in basic eating
habits rather than the supplementation of
accepted foodstuffs. We are not sanguine
about inducing people to consume peanut flour
as a major portion of a staple item in the

diet (why not, for that matter, a few grams of
fish meal per day?).

Fortification with synthetic amino acids
often shows impressive cost advantages where
populations consume diets consisting entirely
of a staple item in which a single amino acid
is limiting. But, these advantages may well
disappear in the more common cases where diets
are mixed, especially where diets vary widely
among individuals in the same population.
They are even less likely to be of practical
significance in economies characterized by a
large subsistence sector.

Recent increases in world dairy product
prices have severely impaired the competitive
position of NFDM in the family of protein
supplements. Although their future course is
uncertain, it seems unlikely that prices will
fall to levels which would make NFDM competitive with other established protein sources
for supplementation in developing countries.

In cases where diets are mixed (as they
seem to be virtually everywhere), it appears
that soy flour is the best prospect among oilseed proteins on the basis of cost and other
factors considered (acceptability, availability of protein in foods, etc.). This conclusion is drawn from very limited information,
however, and should be viewed as tentative.
Analysis of supplementation schemes indicates
that FPC in the price range of 16¢ per pound
to 18¢ per pound f.o.b. point of manufacture
plus 1¢ per pound shipping cost could be
competitive with soy flour in many areas.
This coincides with estimates of FPC production cost in an efficient location (Peru);
i.e., if our cost information is reasonably
accurate, IPA-FPC will be able to compete with
soy protein in cases where both supplements
must be imported. If FPC can be produced
efficiently in the target country (for a unit
cost lower than the value of foreign exchange

needed to import), it may well have a cost
advantage over soy flour and other protein
supplements considered.

We have been led to the conclusion that
general statements regarding the desirability
of alternative protein sources for supplementation are difficult to defend. The variety
of dietary patterns across populations, as
well as variances among individuals in a given
population, indicate that no single supplement
will be preferred in all cases. This empha-
sizes the importance of considering a variety
of FPCs in the effort to combat malnutrition.
The insistence on bland taste in the IPA processed FPC may be a distinct and needless
disadvantage in areas where the flavor of fish
is appreciated.

Any conclusions about the future role of
FPC in the U. S. food industry are premature
for several reasons. Foremost is the fact
that the FDA presently prohibits supplementation of other foods with FPC. (It should be
noted that a petition has been filed with FDA
to permit the use of FPC in manufactured
foods.)* The present regulations amount to a
de facto ban on the use of FPC for human consumption in the United States. It is difficult to see how an agency acting in the public
interest could defend such a policy, especially in light of the stringent specifications placed upon IPA-FPC and the scientific
information provided from nongovernment
sources. If FDA feels that products meeting
its own standards are unfit for human consumption then the standards should be changed;
otherwise, consumers should be allowed to decide which proteins they wish to buy.

Recent evidence indicates that the most
crucial of these standards, pertaining to
fluoride, may be unduly restrictive. Zipkin
et al. conducted rat feeding experiments to
determine the availability of fluoride (the

----

*In July, 1973 FDA approved the use of FPC in
manufactured foods.

amount retained and accumulated during a
prolonged period of daily intake) in diets
containing IPA-FPC.[59] They found that, in
general, less than half of the fluoride in FPC
was accumulated in the body. Present standards were set primarily to avoid mottling of
teeth that occurs when 4 to 8 milligrams of
fluoride are ingested daily. The above study
indicates that FPC meeting current standards
(100 ppm of fluoride) could be consumed at a
rate of well over 20 grams per day (over twice
the rate found necessary to supplement low
protein diets) before mottling of teeth vs.
death or physical impairment from malnutrition). This new information is especially
important since present FDA standards necessitate deboning raw fish, a costly procedure
which removes as much as 15 percent of the
protein before processing.

Second, the problem of marketing products
labeled "with fish protein" may impair the
position of FPC vis-à-vis other protein
sources in U. S. markets even if its price is
competitive. At least one industry expert
feels that this is fish protein's greatest
liability.[60] Finally, the fact that commercial processes have not been developed for
producing FPC with functional properties
desired by the food industry makes definitive
comparison with other protein sources on the
basis of cost impossible at present.

In spite of this, some of the work done on
introducing IPA-FPC into candies, snack foods
and processed meats is encouraging. As
Hammonds and Call point out, "elimination of
disagreeable flavor is the single most important factor for stimulating the sale of a new
protein ingredient."[5] Final solution of this
problem may allow presently produced FPC to
compete in uses where nutritional quality is
important: e.g., baby foods, breakfast food,
and canned and processed meats. These uses

are presently supplied by NFDM (costing 40 to
50¢ per pound of protein) and soy concentrates and isolates (costing 27 to 42¢ per
pound of protein).

With regard to functionality, several researchers have suggested that functional properties should be built into final FPC
products, noting that unprocessed fish protein
possesses functional properties not found in
the IPA extracted product. This re-emphasizes
the importance of investigating a variety of
FPCs.

It is clear that more effort is needed to
involve the food industry in the application
of FPC technology to uses in domestic markets. The apparent lack of communication may
be the result of FDA regulations or preoccupa-
tion of government researchers with development of the IPA process. Whatever the reason,
a mark of successful government research is
application of the knowledge gained by firms
in the private sector, and success is more
likely where industry becomes involved at a
fairly early stage. Mechanisms for the transfer of information and technology on a two-way
basis can and should be improved.

Our analysis of engineering cost estimates
points out the importance of the raw material
source in deciding where to locate FPC production facilities. Among the most crucial factors are, of course, the cost and regularity
of supply of fish, although the oil content of
the species utilized is potentially very
important. Our investigation of two likely
locations indicates that production costs
(before crediting for the sale of by-products)
in the range of 16 to 18¢ per pound in Peru
and 24.5 to 26.5¢ per pound in California are
attainable. Other areas with abundant
supplies of clupeoids may become equally
attractive.

Other factors of importance in choosing an

efficient location are a labor pool possessing
necessary skills; and back-up facilities
needed to maintain the fishing fleet and the
FPC plant and to recover by-products. None of
the cost estimates examined included a potentially important component: equipment needed
to control emission of pollutants into the air
and water. It is probably appropriate to
minimize this cost when considering production
in most developing countries, but a plant
located in the United States (especially in
Southern California) must take these costs into account.

The value of by-products (fish oil and condensed fish solubles) and the technology for
their recovery are of vital importance to the
commercial feasibility of FPC. Furthermore,
this factor will increase in importance as the
trend toward increased utilization of lean
fish for direct human consumption forces reduction operations (FPC and fish meal) to rely
more and more upon clupeoids.

The following are recommendations for further research on the IPA process (with implications for use of the Aberdeen installation):

1. A more thorough investigation of producing
FPC from (fresh) anchovies and other fatty
fish at the pilot plant level is required.
Unfortunately, the present location of the EDP
precludes such investigation at this facility.

2. Recovery of by-products at the pilot plant
level should be attempted to shed light upon
the technical and economic feasibility of this
aspect of production.

3. Researchers studying functionality and use
of FPC in foods have noted that the present
extraction process appears overly hars.
Experimentation with extraction temperatures,
solvent ratios, etc. may reveal ways to

minimize adverse effects in the functionality
of the final product. It is not clear whether
the pilot plant or bench scale would be the
appropriate level for such testing.

4. Solvent losses are a potentially important
component of production cost. At the Aberdeen
installation such losses have been high, primarily because of the experimental nature of
the operation. Operation of the plant on a
commercial basis (i.e., continuously) for a
sufficient period of time is necessary to
develop information on the attainable lower
limits of solvent loss.

   The effect of storage of fish upon the behavior of protein in process and upon FPC
yields in general needs investigation.
Whether such analysis is best carried out in a
pilot plant or at the bench scale is unclear.
   Finally, one of the most severe impediments
to determination of FPCs role in world protein
markets is the lack of even rough estimates of
processing costs based on actual production
experience. In spite of the fact that the
Aberdeen plant may not closely resemble a
commercial facility, information on processing
costs (or even some components of processing
cost) derived from continuous operation on a
commercial basis would be very valuable.

References

1. Schertz, L. P. 1971. Economics of protein improvement programs in lower income
countries. USDA Foreign Economic Development
Report No. 11, July.

2. Roemer, M. 1970. Fishing for growth.
In Export-led Development in Peru, 1950-1967.
Cambridge: Harvard Univ. Press.

3. Personal communication. Mr. Burkett,
Archer Daniel Midlands, Decatur, Ill.

4. Weisberg, S. M. 1971. High nutrition
foods for developing countries. League for
International Food Education, June.

5. Hammonds, T. M. and Call, D. L. 1970.
Utilization of protein ingredients in the
U. S. food industry. Dept. of Agricultural
Economics, Cornell Univ. Agricultural Experi-
ment Station, Cornell University.

6. Gallimore, W. W. 1972. Synthetics and
substitutes for agricultural products:
Projections for 1980. USDA Marketing Research Report No. 047 E.R.S.

7. Personal communication. Traders Oil Mill,
Inc., Fort Worth, Texas.

8. Personal communication. John Hussey,
Quaker Oats Co., Chicago, Ill.

9. Personal communication. Mr. Hauzer,
Plans Cooperative Oil Mill, Lubbock, Texas.

10. Miller, R. R. 1972. Review of casein
situation. Dairy Situation, USDA, Economic
Research Service, DS-338.

11. Miller, R. R. and Crockett, S. L. 1972.
World dairy situation and outlook. Dairy
Situation USDA, Economic Research Service,
DS033E.

12. Personal communication. Jack Rush,
Merck and Co., Inc., Rahway, N. J.

13. Personal communication. Dr. Olcott,
Univ. of Calif., Davis, Calif.

14.   Chemical Abstracts, 1970.   Vol. 73, No.
54637.

15.   Devanney, J. W. et al.   1970.   The
economics of fish protein concentrate.   M.I.T.
Sea Grant Program, Report MITSG 71-3 M.I.T.

16.   Berg, A.   1972.   Industry's struggle with
world malnutrition.   Harvard Business Review
Jan.-Feb.

17.   Simons, J. L. and Gardner, D. M.   1969.
World food needs and new proteins.   In Econo-
mic Development and Cultural Change, Vol. 10,
No. 4.

18.   Odendaal, W. A.   1966.   Experience in
development of Pro-Nutro in South Africa.   In
Preschool Child Malnutrition, National Academy
of Sciences.

19.   Platt, S. B. and Stewart, R. J. C.   1971.
Reversible and irreversible effects of
protein-calorie deficiency on the central
nervous system of animals and man.   In World
Review in Nutrition and Dietetics, Vol. 13.

20.   Cravioto, J.   1966.   Malnutrition and
behavioral development in the preschool
child.   In PreSchool Child Malnutrition,
National Academy of Sciences.

21.   Foster, G. N.   1966.   Social anthropology
of the preschool child.   In Preschool Child
Malnutrition, National Academy of Sciences.

22.   Swaminathan, M.   The nutrition and feeding of infants and preschool children in
developing countries.   World Review in
Nutrition and Dietetics, Vol. 9.

23. Yanez, E. et al. 1967. Quintero fish protein concentrate: Protein quality and use in foods. Food Technology 21: 1604.

24. Stillings, B. R. et al. 1971. Nutritive quality of wheat flour and bread supplemented with either fish protein concentrate or lysine. Cereal Chemistry Vol. 8, No. 3.

25. Sidwell, V. D. Unpublished research reports. U. S. Dept. of Commerce, National Marine Fisheries Service, National Center for Fish Protein Concentrate, College Park, Md.

26. The State of Food and Agriculture: 1971. FAO: Rome.

27. Kwee, W. H. et al. 1969. Quality and nutritive value of paste made from rice, corn, soya, and tapioca enriched with fish protein concentrate. Cereal Chemistry, Vol. 46, No. 1.

28. Bass, J. L. and Caul, J. F. 1972. Laboratory evaluation of three protein sources for use in chapati flours. J. Food Sci. Vol. 37.

29. Thomson, F. A. and Merry, E. 1962. Weight increase in toddler children in the Federation of Malaya: A comparison of dietary supplementation of skim milk and fish biscuits. Brit. J. Nutrition 16: 175.

30. Hyder, K. and Cobb, B. F. 1972. Development of a process for preparing a fish protein concentrate which can be reconstituted into a meat-like product. TAMU-SG-72-201. Texas A & M Univ.

31. Roels, O. A. 1969. Nutrition Reviews 27: 35.

32.   Hale, M. B. 1969. Food Technol. 23:
107.

33.   Cheftel, C. et al. Enzymatic solubilization of fish protein concentrate: batch
studies applicable to continuous enzyme re-
cycling process. J. Agric. and Food Chem. 19:

34.   Tannenbaum, S. R. et al. 1970. Food
Technol. 24: 604, 607.

35.   Spinelli, J., Koury, B., and Miller, R.
In press. Approaches to the utilization of
fish for the preparation of protein isolates.
II. Enzymic modifications of myofibrillar
fish proteins. J. Food Science.

36.   Personal communication. A. F. Anglemeir,
Dept. of Food Science and Technology, Oregon
State University, Corvallis, Oregon.

37.   Knobl, G. M. 1967. The fish protein
concentrate story-Part 4. Food Technol. Vol.
21, No. 8.

38.   Knobl, G. M. et al. 1971. Fish protein
concentrates. Commercial Fisheries Review
July-Aug.

39.   Finch, R. 1969. The U. S. fish protein
concentrate program. Commercial Fisheries
Review, Jan.

40.   Finch, R. 1970. Fish protein for human
foods. CRC Critical Reviews in Food Technology Dec.

41.   Spinelli, J. et al. 1971. The fish
protein concentrate story-Part 13. Food
Technol.

42. Anonymous. 1966. Extraction process wins protein from fish. Chem. Engin. Feb.

43. Ocean Harvesters, Inc. 1971. Summary report of the hake run. Prepared for National Marine Fisheries Service.

44. Ernst, R. C. 1971. The NMFS experiment and demonstration plant process. Commercial Fishery Rev. 33: 22.

45. Personal communication. Dan Lang, SWECO.

46. Anonymous. 1970. The superfood from the sea. Business Week Nov.

47. Tenner, J. 1969. Canadian FPC plant nears reality. National Fisherman Nov.

48. Philips, R. H. 1969. Peruvian firm making FPC and using it in other foods. National Fisherman Nov.

49. General Oceanology, Inc. 1970. Commercial feasibility of producing fish protein concentrate in developing countries. Prepared for Office of Agriculture and Fisheries, Agency for International Development.

50. Crutchfield, J. A. et al. Present and potential pellagic fisheries for reduction: A world survey. Unpublished report, Univ. of Washington.

51. Paulik, G. 1971. The anchoveta fishery of Peru. Center for Quantitative Sciences, Univ. of Washington.

52. Instituto del Mar del Peru. La Pesqueria Maritima Peruana Durante 19__. Lima, Peru.

53. Personal communication. Gordon
Broadhead, Living Marine Resources, Inc., San
Diego, Calif.

54. Roemer, M. 1970. Fishing for Growth,
Export-led Development in Peru. Cambridge:
Harvard Univ. Press.

55. Tillman, M. F. and Paulik, G. J. 1971.
Biological analysis of the northern anchovy
and its fishery system. Center for Quantitative Sciences, Univ. of Washington.

56. Perrin, W. F. and Noetzel, B. G. 1969.
Economic study of the San Pedro wetfish
boats. Bureau of Commercial Fisheries.

57. Paulaha, D. F. 1970. A general economic model for commercial fisheries and its
application to the California anchovy fishery. Unpublished doctoral dissertation,
Univ. of Washington.

58. Sidwell, V. D. et al. 1970. U. S.
Bureau of Commercial Fisheries fish protein
concentrates: Nutritional quality and use in
foods. Food Technol. Vol. 24, No. 8.

59. Zipkin, Zukas, and Stillings, B. 1970.
Nutritional Rev. Sept., pp. 235-236.

60. Champagne, J. R. 1972. Some aspects of
the fish protein market in industrialized
countries-A view from private industry. The
Nestle Company, Inc.

XXIII
MARKETING AND ECONOMICS: PERU, FISH MEAL AND FPC

G. Pontecorvo
Columbia University, New York, New York

Introduction

There are certain tentative hypotheses that should be investigated in any complete analysis of the appropriateness of the location of FPC manufacture in Peru. The inquiry will be limited to conditions favorable to the welfare of Peru.

Given that Peru has a mature fish meal industry, it is important to distinguish between two assumptions. The first is that the fish meal industry based on the anchoveta resource is fully developed; that the resource is exploited at or beyond the MSY (Maximum Sustainable Yield); and that there is excess capacity (capital and labor) both in the primary (catching) and secondary (processing) sectors. The second and less restrictive assumption is that, while the existing industry is mature, expansion may be possible through exploitation of stocks of hake, squid, mackerel and other fish which are currently underutilized off the coast of Peru.

A measure of the opportunity cost of producing FPC in Peru is the loss of foreign exchange generated by fish meal production. Since Peruvian fish meal is approximately two-thirds protein and FPC is at least four-fifths protein, the value added in FPC manufacture would have to compensate for the lower conversion ratio. Hopefully, the output of a Peruvian FPC industry would be exported and the world market for FPC would absorb all of Peru's output at or near the existing world price.

The Fish Meal Industry in Peru
Primary Production. Although a great deal of
biological research by the Instituto del Mar
in Lima and those associated with it has been
directed toward establishing the MSY for the
anchoveta stock, there are a number of serious
questions about its biological condition. As
has been true in so many other fisheries, the
regulatory authorities have a severe administrative problem if they are forced to act to
protect the stock while justification for
their action rests on insufficient biological
knowledge. This problem is compounded by the
economic and political pressures created by
excess capacity in the catching and processing
sectors.* This suggests that, in spite of the
strenuous efforts made by Peru to rationalize
the biological side of the fishery, the stock
of anchovetas is at the present time in danger
of being overfished, and indeed, this may have
occurred already.

Another factor affecting the stock is natural variation. Under certain natural circumstances, Clupeidae are subject to wide swings
in abundance. It is likely, therefore, that
the supply will vary greatly in certain years
(as has been true in 1973) even if no overfishing occurs.

The response of those regulating the
fishery in Peru has been typical of the response of fishery managers concerned primarily
with the biological condition of fish stocks
in the face of increased fishing effort, a
closed season was established; and the season
has been extended as fishing effort has increased. The reduction in the amount of time
each year during which fish may be caught and

----

*Many writers have questioned the utility of
the MSY as an operating tool in fisheries
management.

processed has significant economic consequences. The rate of utilization of both capital
and labor is affected: Overhead costs must be
covered within a shorter period; the cost of
temporary breakdowns during the operating
period increases sharply; and the shorter season also contributes, in all probability, to
the financing of the excess capacity in primary production by the processors.

If the industry were to convert from the
production of fish meal to FPC, the costs of
conversion would be higher than if there were
a more even flow of the resource to the processing plant throughout the year. Therefore,
the implications of a continuous or nearly
continuous supply of fish should be investigated. It is interesting to note that there
is a continuous fishing season at the Port of
Illo in southern Peru where Chilean and Peruvian fisheries overlap. Since the Chileans
have not established a closed season, the
Peruvians have chosen to allow their fishery
at Illo to operate on the same basis as their
Chilean competitors.

The rapid development in Peru of the fish
meal industry with only very modest foreign
assistance clearly suggests, that given a market for the end product, Peruvian interests
could convert the industry from the production
of meal to FPC.

However, the process of conversion would
raise a number of problems. The market for
raw fish is largely in the hands of existing
meal producers who finance a significant part
of the catching capacity. A rough estimate
is that two-thirds of the fleet is owned by
the processors. Of the remaining one-third,
who are independent vessel owners, approximately one-half are under contract to the processors. While the terms of these "contracts"
are not public knowledge, it is reasonable to
hypothesize that the financing of the vessels

and gear is involved. This leaves one-sixth
of the capacity independent of direct ties to
the processors which presumably could provide
the supply for a new FPC plant or plants
(although what portion of the catch comes from
this one-sixth is unknown). However, this
fraction of capacity that is not tied to the
producers has had a tendency to "follow the
fish", i.e., to more along the coast to take
advantage of the relative availability of the
stocks. This capacity would, therefore, have
to be bid away from its current patterns of
activity by the FPC producers. Given the intense competition for fish which results from
exploitation of the stock at or beyond the MSY
and excess capacity in processing, it seems
likely that a new plant would have some supply
problems. Clearly these would be alleviated
if fish stocks other than anchoveta could be
used.

     To summarize the problems at the level of
primary production, we note: 1. If the industry is limited to exploiting the anchoveta
stocks, supply may vary due to wide swings in
abundance as a result of natural population
variation.   2. The existing pressure on the
stock and the regulatory response to that pres
pressure means in all probability a tendency
to ever shorter fishing seasons. This, in
turn, poses problems for the processing sector, and these problems will be exacerbated if
the processing sector becomes more capital
intensive.   3. The current structure of the
industry with excess capacity both in catching
and processing suggest that new plants will
have additional difficulties in obtaining a
reasonably secure supply of raw fish.

Processing and Transportation. The most
important of the several reasons for excess
capacity both in harvesting and processing is
the common property condition of the resource.

Whatever the root causes, however, the
existence of excess capacity presents a significant problem for the entry of new plants to
produce FPC or for the transformation of
existing plants from meal to FPC production.
The impact of any change on employment and
capital values requires careful consideration. For example, if an FPC plant is more
productive than a fish meal plant, (requires
less labor input per unit of output) then,
given the fixed supply of fish, the transformation of the processing sector may displace a
significant amount of labor. Furthermore,
since the FPC industry is more capital intensive, it may evolve a different structure than
the existing fish meal processors, and therefore, force other changes. For example, a
collusive oligopsony among FPC producers could
drive the prices of raw fish down and rationalize primary production by driving out the
excess capacity, thereby displacing skilled
labor and capital. In a developing country
with already high unemployment, any industrial
change that tends to increase unemployment of
skilled labor would be questionable.
    A similar situation would apply to the
existing meal plants and vessels. A significant portion of this equipment was purchased
with foreign exchange, and to the extent that
it is not fully depreciated, its displacement
would represent a capital loss in a country
with an acute capital shortage and small
foreign exchange reserves.* This reasoning

----

*Economic analysis, with its usual assumptions
about factor mobility, price flexibility and
sunk cost suggests these capital losses and
the labor displacement would be short-run
phenomena. And while the theoretical long-run
equilibrium solution and the relevance of the
underlying assumption for the Peruvian

strongly suggests the desirability of expansion of the resource base if the industry is
to be transformed. Given more fish to process, and sufficient time to depreciate existing capital and retain labor, it should be
possible to shift from meal to FPC production
with few adverse welfare effects.

As indicated above, we are assuming that
the conversion of fish to FPC is approximately
five-sixths of the conversion of fish to fish
meal. Transportation costs for fish meal from
Peru to the North American and European markets are between $22 and $25 per metric ton in
bags, and $12 to $14 per ton in bulk (with the
price of the fish meal may be $180 per ton).
This differential is significant, and it suggests the need to investigate the conditions
under which FPC could be shipped. A priori,
it might be that the sanitary requirements
imposed upon FPC would add significantly to
handling and transportation costs, and therefore, play an important part in the analysis
of the desirability of switching in Peru from
the production of meal to FPC.

Any analysis of a shift in production
should include the effect of a loss in foreign
exchange if a portion of the output is shifted
from the export to the domestic market. This
does not appear to be an important consideration in the case of Peru, but it should be
investigated.

Conclusions
It seems clear that Peru could technically
convert from the production of meal to FPC if
it were economically advantageous to do so.

----

situation should be evaluated in any formal
analysis, here we will consider only short-run
disequilibrium conditions.

And more important, not only could Peru convert its meal industry, but there is every
reason to believe it would do so if the market
demand was present. However, given the
structure of the existing meal industry, the
transition would be easier if the resource
base of the industry could be expanded.
Transport and handling are also difficult
problems, but again, they do not appear to be
limiting factors.

   Finally, it should be noted that Peru is
already experimenting with FPC production. A
new plant for the production of FPC has been
put in operation in 1972. It will produce 100
metric tons per day of FPC, which will contain
0.5 percent fat. It will be used primarily
for calf and mink feed, but presumably could
be used for human consumption.

References

1. Crutchfield, J. and Pontecorvo, G.   1969.
The Pacific Salmon Fisheries Chap. 5.   Baltimore: Johns Hopkins Press.

XXIV
FACTORS AFFECTING THE ECONOMICS OF AN FPC
MANUFACTURING OPERATION

E. R. Pariser
Massachusetts Institute of Technology,
Cambridge, Massachusetts

The major economic factors determining the
production cost of fish protein concentrate by
IPA extraction are functions of a number of
interdependent parameters. There are technical problems still to be resolved; practical
choices that have to be made to put an operating plant together; sanitary, safety,
nutritional, and esthetic requirements to be
met; and constraints within which a manufacturer of FPC must elect to operate.
Let us assume that, as a private enterprise or
under government contract, an industrialist
decides to build a plant for the utilization
of marine resources by manufacturing dietary
protein concentrates to be used as inexpensive
dietary supplements, at home or abroad. Let
us furthermore assume that our hypothetical
industrialist is assured a reasonably large-
scale market (of, say, 20,000 tons of FPC per
year) for a product with properties that are
similar to those of the FPC produced by one or
the other of the presently available processing methods. As to cost, the only condition
that he has to meet is that his product is no
more expensive, on a weight for weight
basis, than casein traded on the world market.
    We have chosen for discussion some of the
major areas an industrialist would have to
consider in order to meet his goal.

Definition of Product Characteristics and
Production Volume
The goal is to manufacture a product that is a

stable, wholesome protein concentrate without
appreciable odor or taste with an off-white or
white color. It should have a total lipid
content of less than 0.2 percent; a protein
content of no less than 75 percent; a nutritive value consistently and significantly
better than that of casein; no coliform or
salmonella organisms; and a total plate count
of less than 10,000 microorganisms per gram.
For the purpose of this discussion, functional
properties of the product are considered to be
of less importance than nutritional value,
digestibility, safety, and storage ability.

The plant should be capable of processing:
a) 200 tons (per 24 hour working day) of whole
lean or fatty fish of edible species, yielding
at least an average of 14 percent of a 75 percent protein FPC; and b) 100 tons (per 24 hour
working day) of filleting trimmings, yielding
at least 8 percent of an 85 percent protein
FPC. The plant should operate for at least
200 days per year and produce about 4500 tons
of FPC during that period, utilizing 30,000
tons (60 million pounds) of whole fish and
5000 tons (10 million pounds) of filleting
trimmings.

Raw Material Availability and Procurement

In order to satisfy the plant's demand for raw
material, it is necessary to insure that
edible species of fish are landed regularly
over the course of the year. Suitable species
for utilization are, for instance, fish from
the herring, hake, and capelin families. Although edible, they are not often caught except for the manufacture of fish meal. It is
also important, especially when easily vulnerable and oily fish such as herring and
menhaden are considered, to know the time
intervals within which a load of fish must be
processed to avoid spoilage under different
climatic conditions. A herring seiner may

land as much as 250 to 500 tons of round
herring at a time; this load must be processed within four hours in the summer and one
day in the winter. The receiving potential of
the plant is therefore severely limited unless
refrigeration is provided, and it is also con-
tingent upon the capacity and nature of the
fish unloading system at the plant site.

A reasonably good fishing vessel of 110 to
130 feet may catch 30 million pounds of
herring a year or 4 to 5 million pounds of
ground fish. The yearly operating costs of
such a boat on the North Atlantic seaboard
will be between $300,000 and $400,000. The
costs vary greatly, however, from country to
country, and are especially unpredictable in
less industrialized areas of the world. Purchase of a modern trawler capable of catching
6 million pounds per year of various edible
species would cost today between 10^6 and
2×10^6.

Plant Location
It is vital that a filleting and fish meal
plant be in close proximity to the FPC
installation since filleting waste cannot be
transported safely for any length of time
without spoilage occurring. The plant would
also have to guarantee that waste from the FPC
installation is routinely removed.

The plant should be close to a harbor that
is ice-free most of the year, preferably not
in a tropical area where toxic fish are more
frequent than in temperate zones. It should
be located close to a town that can provide
skilled and unskilled labor, repair shops,
hospitals, and schools. Fresh water, electric
power, and sewage systems should be available
on the site. Roads and/or railways should be
easily accessible.

Precise knowledge is required of the legislation in the country where the plant is to be

built concerning sanitary, food safety, and
processing standards. Some countries permit
the use of only certain raw materials for the
manufacture of FPC; others are more liberal;
still others may not have any regulations at
all. The same applies to the legislation concerning the composition of the final product,
and the way it is labeled, packaged, and sold.

Manufacturing Process and Equipment
Next, a series of decisions have to be made to
select thé most suitable process and equipment
to realize one's production goals. These
decisions, like those that were alluded to
above, have far-reaching consequences concerning production costs, requirements for sanitation, safety and quality control, and
especially for the disposal of by-products and
waste products.

    While there are at least 50 documented pro-
cesses for the manufacture of FPC presently on
file, those that employ straight solvent
extraction are probably the most thoroughly
tested. Within this category, the Halifax-BCF
method appears most attractive (and most
conservative) because of the detailed scrutiny
that it and the resulting products have undergone in all respects. If our hypothetical
entrepreneur is neither willing to wait until
some of the other promising processes have
been sufficiently tested to give him enough
confidence to opt for one of them, nor willing
or capable of financing his own research, he
might be tempted to adopt the Halifax-BCF extraction procedure (with IPA as the solvent)
because of the method's relative safety,
simplicity, and flexibility. He would be
wise, however, to make quite sure that his
plant is laid out in such a manner that processing changes can be made and equipment
added when the functional properties of the
end product must be upgraded to compete with

other products.

It must be decided whether the process
should be of the co- or counter-current type
and whether it should be a batch or a truly
continuous one. Experience has shown that
only counter-current extraction is suitable
for the present purpose. The answer in favor
of a batch or a truly continuous process, on
the other hand, is not as simple as it might
appear. Raw material arrives in unpredictably
different size batches and can be expected to
vary considerably in composition, particularly
in oil content and characteristics. These
batches must be processed under different
conditions because of the variety of solvent
to solids ratios and solvent contact times.
Different raw materials also yield differently
colored end products, depending upon the
muscle and skin pigmentation of the animals.
Raw material batches that produce a darker
colored product should be mixed with a lighter
colored product to maintain color uniformity.

Furthermore, IPA extraction of water,
glycerides, nonglyceride lipids, and small
molecular odor bodies appears to proceed in
discrete stages, the extraction efficiency of
one stage depending largely upon the lipid and
water content of the miscella contacting that
stage. For each stage of the extraction process, there exists, in contrast to the situation in vegetable oil extraction, an optimum
water and lipid content of the extracting
stream. With the solvent to solids ratio
appropriate to a particular raw material, it
appears that under suitable extraction conditions, extraction equilibrium occurs very
rapidly at every stage, probably within one
minute or so. Therefore, the most flexible
and safest method to adopt is a counter-
current, semi-continuous extraction process,
articulated in independently adjustable
stages.

Phases of the Process Requiring Special Equipment

There are several considerations to be taken into account when choosing equipment. These include the difficulties of transport and storage as well as the choosing of suitable sanitary equipment for use in each stage of the process.

Let us assume the following material flow: On arrival at the plant the raw material is washed, culled, and then prebroken in a hammer mill to be either fed to the deboners or stored in IPA in the raw material storage tanks. The bone, skin, and scales from the deboners go to the fish meal plant, and the muscle protein is homogenized in a large-capacity Waring-type blender with the addition of IPA, and is then pumped to the extraction vessels. Here the material is extracted in stages by counter-current solvent flow; each stage is followed by centrifuge separation of the solids and liquids. The fully extracted concentrate is next desolventized, gound to the required particle size, and stored for blending and packaging.

Transport. Special care must be taken in transporting both filleting waste and whole fish. Filleting waste must be washed with chlorinated water and transported from the filleting stations to the storage bins or the processing area of the FPC plant either in fully enclosed stainless steel conveyors of sanitary design, or in sanitary flumes constructed of noncorrodible material other than wood where clean (treated) water is used as the conveying medium.

Whole fish must be unloaded from the boat, preferably in covered, iced boxes, and transported to the plant. Unloading bulk fish from boats by pumps utilizing sea water, as is usually done in the fish meal industry, is

quite unsuitable. Since the raw material must
be of edible grade, i.e., unbruised, it is
essential that the fish be kept in ice or
otherwise refrigerated in the ship's hold.
The requirements for handling raw material in
large quantities present serious and expensive
problems that have not yet been satisfactorily
and economically solved except, perhaps, by
the expedient of culling, prebreaking, and
storing the fish on board ship in IPA.

Storage of raw material. The problem of storing raw material is as thorny as it is
unavoidable. Delivery of fresh fish is usually unpredictable, and so is the variety of
landed species. To insure continuous operation, storage facilities for a minimum of
several days must be provided. The only way
the fish could be safely stored in the round
for any length of time is by blast freezing it
either at sea or on land. This method,
coupled with the necessity of thawing the fish
later, is prohibitively expensive. The best
solution is to store the fish in IPA after
inspection and prebreaking.

Culling. When unwanted fish are eliminated
and conveyed to the fish meal plant, care must
be taken to remove stray metal (ferrous and
nonferrous) and stones, since both components
can cause great damage in the course of the
subsequent operations. Visual inspection and
hand sorting are believed to be the only
methods presently available.

Deboning. There are several Japanese deboning
machines operating on similar principles, but
with different installation and spare part
requirements. It is important to bear in mind
that the machines have to be kept particularly
clean since no IPA is present here as a disin-
fectant. As a result, they require

considerable working space so that they can be
completely dismantled from time to time. The
Japanese machines have operated successfully
in Japan's multimillion dollar fish sausage
and emulsion industry, and their operating
conditions are well known. Successfully
operating American and European deboning
machines are also on the market, but their
characteristics are not as well documented.
Performance tests should be carried out with
actual raw material to decide which type to
choose and whether to install a single- or
multiple-pass deboning line. Little information is available on the performance characteristics of any machine processing a variety
of raw materials.

Extraction and separation. A conventional
jacketed and covered extraction vessel,
equipped with variable speed agitators for
controlled contact of the raw material with
the solvent (Fig. 1A, 2, and 3) is satisfactory. No truly continuous, compact extrac-
tion-separation device has been developed. It
is important to determine what the optimum
solvent to solids ratios, contact times,
extraction temperatures, and number of extraction stages are for the satisfactory extraction of different species of lean and fatty
fish, for fish of one species that are caught
at different times of the year, at different
stages of maturity, and on different fishing
grounds. This body of knowledge, which is
only sketchily available in the literature, is
essential to permit calculations of optimum
vessel capacity, holding time, and temperature
control requirements.
     For liquid-solid phase separations, the
relative advantages of shaker screens and
centrifuges have to be weighed against each
other. Properly comminuted and extracted raw
material can be desolventized by

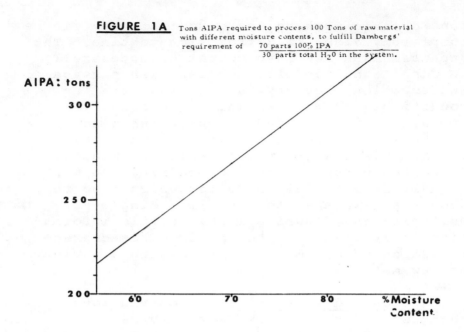

FIGURE 1A Tons AlPA required to process 100 Tons of raw material with different moisture contents, to fulfill Dambergs' requirement of $\frac{70 \text{ parts } 100\% \text{ IPA}}{30 \text{ parts total } H_2O \text{ in the system.}}$

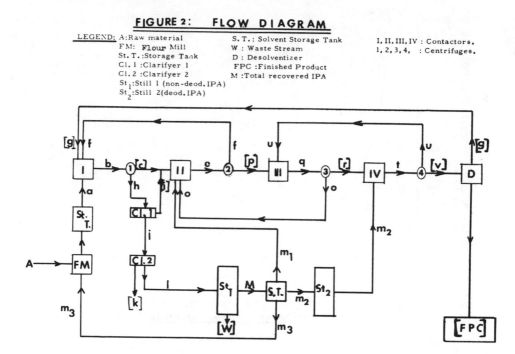

FIGURE 2:   FLOW DIAGRAM

LEGEND: A:Raw material   S.T.: Solvent Storage Tank   I, II, III, IV : Contactors.
        FM: Flour Mill   W : Waste Stream   1, 2, 3, 4,   : Centrifuges.
        St.T. :Storage Tank   D : Desolventizer
        Cl.1 :Clarifyer 1   FPC :Finished Product
        Cl.2 :Clarifyer 2   M :Total recovered IPA
        St₁:Still 1 (non-deod. IPA)
        St₂:Still 2(deod. IPA)

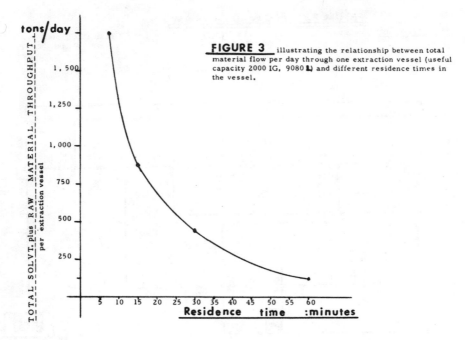

FIGURE 3 illustrating the relationship between total material flow per day through one extraction vessel (useful capacity 2000 IG, 9080 L) and different residence times in the vessel.

centrifugation to a residual content of less
than 35 percent by weight, which usually means
that the material is almost free-flowing and
will not compact when fed into the next stage
in the process, desolventization. Equally important to determine, and mostly unpublished
are data on the physical characteristics of
oil-IPA-water mixtures with different fish
oils. The physical and chemical characteristics of fish oils vary with species, seasons, and feeding grounds, resulting in different oil-IPA-water solubility distribution at
different temperatures. This, in turn is
particularly important for the separation and
recovery of the extracted lipids by centrifugation.

Desolventization. Evaporation of free solvent
from the extracted solids down to a residual
solvent content of 1 or 2 percent by weight
appears to be relatively easy by conventional
methods, preferably under vacuum to insure low
processing temperatures. It is very difficult, however, to arrive at a solvent content
in the vicinity of 100 ppm required under most
commercial conditions for organoleptic, economic, and legal reasons. IPA is a highly polar
substance and the fish solids to which it is
adsorbed have considerable surface, capillar-
ity, and heat sensitivity. Desolventization
is, therefore, a special problem that has
often been neglected within this context.
    Experience has shown that, whereas the
first stage of this operation is best carried
out under reduced pressure, the second requires the introduction of steam under pressure. Excess steam, however, induces
undesirable color changes in the final product. Color changes are also caused by exposure to temperatures above 200° F for more
than a few minutes. We are faced with the
prospect of installing a three-component

assembly in which the solvent content of the
violently agitated concentrate particles is
first reduced from about 35 to 2 percent under
vacuum, from 2 percent to a few parts per
million with steam under pressure, and then
cooled.

Final grinding. It has been shown that, for a
number of food supplementation purposes, the
protein concentrate should be available at a
particle size of about 300 mesh. Although
size reduction belongs to one of the oldest of
the mechanical arts, FPC presents special
challenges of its own. The material's heat
sensitivity, mechanical elasticity, electro-
static properties, and over-all structure make
it particularly difficult and expensive to
grind satisfactorily. Special attention must
be given in the selection of equipment to the
needs of cooling the grinding surfaces, to the
erosive properties of the material, to the
nature and composition of the metal parts with
which the FPC comes in contact, and to the
cost and availability of spare parts.

Solvent recovery. Apart from the cost of the
raw material, the most important economic
factor is the reduction of solvent losses to
the lowest possible level. Major solvent
losses can be due to solvent vapor leaks in
the still bottoms, as dissolved in the extracted fish oils, and in the final steam
stripping stage of the desolventizing operation. Techniques such as refrigerated vapor
traps used in the hexane extraction of vegetable oil seeds can be employed to minimize
these losses, although IPA, unlike hexane, is
water soluble in all proportions.
    To gain some insight into the problems of
IPA purification, the reader is referred to
the observations and results obtained by the
Esso Research and Engineering Company which

conducted a project under contract with the
Department of the Interior on the purification
of IPA. Some relevant passages from the report are quoted below.

   "Studies of recovered azeotropic isopropyl
alcohol solvent showed that basic amine contaminants are a major source of odor. In
addition, the presence of residual odor,
traceable to nonbasic contaminants, has also
been detected. Because the recovered azeotropic isopropyl alcohol is recovered by
distillation processes, the contaminants probably have boiling points close to that of the
pure azeotropic IPA (80.4° C). A number of
potential contaminants are listed in Table 1.

Table 1: Potential Contaminants with Boiling
Points Near Azeotropic Isopropanol

Contaminant	Boiling Point at 760 mm Hg, °C
n-Butyraldehyde	74.7
Ethyl Acetate	77.1
n-Butyl Amine*	77.8
Ethyl Alcohol**	78.4
Methyl Ethyl Ketone**	79.6
Methyl Propionate	79.7
Isopropyl Alcohol-Water Azeotrope (AIPA)	80.4
Dipropyl (n, iso) Ether	82.5
t-Butyl Alcohol**	82.6
Ethylene Glycol Dimethyl Ether	83.0
Triethyl Amine*	89.4

*Observed in analyses on FPC and recycled IPA.
**Occasionally present in commercial azeo-
tropic IPA, including:

Acetone   56°C
Diisopropyl Ether   69°C
n-Propyl Alcohol   97°C

The list of potential contaminants must be broadened to include compounds that form azeotropic mixtures with water or azeotropic IPA."

The Esso researchers found that a dual dis-distillation system consisting of an azeotrope and a deodorizing column could produce an odor-free azeotropic alcohol containing only 4 ppm of amine hydrochloride with a loss of less than 1 percent alcohol.

By-product Disposal

Reliable and sanitary methods for the disposal of the following by-products must be provided as a conditio sine qua non for operating the plant.

Unused fish and fish waste. Undesirable spe-cies of fish separated during the inspection and culling operation must be disposed of by conveyance to a nearby plant for processing into fish meal. A similar link is necessary for the removal of bone, scale and skin com-ponents obtained from the deboning operation. Depending on the composition of the raw material, the waste-product stream can vary considerably in volume. It is mandatory that both the FPC and fish meal plants be flexible and well co-ordinated, since the arrival and nature of raw material are largely unpredict-able.

Fish oil. With an assumed raw material pro-cessing rate of 200 tons per day, the amount of extracted oil can be expected to vary from one ton per day, when only lean fish are pro-cessed, to up to 20 tons per day, when only

fatty fish enter the plant. Storage and
shipment of crude oil in barrels is appropriate.

Waste water. At a processing rate of 200 tons
of fish per day, an FPC yield of 28 tons per
day (14 percent) and an oil yield of one ton
per day (0.5 percent), a total of at least
14×10^3 pounds per hour of waste water containing about 700 pounds of protein and oily
material would be discharged from the plant.
This is a nontrivial quantity both in terms of
financial loss (raw material for the manufacture of fish meal) and in terms of water
pollution. It is, therefore, essential to
pass all the aqueous waste-stream through a
water purification plant in which the organic
material is separated from the inorganic, and
the oil separated from the protein. The fats
can be stored in barrels; the protein sludge,
amounting to as much as seven or eight tons of
dry matter per day, should also be conveyed
to the fish meal plant.

Still bottoms. A final waste product that
should not be overlooked is the distillation
residue that accumulates at the bottom of the
distillation towers. This consists of polymerized, highly viscous organic compounds
that will not reach the aqueous waste-stream
and will have to be removed periodically during general cleaning operations of the solvent
recovery system. Quantitatively, this waste-
product may not amount to more than a few
hundred pounds from each cleaning operation;
it may prove to be a valuable raw material for
the chemical and flavor industry.

Sanitation, Safety, and Quality Control
The present remarks would be incomplete if the
absolute requirements for in-plant laboratory
control were not at least briefly mentioned.

Few raw materials provide such an excellent
medium as fish for the growth of potentially
harmful microorganisms. Although IPA is an
excellent bacteriostat over a wide dilution
range, and the fully extracted material is
practically sterile on emerging from the
desolventizing stage, recontamination through
subsequent handling is possible and must be
controlled. Quite apart from the health
hazards of microbial infection, very small
amounts of putrefying fish tissue produce
enormous volumes of odor bodies that can per-
meate entire buildings and once established,
are difficult to eliminate. Sanitary control
of the workers is also essential.
     The fire and health hazards of IPA vapors
are well-known, and automatic monitoring and
warning devices controlling IPA air mixtures
in working areas must be used. Necessary
precautions must be taken to avoid sparks,
the accumulation of static electricity, and
the possibility of accidental fires.
     The most taxing duties of the plant
laboratory are the continuous testing of raw
material, intermediate and final products for
proteins, lipids, water, IPA, microorganisms,
and so on. Very small IPA residues in the
final product and the purity of the deodorized solvent must be rapidly determined. It
may be necessary to install an experimental
rat colony to conduct nutritive studies of
FPC samples. Initially, a staff of at least
three experienced, full time chemists per
shift will be required to control the plant
operations.

Cost Estimates
Some rough cost estimates of the equipment
that was discussed above together with an
overview of selected operating costs will be
found in Table 2. All costs are approximate
and apply to equipment capable of handling

Table 2. Cost Estimates of Equipment,
Processing, and Direct Operating Costs

1. Selected Equipment Items $ (000)
    Raw material transport   65
    Raw material storage   160
    Deboning machines   38
    Extraction vessels   25
    Centrifuges   300
    Desolventizers   200
    Final grinding   30
    Solvent recovery   200
    Water treatment   100
2. Processing Costs
    a) Raw material cost
        Whole fish $60.00 per ton or $.030
        per pound
        Trimmings $18.00 per ton or $.009
        per pound
        Composition of raw
        material   86% whole fish
                                14% trimmings
        Raw material cost $.027 per pound
    b) Yield of FPC
        Whole fish   14% FPC
        Trimmings   8% FPC
        100 pound raw material will yield 13.2
        pounds FPC
        1 pound FPC
        requires $.205 raw material
    c) IPA loss
        Cost of IPA (99%) $.082 per pound
        (89%) $.074 per pound
        Assume a use of 1.75 parts by weight
        of 80% IPA: For 200 tons raw material
        use 350 tons IPA per day
        Loss of 1 percent of solvent, or 3.5
        tons per day-7000 pounds per day
        Cost of 7000 pounds
        89% IAP $518.00 per day
        Daily production of
        FPC   52,800 pounds

                    Therefore: solvent loss
                    loss $.01 per pound FPC
          d)   Power require-
                    ments $.011 per pound
                                                FPC
          e)   Water require-
                    ments $.003 per pound
                                                FPC
3.   Summary of Direct Operating Costs: Cents
      per Pound FPC
      Raw material $.205
      IPA $.010
      Steam $.030
      Power $.011
      Water $.003
      Labor $.050
      Miscellaneous $.027
                                $.336

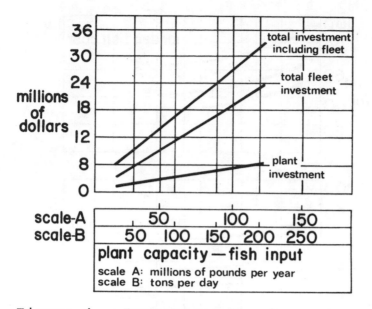

Figure 4. Investment Requirements
(C. D. Holder, K. H. Kidel, W. B. Magyar,
and D. S. Ross. Conference on FPC, Ottawa,
Oct. 24-25, 1967.)

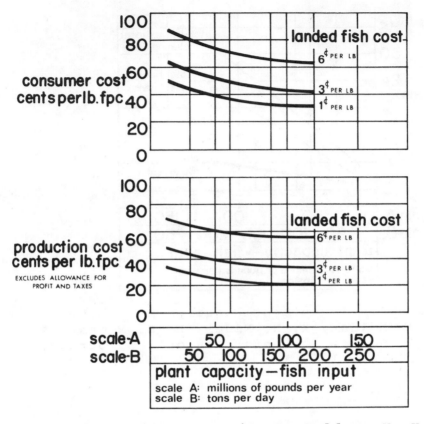

Figure 5. Unit Costs (C. D. Holder, K. H. Kidel, W. B. Magyar and D. S. Ross. Conference on FPC, Ottawa, Oct. 24-25, 1967.)

200 tons of raw material per day. (See
Figures 4 and 5.)

Summary

The above remarks and figures were selected
for discussion to serve as examples of some of
the technical problems that require answers
and as indices for some of the major cost
elements that are involved in the manufacture
of FPC. The figures were arrived at on the
basis of actual equipment, power, water and
other costs in a particular location, the raw
material costs on the basis of actual commercial bids. The latter must, of course, be
expected to fluctuate widely and should not be
taken as generally applicable: There are
locations where whole fish and filleting
waste are considerably below the cost given
here, just as there are many instances where
these costs are far too low.
    The final direct operating cost of 33.6¢
per pound of FPC does not include items such
as interest, amortization and profit; it must,
therefore, be assumed that 10 to 15¢ must be
added to the above figures to arrive at a
realistic sales price.
    The question of whether or not a final cost
of 40 or 50¢ per pound might mean that FPC
can, in a particular country, be manufactured
as an economically viable enterprise, depends
entirely upon the availability and acceptability of other equivalent low cost protein
sources, the extent of malnutrition, the general economic status of the population and most
importantly, the extent to which the local
government acknowledges its obligations to
guarantee a minimal level of nutritional
sufficiency.

XXV
SOME PROBLEMS IN MARKETING FPC

R. Kreuzer
Fishery Products and Marketing Branch, Food
and Agriculture Organization of the United
Nations

FPC (fish protein concentrate) is a nutritive
supplement that has caught the imagination of
many people because of its high food value and
its easy storage possibilities. It is potentially an effective means of overcoming malnutrition in underdeveloped areas and an
excellent protein additive for the food market
of developed areas.

Although there are as yet no FPC products
on the food market, they have recently been
introduced in the animal feed market, mainly
as a protein component in milk replacers used
for calf feeding. It is expected that the
potential of FPC in the feed sector, which is
just beginning to be realized, will stimulate
greater interest in more intensive technical
research in the food sector. A brief survey
of the recent and potential FPC/milk replacer
market may, therefore, be of interest.

FPC in the Animal Feed Market
In 1971 about 2,228,000 tons of milk replacer
were used for calf meat and beef production;
910,000 tons for red meat, and 1,318,000 tons
for white meat. Of this amount, 1,570,000
tons were marketed in Common Market countries; 650,000 tons in France, 35,000 tons in
the Netherlands, 270,000 tons in Italy, and
225,000 tons in the Federal Republic of
Germany.

Milk replacers presently used for meat
production contain skim milk, soya, yeast, or
starch as protein sources. FPC is now used to

a very limited extent in these preparations;
the extent to which it will be used in the
future depends on the availability of suitable
FPC products and their price, and on the price
of skim milk, soya, and yeast. At present,
three products containing FPC are sold on the
European market: "Protanimal", produced by
Astra, Sweden; "Micronized Protein Concentrate" (MPC), produced in Norway; and "CPSP
90", produced by Sopropeche, France. The former two products are insoluble; the latter one
is soluble.

The market potential in Europe for a milk
replacer for red meat using insoluble FPC is
estimated at 50,000 tons per year by 1980.
The market potential for a milk replacer for
white meat using soluble FPC is estimated at
250,000 to 300,000 tons per year, possibly
doubling in ten years.

Calf feeding tests have been carried out
successfully with the three products containing FPC. The composition of the product containing CPSP 90 is as follows: CPSP 90, 20%;
whey, 53%; fat, 23%; and Premix, 4% (vitamins,
antibiotics, minerals, synthetic methionine,
etc.). The level of iron content in this
product is about 110 ppm; approximately 80
ppm in CPSP 90 and 28 to 30 ppm in whey. The
results of these experiments were that yeast
from oil would be the only serious competitor
to CPSP 90 if the iron content could be
lowered. The iron content in CPSP 90 is 80 to
100 ppm and in yeast from oil (BP); 200 ppm.
Table 1 shows a comparison based on experiments carried out in different laboratories
of the three FPC products mentioned above.

Potential Processing Methods
Present research in several countries is moving rapidly in the direction of developing
processing methods to produce an FPC with more
functional properties. In Sweden, Astra has

Table 1.

Characteristics	Protanimal	MPC	CPSP 90
Solubility	Nil	Nil	90%-100%
Particle size	100-120 micron (μ), suspension not stable, has to be improved by addition of 1% alginate (Gnar gum).	Ca. 35 micron (μ) rather stable suspension, addition of small amount of thickening agent gives required stability.	Similar to skim milk powder-product soluble.
Smell	Practically nil	Slight when mixed with water	Strong, can be masked by special additives
Crude protein	80-85%	78-80%	83-87%
Moisture	5-8%	6-12%	5-6%
Minerals	10-15%	4-5%	6-8%
Iron	500 ppm	250 ppm	80-100 ppm (A product with ca. 40 ppm may be available in the near future.)
Fat (ether extracted)	Less than 0.1%	Maximum 1%	1.89%

Characteristics	Protanimal	MPC	CPSP 90
Biological value for calf feeding			(Skim milk 95)
Digestibility of organic matter	86.6 (mixed with skim milk)		94 (mixed with whey)
Digestibility of protein	93 (mixed with skim milk)	88.5-89.2 (when live weight of calves was 60 & 130 kg, respectively)	91 (mixed with whey) (Skim milk 95)
	87-89 (mixed with whey)		
Digestibility of fat in feed	86 (mixed with whey)		
Average rate of growth	1000 g/day (skim milk 1200 g/day)		900-950 g/day (skim milk 1.125 g/day)
Applications	Only suitable for red meat production and heifer rearing because of high iron content.	Up to 25% in milk replacers for bull & herd calves (red meat production)	15-20% without gelatine agent for red meat production

Characteristics	Protanimal	MPC	CPSP 90
	Maximum incorporated in calf feed 15% (because of high mineral content)	3-5% for veal calves (white meat production) if 15 ppm iron is considered upper limit in a milk replacer	18% with gelatine agent for white meat production
Value for calf nutrition	15% less than control with skim milk		15% less than control with skim milk.

developed a new FPC product made from
eviscerated and deboned fish for the food
market. In Chile, an attempt is being made to
produce FPC for large-scale use in child feeding programs. In France, a soluble FPC is
being produced by enzymatic hydrolysis.

There are, however, a number of technical,
economic and administrative problems involved
in putting FPC to use as human food. It
appears that the concept and strategy hitherto
pursued with regard to the development and use
of solvent extracted FPC requires revision.
For the past ten years, technologists and
nutritionists have focused their attention on
the solvent extracted Type A FPC. The use of
this product, however, is limited. It can be
incorporated without difficulty only into
stews, soups, and those foods which involve
the preliminary formation of a dough or
paste; and the amount that can easily be
incorporated is only about 5 percent. It remains useless, for example, to the millions
who eat rice as a staple food. Processing
costs are relatively high and economic production requires a plant capacity capable of
processing 200 to 500 tons of raw material
daily.

To be useful to developing countries, FPC
processes should be applicable to small fishery resources. In this respect, the FPC process being developed in France is of interest
for many developing countries as it enables
fresh fish from shrimp trawlers to be used for
the commercial production of FPC. The first
step of the process, fermentation, takes place
on board the fishing vessels. The subsequent
steps, purification and spray drying, are
carried out on shore. The shore installation
can process the fermented products from up to
twelve shrimp trawlers.

In order to expand the use of FPC to human
needs, it will be necessary to develop a

broader range of products at a higher
percentage of acceptability. For use in
developing countries where the problem of
malnutrition flourishes, the production of
FPC should be economically feasible in smaller
quantities.

XXVI
SOME ASPECTS OF THE FISH PROTEIN MARKET IN
INDUSTRIALIZED COUNTRIES: A VIEW FROM
PRIVATE INDUSTRY

Joseph R. Champagne
The Nestle Company, Inc., White Plains, New
York

There are several general assumptions which
should be made by the commercial community
when considering the market for fish protein.
First, private industry will wish to maintain
its profit objectives when marketing fish
protein and/or foods containing fish protein.
Second, private industry groups manufacturing
the protein will either market fish protein as
an industrial product to be sold to other food
companies, or they will incorporate the fish
protein in their own consumer food products.
Third, fish protein products must be competitive functionally and economically with other
well accepted protein ingredients; for
example, soy, egg, and milk proteins.
     The critical factors which private industry
must consider are technical feasibility,
economic feasibility and marketability.

Technical Feasibility

In order to compete with other protein ingredients, the manufacturer should be able to
produce fish protein products which function
in several different ways. At present, soy,
milk, or egg protein ingredients perform these
functions. Table I describes some of the
major characteristics and gives a brief description of what kind of functionality fish
protein products should possess.

Economic Feasibility

Assuming that the products are technically

Table I. Ideal Properties for Protein
Ingredients for Industrialized Countries

Ideal Product	General Characteristics	Market
I	Low pH solubility, clarity in solution. No thermocoagulability.	Beverages,* soups
II	Overall compatibility in baked goods. No effect on loaf volume, white color, etc. and/or Good water and fat absorption properties. Thermocoagulability.	Baked goods** and/or Meat Products
III	Egg white replacements.	Broad usage**

----

*Assumes at least a 90% protein product.
**Assumes at least a 70% protein product.

feasible, they will then have to compete with
soy, milk, and egg proteins economically. The
fish protein manufacturer would have to price
them to the food industry as seen in Table II.

These prices would make fish proteins
relatively competitive with existing protein
ingredients during the period of 1972-1975.

If the manufacturer prefers to use his fish
protein ingredients in his own products, the
feasible prices become the upper limits as
stated above. Since he would not be concerned
with in-house profits, he would have greater
room for processing costs.

If the manufacturer wishes to market the
fish protein as an industrial product to
another food manufacturer, his maximum cost
limit must be lower than the above figures
since he must sell his product at those ranges
in order to be competitive. To make a profit,
and incur selling costs and so forth, the
upper limits would be something like the
following in Table III. These figures are
based on the rule of thumb that the total
manufacturing cost is one-half the selling
price for an industrial ingredient of this
kind.

Marketability

Given, then, that the product is technically
and economically feasible, the question remains, is it marketable? Let us assume that
the manufacturer will develop several high
protein consumer products containing fish
protein. If he has Type I, the soluble protein, he will put it in a beverage and market
it as a nutritious high protein beverage to
sell. The consumer must be convinced that it
is worth it to pay 10 to 25¢ more for a 6-pak
of high protein beverage. This will involve
consumer education, and heavy advertising and
promotion costs. The manufacturer will have
to overcome the relatively unattractive label

Table II. Targeted Protein Products: Ideal
Pricing as Industrial Products

Ideal Product		$/lb.		Market
		Mini-mum	Maxi-mum	
I	Beverage-type isolate (100% soluble at low pH)	.50	.80	Beverages, soups
II	Low-medium functionality concentrate	.15	.30	Baked goods
III	Egg white replacement	.80	1.20	Broad usage

Table III. Targeted Protein Products:
Theoretical Maximum Manufacturing Cost Limits
for Ideal Protein Products

Ideal Product	Maximum Cost Limit ($/lb.)	Market
I	.25 - .40	Beverages, soups
II	.08 - .15	Baked goods
III	.40 - .60	Broad usage

declaration "with fish protein" on his
beverage bottle. In the U. S. this is probably fish protein's greatest liability.
Furthermore, there is the possibility that
breakthroughs in soy or milk protein chemistry
will result in cheaper products.

These are but a few of the many critical
factors which must be evaluated before entering into a fish protein enterprise. And we
have not gotten involved in what is perhaps
the key point in relation to fish proteins--
the supply of raw material. Nor have we discussed the effect of regulatory limitations
on the marketability of fish proteins.

If our theoretical manufacturer's beverage
becomes as popular as Dad's Root Beer, which
has only about 0.5 percent of the soft drink
market, and he uses 3 percent fish protein,
can he make 14 MM pounds of fish protein? If
he is lucky enough to capture 2 percent of the
soft drink market, like Fresca, for example,
can he make 56 MM pounds of fish protein? The
amounts of fish protein potentially required
equate to huge quantities of fish and preferably fish trimmings, which should be available
at low prices with only minimal variations
year in and year out.

The challenges are certainly significant
ones.

XXVII
NOTES FROM NABISCO-ASTRA

H. J. Watson
Nabisco-Astra Development Corporation

On February 17, 1970, the Nabisco-Astra
Nutrition Development Corporation was formed
with the intent of developing and marketing
food products with high protein levels. The
corporation is in a unique position, being the
only privately funded organization in the
United States working to market foods containing fish protein. In our effort to market
Astra Essential Fish Protein (EFP 90), we have
conducted consumer research in the United
States, and research projects under grants
from USAID and the Overseas Private Investment
Corporation. Our experimental products have
been exposed to a wide variety of tastes and
consumer levels ranging from Congressional
dinner parties to sampling at trade shows, and
scientific and commercial conventions. We
have found no problems in formulating
organoleptically appealing products containing
Astra EFP 90.
    While the consumer is more than ever aware
of the need for higher protein intake, fish
protein usually places last in interview ses-
sions as an acceptable source of protein
fortification. One of the ways Nabisco-Astra
is approaching the problem of consumer education domestically is through the mass feeding
market, for example, the School Lunch and
Breakfast programs. Product testing in grade
schools has revealed a rating of above 7 on a
scale of 1 to 10. Three products will be provided for a Pilot Program of child feeding at
Recreation Centers in Cincinnati where a total
of 10,000 children per day will be fed a snack
or lunch for ten weeks. If children can

accept the foods knowing they are fortified
with fish protein, and it is assured that the
product is pure, tasteless, and odorless, a
great step toward public acceptance will have
been made.

Acceptability, 380, 425
 of anchovy-FPC, 410,
   424-426
 in children, 347, 369,
   481
 problem of, 302, 426
 tests of, 312-313
Acceptability studies,
   278, 348-349, 382, 385
Ackman, R. G., 78, 80
Actomyosin, 122
Adsorption, enzyme, 284-
   290, 298
Africa, FPC in, 302-304
 subsistence economies
   in, 387
Aftertaste, 256
Agency for International
   Development (AID), 358,
   360
Aggregation, 152
Albumin, 122, 228, 342
Alewife, FPC from, 175t
Allison, J. B., 195, 196t
Alpine Marine Protein In-
   dustries, Inc., 78, 397
Alverson, G., 27
Amino acids, costs of,
   363, 365t
 in FPC, 167, 168t, 181,
   234
 in FPH, 155
 in LFP, 131t, 132, 133
 and nitrogen, 238t
 obtaining, 149
 preservation of, 200
 during processing, 379
 synthetic, 363-364, 370
Anchovy, 13, 42, 47, 68
 Argentine, 51
 Californian, 42, 420t-
   421t, 423
 in Central Pacific, 49

FPC from, 69t, 175t, 402,
   415t, 424-426
 harvest of, 15t
 northern, 416, 424
 Peruvian, 15t, 39, 41,
   51, 407, 412t, 414, 440
 in South Atlantic, 48
 in South Pacific, 49
Anglemier, A. F., 83, 321,
   392
Animal feed, 27, 357, 362,
   468-469
Aquatic animals, catch of,
   10, 18t
Aqueous processes, 111,
   113, 117f, 394
Aqueous-solvent processes,
   111-113, 115-116, 118-
   119
Arnold, J., 33
Aroma, FPC, 256. See also
   Odor
Arsenic, 65
 in FPC, 106
 in LFP, 130t
 in swordfish, 66t
Ash, C. S., 75
Ash, in FPH process, 144t.
   See also Minerals
Asia, subsistence econo-
   mies in, 388
Astra Nutrition Corp. of
   Sweden, 85, 87, 116,
   178, 397, 469
Astra process, 73, 212
Australia, 362

Baby foods, 368, 429
Bacillus, in FPC, 67
Baertl, J. M., 269
Baleen whale, 29
Barnes, R. H., 185, 186
Bass, Janet L., 266, 384

Beef, 173t
Berg, A., 366, 367
Bertullo, V. H., 86
Beverage, FPC in, 276-
    277, 479
Biological value (BV), of
    FPC, 235, 245-249
  and nitrogen balance,
    246t
  and NPU, 248t
Biscuits, FPC in, 267-
    268, 304
Bitterness, in LFP, 132
Blaw Knox Co., 76
Bleaching, 333
Boerema, L. K., 44
Bombay duck, FPC from,
    176t
Brazil, FPC in, 269
Bread, enrichment of,
    303
  FPC in, 69t, 194, 195,
    256, 258t, 259t, 261-
    266, 308-310
Bressani, Richardo, 192
Brinkman, G. L., 221
British American Hospital,
    Lima, 223
Broadhead, W. C., 27
Burd, A. C., 44
Bureau of Commercial
    Fisheries (BCF), 212,
    394
By-products, disposal of,
    460
  from FPC processing, 415
  recovery of, 396, 416,
    424, 431
  value of, 422

Cadmium, 130t
Calcium, 130t, 170, 171t
Calf feeding tests, 469,

471t
California, FPC production
    in, 417, 419
Call, D. L., 113, 373
Call, T. M., 359, 389,
    429
Calloway, D. H., 245
Canada, 59, 102, 167
Capelin, 447
  Arctic, 13
  harvest of, 14t
  North Sea, 41
  Norwegian, 40
Carbohydrates, 140
Carbon dioxide, 71
Carcinogens, 335
Cardinal Proteins, 397
Caribbean, 47
Casein, vs. FPC, 185,
    186, 191, 199
  PER for, 178
  prices of, 363, 365t
  protein repletion with,
    190f
  supply of, 362
Cash crops, 387
Catch Per Unit (CPU), 418
Caul, Jean F., 266, 384
Central Atlantic, 47
Central Food Technologi-
    cal Research Institute,
    Mysore, 217
Central Pacific, 48-49
Centrifugation, 112, 298,
    332, 457
Cephalopods, 42
Cereals, 308
  FPC in, 213-227, 316
Chapati, evaluation of,
    384
  FPC in, 266
Chapman, W. M., 13, 17
Cheftel, C., 392

Children, high protein
  mixtures for, 313
  malnourished, 338
  PCM in, 426
Chile, FPC in, 308, 398,
  399t, 405t
  FPC production in, 403,
  411, 412
  nutrition programs in,
  139, 370
  protein sources in, 135
Chlorocholine chloride
  (CCC), 182
Christian Medical College,
  South India, 223
Chromatographic analysis,
  332
Chromium, 66t, 171t
Ciguatera, 38
Clarke, M. R., 23
Clinics, 388
Clupeidae, 404, 440
Coagulation, 112
  of fish protein, 122
  protein, 104
Cobalt, in swordfish, 66t
Cod, FPC from, 176t, 179t
  polar, 46
Color, of anchovy-FPC,
  425
  and desolventization,
  326
  experiments on, 332-333
  of FPC, 256
  of PH-65, 157t
Comminution, 72-74
Committee on Aquatic Food
  Resources, NAS/NRC,
  227
Common Market, 468
Concentration, process of,
  60, 64
Condensation, 129t

Conservation, 39
Consumer acceptability,
  136, 137, 141t. See
  also Acceptability
Consumer education, 480
Consumers, "captive," 388
Contaminants, potential,
  459-460
Contasso, Gustavo, 277
Conveyor systems, 78
Cookies, enriched, 314
  FPC in, 69t, 256, 258t,
  259t, 312-313, 346t
Cooking, and leaching,
  271
  protein losses due to,
  380
  and supplements, 379
Cooling, 38
Copper, 171t
  in FPC, 106
  in LFP, 130t
  in swordfish, 66t
Corn, basal diet of, 375,
  377
  FPC fortification of,
  380
Costs, estimates of, 462,
  463t-464t
  of fishery products, 42-
  43
  "fixed," 398
  of FPC, 58-59, 88, 124,
  399t
  of FPC production, 90f
  "nonvariable," 401
  operating, 467
  overhead, 441
  of raw material, 39, 67,
  87
  unit, 466
Cottonseed flour, 345,
  374t, 376, 381t

Cottonseed products, 360, 361, 365t
CPC, 384
CPSP 90, 469, 470t, 471t, 472t
Crackers, FPC in, 275
Cravioto, J., 368
Crisan, Eli V., 269
Crustaceans, 37
Crutchfield, James A., 404
CSM (corn-soy-milk), 367
Culling, 452
Cysteine hydrochloride, 65
Cystine, 168t, 169t

Dairy products, 391
  marketing of, 361
  price of, 365t, 427
Dambergs, N., 63, 102
De, H. N., 178
Deboning, 72-74, 395, 452-453
Deficiencies, calorie, 364
  protein, 187, 188t, 328. See also Protein-calorie malnutrition
Dehydration, 293, 300
Delfino, A. H., 227
Delivery, problem of, 387-388
DeMaeyer, E. M., 215
Demand, for fish meal, 25
  for meals, 27
  world fish, 53
Denaturation, 152
Dental caries, 227
Dental survey, 345
Deodorization, 129t
Department of Agriculture, Canadian, 104
Department of Industry, Trade, and Commerce, Canadian, 103

Depreciation, 401, 422
Deproteinization, 122
Design, of FPC process, 295-298
Desolventization, 76-79, 321-326, 457-458
Deuel, Harry J., Jr., 185
Devanney, J. W., 3, 137, 367
Developed countries, protein supplements in, 388-389
Developing countries, 356
  delivery systems in, 387
  dietary habits in, 369-370
  foreign exchange in, 403
  FPC for, 473, 474
  supplementation programs in, 364, 426
Dialysis, 82
Diammonium citrate, 240, 241f, 242, 243t, 244t, 249
Diet, FPC supplemented, 193f, 194
  mixed, 370, 427
Dimethylamine (DMA), 332, 335
  in FPC, 335
Distribution, government, 367
Donuts, FPC in, 275-276
Doraiswamy, T. R., 217
Dough, FPC in, 270
Dreosti, D. M., 114, 196t, 200
Dried skim milk (DSM), 214, 226, 227, 374t
Drozdowski, B., 80
Drying, 76-79, 321
Dry solids, desolventizing of, 324t

DSM. See Dried skim milk
Dubrow, D. L., 64, 71,
    76, 77, 84, 172

East Central Pacific, 53
Economics, 136, 141t, 387
EDP (Experimental and
    Demonstration Plant),
    395
Education, consumer, 480
  nutritional, 375
Emulsion, stability of,
    319
Engineering, cost esti-
    mates for, 397
Enzymatic processes, 83,
    85-87, 150f
Enzymes, deactivation of,
    300
  hydrolysis of, 153f
Equipment, costs of, 463t-
    464t
  for FPC processing, 451
  manufacturing, 449-450
Erdman, Anne Marie, 269
Ernst, R. C., 74
Essential Fish Protein
    (EFP 90), 480
Esso Research and Engin-
    eering Co., 458
Ethylene dichloride, 59,
    182, 184
Euphasia superba, DANA,
    20
Exports, 403
Extenders, meat, 393
Extensigraph studies,
    262
Extraction, 67, 74-76,
    111, 143, 302, 392,
    453-457
  alcohol, 397
  counter-current, 450
  and deboning, 177

and drying times, 323t
  ethylene dichloride, 181,
    201
  isopropanol, 102
  isopropyl alcohol, 80,
    83, 85, 174, 175t, 179t,
    184, 320f, 385
  solvent, 119, 318
  stages of, 409-410, 450
  straight solvent, 449
  tertiary butanol, 181
  trimethylamine, 148f
  water, 145f, 148f
Extracts, toxicity of, 197

Farinograph studies, 262
Fatty acids, 62
Fatty fish, FPC from, 68,
    112, 431
Fermentation, 473
Fillets, composition of,
    61t
  FPC from, 177
Finch, R., 112, 165
Fish, composition of, 61t
  fat in, 60
  freeze-dried, 64
  for pets, 306
  price of, 407
  unused, 460
Fisheries-agriculture-
    protein complex, 255-
    259
Fisheries commissions,
    international, 34
Fisheries Research Board
    Laboratory, Halifax,
    104
Fisheries Service, Canad-
    ian, 105
Fishery, bottom trawl, 41
  clupeoid, 404, 440
  coastal, 34
  management of, 33

Fishery (continued)
 midwater trawl, 40
 Northern anchovy, 418
 purse seine, 40
 seasonal considerations
  in, 51-52
Fishery Products Technol-
  ogy Laboratory, NMFS,
  318
Fish fingers, 391
Fish flour, 213, 215, 315t
Fishing Industry Research
  Institute (FIRI), of
  South Africa, 218, 304,
  305
Fish meal, 12, 123
 consumption of, 17
 FPC from, 257
 in Peru, 439, 440-442
 price of, 408
 production of, 26, 27,
  54, 305
Fish protein, 91, 165,
  173t, 175t, 185
Fish protein hydrolysate
  (FPH), industrial com-
  plex for, 158f
 lipids in, 154
 nutritional quality of,
  178, 180t, 181, 183t
 processing of, 140-141t,
  142f. See also PH-65
Fish pulp, 146f, 147
Flavors, 79, 87, 256-261
 fishy, 147
 masking of, 255
 residual, 88
Flour, FIRI, 218
 fish, 213, 215
Fluoride, 38, 60, 103,
  170, 227, 228, 229,
  428, 429
Fluorine, 58, 106, 171t

Fluorosis, 345
Food and Drug Administra-
  tion (FDA), on FPC, 428
 regulations of, 78, 105,
  166, 184, 228
 role of, 3
 standards of, 319, 386
Foods, FPC in, 69t, 350
Food Science and Technol-
  ogy Dept. of UCD, 263
Food web, 30
Foreign exchange, 403,
  439, 443
FPC (Fish Protein Concen-
  trate), advantages of,
  468
 aqueous phosphate pro-
  cess for, 117f
 for Bangladesh refugees,
  221
 ban on, 428
 break-even cost of, 372,
  381t, 383t
 BV of, 245-249
 characteristics of, 58
 for children, 343t
 in Chile, 135, 399t
 concentration of, 293-
  295
 costs of, 88, 393-394,
  407-416
 from decomposed fish,
  178
 definition of, 9, 255,
  446-447
 dilution of, 242, 243t,
  244t
 economics of, 376, 402,
  475-477
 emulsifying capacity of,
  322t, 334
 enzymatically-produced,
  178

FPC (Fish Protein
  Concentrate) (continued)
  ethylene dichloride-ex-
    tracted, 184
  evaluation of, 479
  feasibility of, 389, 407,
    475
  flavorful, 278
  FAO guideline for, 59
  from fatty fish, 68, 112,
    431
  functionality of, 330,
    431
  hydrolyzed, 331
  insoluble, 469
  lipid content of, 166
  metabolic evaluation of,
    343t
  mineral composition of,
    170-172
  and nitrogen excretion,
    240, 241f, 242, 243t,
    244t
  and nitrogen retention,
    222
  non-deodorized, 212
  nonextracted, 305-306
  nonspecific nitrogen
    replacement of, 235-
    245
  nutritive quality of,
    176t
  optimum level of, 192
  organoleptic stability
    of, 113
  in pasta products, 273
  PER of, 174, 178, 181
  problems of, 3, 137
  processing of, 87-91
  production of, 90f, 408
  properties of, 283
  protein quality of, 179t,
    234, 235, 249
  protein repletion with,
    190f
  soluble, 124, 290-293
  in staple foods, 374t
  as supplement, 140, 191,
    192
  toxic, 182
  type A, 473
  utilization of, 184-191,
    260
  world market for, 439
Food industry, FPC in, 428
Food supplementation
  studies, 344. See also
  Supplementation
Fortification, effective-
  ness of, 373
  level of, 278
  over-, 371
  with synthetic amino
    acids, 371, 427. See
    also Supplementation
Foster, G. N., 368
France, FPC in, 473
Frange, R., 194
Fricola, 224
Friedman, Leo, 196t, 197,
  198
Fruit, FPC in, 304
Frysztacki, C. A., 184

Gas packing, 305
General Oceanology, Inc.
  (GO), 398, 400, 401,
  414
Glycine, 240, 241f, 244t,
  249
Gomez, F., 213, 266
Gonik, A., 220
Gopalan, C., 223, 225
Graham, G. G., 216, 225
Greenfield, C., 84
Grinding, 129, 458

Grits, FPC in, 256, 258t, 259t
Growth factors, 26
Growth rate, and supple-
  mentation, 219. See
  also Weight gain
Gruel, FPC in, 346t
Gruttner, R., 213
Gulf of Mexico, 47, 53
Gulf of Thailand, 49
Gulland, J. A., 8, 20, 23, 33, 42
Gunnarson, G. K., 102
Guttman, A., 102

Hake, 3, 38, 47, 447
  in Central Pacific, 49
  Chilean, 398, 412t
  Clupeonella, 14t
  enzyme hydrolysis of, 180t
  FPC from, 69t, 175t, 176t, 255, 260, 264t, 268, 330, 395
  migration of, 52
  in South Atlantic, 48
  in South Pacific, 49
Hale, M. B., 86, 392
Halibut, 173t
Halifax-BCF method, 449
Halifax process, 103
Hammerle, Olivia A., 186
Hammonds, T. M., 113, 359, 373, 389, 429
Handling, during FPC pro-
  cessing, 68-72
Hansen, J. D. L., 213, 304
Hariharan, K., 186
Harrington, W. R., 290
Harvest, for FPC, 14t-16t
  fishery, 8, 9
  Peruvian, 442-443

projections of, 17-25
Heavy metals, in LFP, 130t
Hegsted, D. M., 194
Heme pigments, 84
Herring, 3, 38, 42, 45, 68, 447
  Atlantic-Scandian, 51, 404
  conservation of, 46
  Falkland, 48, 49, 50
  FPC from, 69t, 166, 175t, 176t, 402
  harvest of, 14t, 16t
  North Sea, 51
  nutritive quality of, 173t
  thread, 13, 15t, 17, 25, 47, 49
Hettich, F. P., 86
Hevia, P., 76
Hexane, 62
Higashi, H., 125
Higroscopicity, of PH-65, 157t
Histidine, 87
History, of protein sup-
  plementation, 364-369
Hospitals, 388
HTH (heat transfer medium), 84
Hwang, W. I., 217
Hydrolysates, 150f, 151f, 154, 300
Hydrolysis, 331
  cause of, 152, 153f
  enzymatic, 111, 147-154
  fish pulp, 143
  short-time, 151f
Hypersensitivity, in
  children, 347

Ices, FPC-enriched, 344
Imports, 403

Incaparina, 226, 360, 361, 366, 367
Incumbe, 368
Indian Ocean, 50
Indicative World Plan for Agricultural Development, FAO, 45
Industrial Protein Center, Chilean, 135
Industry, fishing, 36
  fish meal, 409
  food, 390, 428
  food processing, 389
  Peruvian fish meal, 445
Infants, and FPC, 212
  high protein mixtures for, 313
Institute of Nutrition of Central America and Panama (INCAP), 221, 361
Instituto de Investigacion Nutricional, 337
Instituto del Mar del Peru, 407, 408, 440
International Conference on Progress in Meeting Protein Needs of Infants and Preschool Children, 213
Investment, requirements for, 465f
Iron, 170, 171t
Isolated soy protein (ISP), 187
Isoleucine, 167, 168t, 169t
Isopropyl alcohol (IPA), 57, 59, 63, 112, 431
  circulation of, 80
  extraction of, 68
  material balance of, 89f
  as solvent, 76

Jaffe, W. G., 196t, 200
Jansen, G. R., 194
Japan, amino acid production of, 363
  catch of, 45
  fish products in, 391, 453
  and lantern fish harvesting, 24
  soy products in, 358
Jeffreys, G. A., 86
Jekat, F., 242
Johnson, B. Connor, 196t, 199

Kansas State Univ., 263
Kapsiotis, G. D., 273
Kinetics, of FPC solubilization, 284-290
Knobl, G. M., 397, 425
Kofranyi, E., 242
Korea, FPC in, 269, 419
Koury, B., 71, 85
Krell, A. J., 86
Krill, Antarctic, 17, 19, 20, 21, 22, 29, 50
  FPC from, 176t
  harvest of, 16t
Kwashiorkor, 215, 222, 303
  and supplementation, 224
  treatment of, 226, 228, 229
Kwee, W. H., 382
Kyowa Fermentation Industry & Co., Ltd., 363

Labor, 410, 431
Lantern fish, 14t, 17, 19, 23, 24, 29, 42
Lasker, Rubin, 424
Law of the Sea Conference, 34

Lead, in FPC, 38, 106
Lee, K. Y., 217
Legumes, FPC in, 316
Lemon sole, 173t
Leucine, 168t, 169t
Lingcod, 173t
Lipid oxidation, 59, 143
Lipids, 62, 140
 addition of, 154
 extraction of, 68
 in FPH process, 144t
 removal of, 81
Liquid cyclone process,
  360
Liquified fish protein
  (LFP), 125
 amino acids in, 131t,
  132, 133
 chloride in, 130t
 mineral content of, 132
 yield of, 127, 129
Livestock, 357
Location, of FPC process-
  ing plants, 408, 431,
  448-449
Losses, solvent, 432, 458
Lysine, 168t, 169t
 costs of, 363
 in FPC, 167
 in FPC-enriched bread,
  310
 prices of, 365t
 in staple foods, 374t
 synthetic, 363, 376

Mackerel, 13, 25, 45
 conservation of, 46
 harvest of, 14t
 horse, 45, 46, 48
 jack, 17, 41
 LFP from, 128t, 129t
 in South Pacific, 49
Magnesium, 170, 171t

 in LFP, 130t
Mahnken, G., 3
Maillard reaction, 377
Maize, diets of, 214
Maize porridge, fortifi-
  cation of, 303
Makdani, D. D., 170
Malaysia, FPC in, 267
Malnutrition, 136, 139,
  303
 clinical evaluation of,
  338, 340t
 and FPC, 185, 186, 341t
 treatment of, 339
Management, of fishery
  harvest, 9
 of marine resources, 27-
  30, 33
Manganese, in swordfish,
  66t
Manufacturing, of FPC, 38,
  39, 449-450
 of LFP, 125-132. See
  also Processing; Production
Marasmus, 225
Margen, S., 245
Marine Protein Concen-
  trate, 328
Market, for fish protein,
  475
 food-use, 104
 for FPC, 355, 429, 468,
  477
 potential, 389
 requirement of, 120
 world, 355
Marraqueta, 377
McLaughlan, J. M., 178
Meals, consumption of, 27.
  See also Fish meal
Meat analogs, 393
Medwadowski, Barbara, 166

Meinke, W. W., 87
Menadione, and FPC supplement, 198
Menhaden, 3, 38, 68
 FPC from, 69t, 166, 175t, 179t, 198, 260, 402
 harvest of, 15t
 U.S., 39, 41
Merck and Co., 363
Mercury, 64-65
 in swordfish, 66t
Merry, E., 216, 267, 386
Metabolic studies, 338
Methionine, 168t, 169t
 in FPC, 167
 price of, 365t
 in staple foods, 374t
Mice, experiments with, 197
Microbiology, of fish protein hydrolysis, 154
Micronized Protein Concentrate (MPC), 469, 470t, 471t, 472t
Microorganisms, for FPC processing, 86
Migration, 51
Mihalyi, E., 290
Milk analogs, 140, 155
Milk powder, 315t
Milk products, 391
Milling, 79
Minerals, in FPC, 201, 333
Mixtures, protein-rich, 315t
Model 60 ACM Mill, 79
Molluscs, 37
Monckeberg, Fernando, 219
Monsanto Co., 283
Monzyme, 283, 284-287
 distribution of, 289t
 thermal denaturation

 curves for, 300
Moorjani, M. N., 223
Moroccan sardine, FPC from, 175t
Morrison, A. B., 178
MSY (maximum sustainable yield), 439, 440
Myctophids, 46

Nabisco Astra Nutrition, Inc., 87, 480
Nath, R. L., 267
National Academy of Sciences, 1
National Center for Fish Protein Concentrate, 78, 330
National Institute of Nutrition, Hyderabad, India, 223
National Marine Fisheries Service, 33, 35-36, 65, 103, 198, 283
National Nutrition Research Institute (NNRI), in Pretoria, 303
Net protein,utilization (NPU), and BV, 248t
 of FPC, 235
Newberne, P. M., 196t
New Zealand, 362
Nitrogen, and amino acids, 238t
 nonspecific, 235-245
 urinary excretion of, 237, 239
Nitrogen balance, 246, 340t
Nitrogen retention, 342, 343t
Nitrosamines, 335
Noetzel, B. G., 417
Nonfat dry milk (NFDM),

Nonfat dry milk (NFDM),
  361-363
 costs of, 362, 363, 427
 and FPC production, 409
 prices of, 365t
Nonheat coagulable nitro-
  gen compounds (NCN),
  149
Nonprotein-nitrogen (NPN),
  147
Nonsolvent processes, 81
Noodles, enriched, 344
North Atlantic, 46
North Pacific, 48
Norway, FPC in, 122, 123-
  124
Nutrition, 136
 of FPH, 141t
 human, 37
 problem of, 380
Nutrition Dept. of Coun-
  cil for Scientific and
  Industrial Research,
  265
Nutrition Development
  Corp., 480

Ocean Harvesters, Inc.,
  74, 79, 394, 409
Ocean perch, FPC from,
  181
Ocean pout, FPC from,
  175t
Odense, P. M., 78
Odor, 79, 256-261
 experiments on, 332-
  333
 of PH-65, 157t
 residual, 88
Office of National Stu-
  dent Auxiliary and
  Scholarships, 312
Oil, fish, 460-461

of Northern anchovies,
  424
recovery of, 80-81
yield of, 414
Oilcake meal, world pro-
  duction of, 28f
Oilseeds, marketing of,
  357-361
Oligopsony, collusive,
  443
Oregon State Univ., 330
OVAPIRU, 215
Overfishing, 442
Overseas Private Invest-
  ment Corp., 480
Oxidation, lipid, 59, 143

Packaging, 4
Pakistan, supplementation
  in, 366
Palatability, of FPC, 223
Particle size, 149
Pasta, enriched, 379
 fortified, 271, 272t,
  274
 FPC in, 69t, 195, 255,
  268-270, 310, 344, 425
 supplementation of, 273
Patients, protein supple-
  ment for, 304
Paulaha, D. F., 417
Paulik, G. J., 404, 417
Peanut flour, 191, 373,
  374t, 381t
Pelagic species, 44, 45,
  47, 48, 50
Pereira, S. M., 223, 224
Perrin, W. F., 417
Peru, FPC in, 269, 351,
  412, 413t, 427, 430,
  439, 445
 fish meal industry in,
  440-442, 439

Peru (continued)
  supplementation program
    in, 337
Pesticides, 58, 65
PH-65, 154, 155, 156t,
    157t
Phenylalanine, 168t, 169t
Phosphate, condensed, 116-
    118
Phospholipids, 62, 80
Phosphorus, 170, 171t
  in LFP, 130t
Pigott, G. M., 82
Pigs, experiments with,
    187
Pilchard, 15t, 45, 48
Plant, fish meal, 443
  for FPC processing, 402,
    404, 443, 447-449
Pollack, LFP from, 128t
Pomeranz, Y., 262
Pond, Wilson G., 185, 186
Porridge, enriched, 304
Port of Illo, 441
Potassium, 171t
Poultry, 357
Power, H. E., 177
Precooking, 127
Preferences, dietary,
    304-305
Preparation, for FPC
    process, 68-72
Preservation, 38, 39
Press cake, 257, 306
Pretorius, P. J., 218
Pricing, of protein pro-
    ducts, 478
Prisons, 388
Processing, 57, 87-91
  batch, 450
  contaminants in, 459-
    460
  continuous, 450

costs of, 432, 463t-464t,
    473
  facility for, 402
  flexibility of, 118-119
  losses from, 379-380
  in Peru, 442, 443
  phases of, 451
  potential methods of,
    469-474
  simplification of, 83-85
Production, of Calif. an-
    chovy FPC, 420t-421t,
    423t
  costs of, 400, 404, 405t,
    406, 413t, 414, 415t, 430,
    446
  of fish meal, 26, 27
  of FPC, 44, 90f, 408
  in Chile, 410
  of Northern anchovy FPC,
    416-424
Proflo, 360
Programs, food supplemen-
    tation, 369
Pronase, 127
Pro-Nutro, 303
Protanimal, 469, 470t,
    471t, 472t
Protein, 140
  alternative, 25-27, 428
  connective tissue, 63
  extraction of, 82
  fish, 91, 165, 173t, 175t,
    185
  in FPC, 174, 333
  in FPH process, 144t
  ideal properties for, 476t
  markets for, 355, 356
  muscle, 62-63
  need for, 2, 4
  processing loss of, 70-
    71, 195
  repletion of, 189, 190f

Protein (continued)
  salt soluble, 319, 322t
  sarcophasmic, 63
  soy, 359
  sulfhydryl groups of, 181
  vegetable, 229
  whole egg, 235
Protein Advisory Group, 70
Protein-calorie malnutri-
    tion (PCM), 228
  in children, 426
  and supplementation, 224,
    225
Protein deficiency, and
    FPC, 187, 188t
  problem of, 328
Protein efficiency ratios
    (PER), 86
  during drying process,
    76
  of FPC, 63-64
Protein sources, BV of,
    247
Proteolysis, 86
Publicity, about FPC, 2
Purification, IPA, 458
Purified fish pulp pro-
    cess, 145f
Purse seine, 40
PVM (Proteine Verrykings-
    medium), 303

Quality control, 461-462
Quality of life, 29
Quintero-FPC, 197, 218
Quintero plant, in Chile,
    377

Rancidity, control of, 123
Rasmussen, A. I., 184
Rats, experiments with,
    185, 193f, 197, 199
Raw material, for FPC, 12,

    37-43, 447
  storage of, 452
Reactor, batch, 295
  enzyme, 290
  FPC solubilization, 292
Reconstitution, of PH--5,
    157
Recreation, 36
Red crab, harvest of, 16t,
    19
Red snapper, 173t
Reflectance scan, 325, 326
Refrigeration, 408, 452
Regulations, for FPC, 107.
  See also Food and Drug
  Administration
Repletion, protein, 187-
    189f, 190f
Requirements, FAO/WHO nu-
    tritional, 384
Research, 430
Residence time, 295-298
Resolubilization, 299f, 300
Resources, underutilized,
    12, 19
Residue, resuspension of,
    298-300
RNV (relative nutritive
    value), 177
Roels, O. A., 392
Roemer, M., 407, 409
Rogers, W. I., 82
Rucker, P. G., 182
Rulkens, W. J., 77
Rusoff, Irving I., 276
Rutman, M., 83, 91, 114

Safety, 58, 461
Salt, accumulation of,
    284
Sand eels, 13, 14t, 46,
    48, 51
Sanitation, 42, 65, 461

San Pedro wetfish fleet,
  417
Sardines, Californian,
  404
 FPC from, 176t, 260
 harvest of, 16t
 in Indian Ocean, 50
 oil from, 15t
Sardinella, 47
 harvest of, 14t
 migration of, 52
 West African, 13
Satiety, in children, 347
Sauces, FPC in, 304
Sauries, 46, 47, 48
Sausage, fish, 391, 453
 FPC in, 393
Sausage test, 105
Schafer, K. H., 213
Schendel, Harold E.,
  196t, 199
Schools, 388
Schweigert, Dr. B. S., 1
Scrimshaw, Nevin, 165,
  226
Seas, potential of, 8
Seiners, Peruvian, 41
Selenium, 66t, 171t
Semolina, 271
Semolina-FPC mixture, 268
Sen, D. P., 266
Senecal, Jean, 214
Sensitivity testing, 422
Separation, 60, 73, 143,
  453-457
Sharks, harvest of, 16t
Shoaling fish species, 44
Shrimp, 20, 47, 49
Sidwell, V. D., 195, 268,
  273, 275, 379, 385, 425
Silvestre, Frenk, 213
Single-cell protein (SCP),
  27

Skim milk, 191. See also
  Dried skim milk; Nonfat
  dry milk
Snacks, FPC in, 273
Sodium, 171t
 in LFP, 130t
Solubility, of FPC, 333
Solubilization, 111, 291f,
  296f, 392
 acid, 114-115
 contamination during,
  283-284
 continuous, 294f
 enzyme levels of, 287
 of FPC, 283
 resolubilization, 299f,
  300
 at various residence
  times, 297f
Solvents, 74
 recovery of, 77, 79-80,
  397, 458-460
Soups, FPC in, 277, 304,
  313-316, 346t
South Africa, FPC in, 265,
  303
South Atlantic, 47-48
South Pacific, 49
Southwest Atlantic, 53
Soy, flavor of, 391
Soybean meal, 25, 26, 28f
Soybeans, marketing of,
  357-358
Soy flour, 373, 374t, 381t,
  386
Soy products, 358, 359,
  365t
Spada, R., 218
Spaghetti, 310, 311, 312.
  See also Pasta
Spain, soy products in,
  358
Spawning, 51

SPC, 384
Spencer, H., 220
Sphingolipids, 62
Spillage, 80
Spinelli, J., 83, 85, 91,
  116, 119
Sprague, L. M., 23, 33
Spray drying, 86, 129t
Squid, 13
  concentrations of, 23
  harvest of, 16t
  oceanic, 17, 19, 23, 29
  potential of, 50
Srikantia, S. G., 223, 225
Staple foods, fortifica-
  tion of, 375
Still bottoms, 461
Stillings, B. R., 76, 84,
  170, 186, 192, 196t,
  198, 275, 377
Storage, 70
  and protein loss, 395–
  396, 409
  of raw material, 452
Subsidies, 36
Sunflower meal, biologi-
  cal quality of, 315t
Supplementation, break-
  even costs of, 377, 378
  in developed countries,
  388–389
  history of, 364–369
  low cost, 426
  need for, 2
  of pasta, 272
  preschool program of,
  345
  universal, 369–376. See
  also Fortification
Supplements, clinical
  testing of, 214, 215,
  216, 217, 218, 219, 220,
  225

concentration ratios of,
  383t
costs of, 372, 381t
functional properties of,
  390
high-protein, 274
prices of, 365t
in staple foods, 374t
Supply, variations in,
  442
Sure, Barnett, 192
Suspension stability, of
  PH-65, 157t
Swaminathan, M., 387
SWECO, 401, 424
Swilling, protein, 104
Swordfish, 66t
Synthetics, fortification
  with, 370
  price of, 365t

Tannenbaum, S. R., 83, 115,
  331, 392
Taste, 86, 391
  of M-FPC, 334
  of PH-65, 157t
Taste panels, at FIRI,
  305
Tavill, F., 220
Technology, 136
  dairy, 143
  FPC, 430
  FPH, 141t
  harvesting, 9, 17, 24
  processing, 19
  product, 12
Temperature, extraction,
  318–321
Testing, clinical, 212,
  214, 215, 216–219, 225
Texture, of PH-65, 157t
Thailand, diet in, 328
Thijssen, H. A. C., 76, 77

Thomson, F. A., 216, 267,
    386
Tillman, M. F., 417
Tortillas, FPC in, 266-
    267
TPC (total plate counts),
    65-67
Toxicity, in children, 347
Toxicological studies, of
    FPC, 195-200
    of FPH, 155
Trace elements, 170
Transportation, 444, 451
Trash fish, 392
Trawl, midwater, 40
Trichloroethylene, 62
Triglycerides, 80
Trimethylamine, 147, 335
Tryosine, 168t, 169t
Tryptophan, 86, 168, 169t,
    242, 363, 365t
Tsen, C. C., 263
Tuna, 47

UNICEF, 84, 267
United Kingdom, catch of,
    45
Universidad de Chile, 155
Urea, 26
USSR, 22, 51

Vacuum-evaporating, 319
Valine, 168t, 169t
Vandenheuval, F. A., 102
Vanderborght, H. L., 215
Vegetable meals, 25
Vergara, Uribe A., 263
Verrando, Carlos, 84, 277,
    397
Verrando process, 212
Vessels, fishing, 448
VioBin Co., 199, 200
VioBin-FPC, 75, 212, 216,

    217, 218, 219, 394, 397
Viscosity, 149
    of PH-65, 157t
Vitamin K, 198
Viteri, F., 222

Wages, 410
Waste, fish, 460
    discharge of, 81
Waste control systems, 82
Waste streams, 81
Waste water, 461
Weaning foods, 328
Weanlings, 388, 426
Wehmeyer, A. S., 218
Weight gain, and supple-
    mentation, 193f, 217,
    340t, 341t
Weiners, FPC in, 321
    supplementation of, 393
Western Central Atlantic,
    53
Wet solids, desolventizing
    of, 324t
Wheat flour (WF), biologi-
    cal quality of, 315
    FPC-90%, 341t
    metabolic evaluation of,
    340t
Whippability, 83
White spring salmon, 173
Whiting, blue, 46
Wikramanayake, T. W., 218
Woo, Choi Haynie, 269
World catches, 10

Yanez, E., 155, 167, 197,
    219
Yeast, 227
Yield, of FPC, 333
    sustainable, 13

Zinc, in FPC, 106, 171t

Zinc (continued)
 in FPC, 106, 171t
 in swordfish, 66t
Zipkin, Zukas, 428